May We Make the World?

Basic Bioethics

Arthur Caplan, editor

A complete list of the books in the Basic Bioethics series appears at the back of this book.

May We Make the World?

Gene Drives, Malaria, and the Future of Nature

Laurie Zoloth

The MIT Press
Cambridge, Massachusetts
London, England

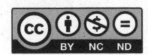
The MIT Press would like to thank the anonymous peer reviewers who provided comments on drafts of this book. The generous work of academic experts is essential for establishing the authority and quality of our publications. We acknowledge with gratitude the contributions of these otherwise uncredited readers.

This book was set in ITC Stone Sans and ITC Stone Serif by Westchester Publishing Services. Printed and bound in the United States of America.

Library of Congress Cataloging-in-Publication Data

Names: Zoloth, Laurie, author.
Title: May we make the world? : gene drives, malaria, and the future of
    nature / Laurie Zoloth.
Other titles: Basic bioethics.
Description: Cambridge, Massachusetts : The MIT Press, 2023. |
    Series: Basic bioethics | Includes bibliographical references and index.
Identifiers: LCCN 2023002847 (print) | LCCN 2023002848 (ebook) |
    ISBN 9780262546980 (paperback) | ISBN 9780262377003 (epub) |
    ISBN 9780262376990 (pdf)
Subjects: LCSH: Malaria—Prevention—Moral and ethical aspects. |
    Malaria—Africa—Prevention. | Gene drives—Moral and ethical aspects. |
    Mosquitoes—Genetic engineering—Moral and ethical aspects.
Classification: LCC RA644.M2 Z65 2023 (print) | LCC RA644.M2 (ebook) |
    DDC 614.5/320096—dc23/eng/20230623
LC record available at https://lccn.loc.gov/2023002847
LC ebook record available at https://lccn.loc.gov/2023002848

10 9 8 7 6 5 4 3 2 1

To my colleagues in science, who bring me their questions.
To my friends, who bring me their discernment,
To my family, who bring me their love.

יָדֶיךָ עָשׂוּנִי וַיְכוֹנְנוּנִי הֲבִינֵנִי וְאֶלְמְדָה מִצְוֺתֶיךָ׃
יְרֵאֶיךָ יִרְאוּנִי וְיִשְׂמָחוּ כִּי לִדְבָרְךָ יִחָלְתִּי׃

Psalm 119:73–74

Contents

Acknowledgments xi

Introduction xv

1 The World as We Know It: Malaria and Its History 1

2 The World as It Is Imagined: Gene Drives for Malaria 77

3 The World as We Order It: A Review of Regulation 113

4 The World as We Speak It: Stakeholder Engagement and African
   Discourses 163

5 The World of Dissent: Listening to Opposition 199

6 The World as We Judge It: Ethical Issues Considered 237

Conclusion: Making the Moral World 299

Notes 323

Index 359

Acknowledgments

My mother, Helen Zoloth, z'l, liked thinking about what she called "my mosquitoes." When I first told her about this project and showed her the website about Target Malaria, she, at ninety-five years old, was fascinated. She followed the news about gene drives, quite proud she knew about them first, before any of her friends, and she never failed to ask me how the work was coming along. And when I was always the first one bitten by mosquitoes on the Californian summer nights when I visited, she would laugh and say, "They know you're out to get them." She liked thinking about what her children cared about, and for me, in her last years, it was what to make about the power of science and about the human presence in the natural world. She was the one who remembered that, at ten years old, I had insisted on returning the grunion that my family and our neighbors had caught on the beach back to the ocean, yelling, "It's not right" as I grabbed their buckets and sent the fish into the surf. I had just learned the words "ecological niche" from my father, Arthur Zoloth, z'l. When I was in middle school, he drove me to the fruit-fly laboratories at the University of California, Los Angeles, where, amazingly enough, I walked alone into the laboratory and found some kind graduate students, who gave a thirteen-year-old girl glass flasks, test tubes, and a great many fruit-fly eggs and showed her how to make the agar to feed them when they hatched. And they did it again when, after I mixed a little dichlorodiphenyltrichloroethane (DDT; which of course we had on hand, pre–Rachel Carson) into the agar, they all died. And they did it again, until I learned how to keep the larvae alive, taking over the kitchen and the pantry with flasks full of fruit flies, which now, as a parent, I find even more astonishing. It was my idea to see if I could adapt the fruit flies to DDT if I did it slowly enough over one winter. It kind of worked, or at least it proved that fruit flies can take even a clumsy middle schooler caring for them and survive. The judges of the LA County Science Fair, Junior Division, at least, liked the concept enough to award me first prize for a project that, oddly enough, would end up being a bit of a prelude to this book, in that what I remember most is one overalled farmer sidling up to me at the county fair, where I stood next to the corn and soybean exhibit, a few wan fruit flies flying sadly in the flasks, and asking me, softly, "Well, little lady, just what are you going to do now with those flies I can't kill?"

So, thanks, first of all, to my parents, Helen and Arthur Zoloth, who taught their children to know the natural world with intensity and care, for exploring the rivers, beaches, hills and arroyos of Los Angeles with us, for showing us where the big frog by the house lived and when the owl returned each autumn, and for showing us how to explore the willows upstream as we followed after them. Thus, my big brother became Professor Zoloth, a scientist, and I became Professor Zoloth, a watcher of science.

This book would not be possible without the extraordinary Brocher Foundation. The Brocher Fellowship in Ethics, in the lovely late summer and fall of 2018 allowed me time to sit quietly and read everything that had been written at that point about gene drives, including the book, *Genes in Conflict*, by Austin Burt and Robert Trivers, twice, and to think hard about it, while eating French bread from just over the border, with Gruyère cheese and fresh tomatoes from the village of Hermance. Over those months, my fellow scholars at the Foundation house interrogated me, challenged me, swam with me in the icy lake, and cheered me on when I printed out the first draft of this book. Thank you to Ali Kazemian, Anna Berti Suman, Bill Ollier, Clare Atterton, John Noel Viana, Julia el Mecky, Lorenzo Alunni, Martin Yuille, Morvan Cook, Ruud ter Meulen, Tereza Handl, Vincent Menuz, and especially Euzebiusz Jamrozik and Prevan Moodley, whose expertise in malaria was so very helpful. Of course, the staff—Anyck Beauvallet-Gerard, Cecile Caldwell, Marie Grosclaude, Sabine Turpin, and Philippe Pellet—make the intellectual work possible with their support and care. The Brocher Foundation continues to be one of the most important and thoughtful locations for the international discourse that is bioethics. I am extraordinarily grateful for this place and for that time. Thank you to the University of Chicago Divinity School and then dean David Nirenberg, who granted me research leave to go work on a project in bioethics at that lovely spot and time to go to the laboratory at Terni and to Ghana for the team meeting.

I am deeply grateful as well to the scientists who, with patience and humility, allow bioethicists like me to question them so persistently. It is a privilege. First of all, thanks to the Target Malaria team, especially to Austin Burt, who brought me the first questions, and to Delphine Thizy, so dedicated to ethics and so committed to engagement; to Karen Logan, Naima Sykes, Isabelle Coche, Camila Beech, John Connolly, Andrew Hammond, Jonathan Kayondo, Mamadou Coulibaly, Abdoulaye Diabate, Fred Aboagye-Antwi, Geoff Turner, Morgane Danielou, John Mumford. Alekos Simoni, Federica Bernardini, Samantha O'Loughlin, Mouhamed Drabo, Adilson de Pina, Lea Pare Toe, Talya Hackett, Frederic Trippet, Eoin Mac Hale, Megan Quinlan, Lucy Oliff, Zaira Lanna, and the lovely team at Terni, whose generosity and warmth over a good meal was remarkable; and to the teachers, laboratory workers, trainers, community organizers, and villagers who work every day in the hope of making the world healthier and more just. I hope this work does justice to your efforts. This manuscript was closely read by the Target Malaria team, for which I am deeply grateful, but the conclusions as well as any errors are entirely my own.

Close behind are my colleagues on the international Ethics Advisory Board where I served for almost a decade: Abha Saxena, Arzoo Ahmed, Claire Divver, Dominic White, Fred Gould, Kent Redford, Lydia Kapiriri, Maja Horst, Noni Mumba, Paul Ndebele, Paulina Tindana, and Rashmi Narayana. You read my work, listened to my arguments, and always taught me a great deal.

I also owe a debt to the members of one of the projects that I worked on as co-PI when I was writing this book. As a scholar of religion, I was interested in thinking about how religious arguments, so important in public life, played a role in our thinking about gene drives for malaria. This question is best answered in collaboration with scholars of many different religious traditions, and our work together has been extremely important to this book. Readers of my work in religious ethics will find that work in the product of that research, a joint paper about religious views on the topic. Thank you to the wonderful Noelle Norona who was the main contributor to this paper; to my co-chair, David Ford, who immediately understood why this project is so important; and to Abdul Hafiz Walusimbi, Alfred Olwa, Arzoo Ahmed, Ben Pazi Hanoch, Christian Wedemeyer, Cornelius Wambi Gulere, David Amponsah, Faustino Orach Meza, Simon Ramde, and Vasudha Narayanan.

Thanks as well to the many other colleagues who listened to me think aloud with them about gene drives, among them David Edelstein, Ethan Bier,

Gaymon Bennett, Jeffrey Bishop, Kevin Esvelt, Megan Palmer, Morty Schapiro, Sam Weiss Evans, Willemein Otten and Marc Berkson. My best conversation partners are anonymous ones: the terrific reviewers of this manuscript, whose suggestions and critiques were very important in creating the book that you have in your hands now. My editor at MIT Press, Philip Laughlin, has been extraordinarily helpful, as was the production team at the Press especially the very patient Rashmi Malhotra. Linda Hallinger, indexer, and editor has been helpful as well. A special thanks to Temima Levy, my scholarly granddaughter, my extraordinary copy editor and my British grammarian.

Finally, thanks to my family, especially to my brother, the scientist, and always to my children, who never doubted me when I explained that all the world could be understood—where humans lived, the Great Migration, architecture in Italy, vaccine policy, Shakespeare, colonialism, World War II, and Dr. Suess—through malaria. Thank you Matthew, Noah, Benjamin, Joshua, and Sarah, and the lovely people whom they love, Saskia, Margaux, Reby, and Josh, and thanks to my smart and savvy grandchildren, Temima, Saadya, Salome, Emuna, Ezra, Zohar, Lola and Ada, who are growing up to ask questions of their own, and into whose world, and whose nature, those questions will unfold.

Introduction

I.1 The Falls of Marmore

You hear the thunder of the waterfalls before you see them. The air is thick with cool, rising mist. The path is fern-lined, impossibly green, lifting first gently, then steeply, from the river Nera below, and the trail winds from a narrow, craggy valley, the falls spilling over the cliffs towering above the trail. This is the Cascata delle Marmore, built by the Romans, and they are beautiful. They cascade down the granite cliffs in three giant steps. Surrounded by dappled forests, the air is laced with bright birds, and there are delicate ferns and wild iris underfoot. The Nera is dark green, trembling with foam, and it runs into the valley folded below us. On a hill beside the river is the ancient market town of Terni, equipped with Roman arches, an amphitheater, tenth-century churches, and cobbled streets with shrines to St. Valentine.

It is the very picture of a natural wonder. Yet, in precisely an hour, the falls will turn off. The water will turn off as surely as the faucet in my Chicago kitchen, because these falls, for all their pristine loveliness, insistent verdant grace, and wild beauty, are entirely man-made. Roman made. They are enormous—541 feet tall. They are the tallest artificially constructed falls in the world and have been for more than 2,000 years.

The reason why they are here, and have been since 271 BCE, is because of the disease of malaria, humankind's oldest foe. The falls were the great technology of Imperial Rome, and they represented the enormity of the human effort to transform creation itself, nature itself, in order to combat the fatal danger of nature, to try to end the deadly fevers and plagues that are a part of the natural world.

This is the subject of this book.

I am in Terni, standing in the middle of the forested cliffs and soaked to the skin, not to see the falls, but because in that town below us is the Polo Scientifico Didattico di Terni-UNIPG, the research laboratory devoted to advanced research on malaria and the insect vector that carries the pathogen that causes malaria. The Terni laboratory is home to the most sophisticated large-cage research on *Anopheles gambiae* mosquitoes in Europe. These mosquitoes, the malaria that they carry, and the desperate human efforts to evade its ravages had all been a part of this Italian forest for as long as humanity has existed. Malaria was not declared eradicated by WHO in Italy until 1970. I am here to see a research project whose ultimate aim is to end the disease globally.

Above me, out of sight, is the large flat farmland of Marmore and the town of Rieti where a river, the Velino, flows from a man-made stone channel into a lake, also man-made, called the Lago de Piediluco, and then out of the lake to spill over the cliff. The stonework is ancient, efficient, and impossibly beautiful, so covered in ferns and wild rosemary that it takes a moment to recognize the hands of the Roman craftsmen who placed it here centuries ago. This rich farmland had once been a fetid swamp, thick with mosquitoes and the organism, the plasmodium, that traveled with them and brought the terrifying, deadly fever the Romans knew well. Thus, in 271 BCE, the Roman consul Manius Curius Dentatus is recorded as ordering the construction of a canal. The Romans who dug the canal, drained the swamp, and claimed the new farmland for themselves simply diverted the river and pushed it over the cliffs onto flat, carved stones. The new falls would flood the towns below, alternating with seasons of low flow that again threatened the town above with emerging swamps. Fights between the towns above and below about how to design nature are recorded in the Roman Senate in 54 CE, and they continued over the next thousand years until, in 1422, Pope Gregory XII ordered a new, deeper canal to be built. A hundred years later, in 1545, Pope Paul III oversaw the construction of a regulating valve to control the flow—a project that took another fifty years to be completed. Two centuries later, in 1787, the stone falls were widened into huge, graduating steps, modified to control the flow even more closely, and used to generate power. In the next century, 1896, came the steel mills of Terni, which stood as Italy's sign of the Industrial Revolution, of modernity itself, and were powered by the falls. In the 1940s—until they were bombed to dust in World War II by Allied planes— the mills were the center of Italian military infrastructure, turning out steel for weapons of war. Now, it is mostly tourists and hikers who come to marvel at a wonder that has stood here since antiquity, as Romans marched north to England; through the medieval period, when plagues came; and through the Renaissance, as the wonders of Rome were built, as the ceiling of the Vatican was painted, as Italians made art and music and fought fierce, endless wars. The Cascata delle Marmore would fall into disrepair and be rebuilt again, rising again through early modernity, and, in the long meanwhile, the Europeans brought malaria to the Americas and brought back tomatoes, corn, potatoes, chocolate, and quinine. The falls still are there, in our contemporary world—this great and beautiful human achievement still stands, wildly audacious, built with simple hand tools. "Let's just move the river over here," some Roman genius must have said, and remarkably, they did. It is the trace of our species in the wide wild world. These projects that shape nature are the first graze of the gesture that will be the Anthropocene. They are as human as speech, as song.

I.2   The Next Technology

The falls made the farmland habitable. They made the town grow. They powered the mills that made the weapons of war. Now, they make Terni a good place for an early phase of a complex project—to test some of the most cutting-edge technology in modern genetic research. Push the water over the cliff and a chain of events follows. After a while, we begin to think of the human gesture as simply part of the landscape: the falls, the absence of malaria in the forest, the ferns grown over the waterworks become—to us— equally unremarkable.

This is a book about the ethical issues that we need to consider when we make the world, or rather when we remake the world, so that it is better, or safer, for humans to live in it. This is, in a way, the story of the long road from the Romans who made the falls to the scientists in Terni, to the laboratories across Africa, who are now working to "make" a mosquito that cannot transmit malaria by using a genetic technique called a "gene drive." In thinking about this new idea, this world-making idea, and the ethical issues it raises, you have to think about a great many things: the history of malaria, the human attempts to stop the disease, the way that mosquitoes live and die, the rules about public health, and the rules about emerging science, how the complicated genetic idea of a gene drive is worked out, how to create experiments to test it, how to understand the people who are doing the work, how to understand risks and failures, the way that communities decide things, the way that people who oppose genetic research argue against it, and the way that the long history of Westerners in Africa has shaped the communities most affected by the disease. To inquire about the ethics of gene drives is not a facile task, but without thinking carefully about all of these issues, one cannot really make a judgment about the moral worth of the project or create normative structures within which it might take place or consider whether it ought to proceed or be halted. These several overlapping discourses are what I will consider in this book. I intend to bring together not only several overlapping conversations—about history, molecular biology, philosophy, and ethics—but also several different audiences.

When the reviewers of the first draft read it, they kept asking about this. Who is this written for? Scientists? Bioethicists? People interested in theories of the natural world? Well, I hope all of you, certainly. The answer is that I am deliberately aiming to create a linguistic "crossroads" where many sorts of people can come to be the audience: people from several different areas of expertise, and people with no particular expertise at all, but who are all interested in a fascinating problem. It is my conceit that this book creates a conversation that welcomes each of you: readers who will perhaps know much about gene drives but not as much about colonialism, or who know about policy but not about philosophy. I believe that books can create what Hannah Arendt calls "the space of appearance," which is a public square where different citizens can make their best arguments and where consensus emerges from justification and debate. Arendt wanted us to think, then to judge moral action, and then to take responsibility for our choices. This type of multivocal thinking, what Arendt called "plurality" in thinking, is complex but, I contend, critical if we are to make fair judgments. And like a real public square, the kind that Arendt had in mind, the chapters bring different voices to the fore. This turned out to be harder in practice than in Arendt's theory, because even the languages of our academic disciplines are so different, something I understood after I sent this book out to be reviewed, with the scientists who first read this manuscript baffled by post-modern philosophy ("imaginary," "apophantic," "synecdoche") and ethicists unable to follow the science ("gRNA," "mutagenic chain reaction," "homozygote"). The language of the policy makers was also specific ("regulatory capture," "equipoise," "community consent") so that ideas and norms that were assumed by one group, and so commonly used that they barely need mention, were completely novel to another group. It requires very close listening to understand that many issues that deeply and fundamentally concern ethicists are simply not a part of scientific expertise, and vice-versa. I have done my best to translate but you, reader, I hope will be patient with arguments that are not in your own language. The public square can be a cacophonous place!

Let me also note something that worried the reviewers, which is that at times, I cite long passages from other scholars who have written before me. This too is a deliberate attempt to allow you direct access to primary source material, for I like text study in my work as a scholar of religion and find that careful reading of texts allows a far richer and thicker sense of the meaning that the author has in mind, often better than my retelling of the argument. In the case of the historical accounts, one can also consider the nuance in the language as the text presents its case. I am asking, in this book, for you, wherever you initially begin, to consider how the different chapters highlight different ethical considerations and, in that collection of ideas, to find new ways to think about my question: whether we, with all of our power and our knowledge, may transform the world, beginning, in particular, with one piece of it—sub-Saharan Africa.

One can tell the story of gene drives for malaria in a number of ways. Here is how I began to think about this complex problem. Like most Americans, until the COVID-19 pandemic, I rarely thought about epidemic infectious diseases and certainly not about malaria. For most Americans, such a thought was relegated, if one thought about it at all, to the vague, reflexive concern that one has for "Africa," a generalized imaginary.[1] There, as in many places far away from Western concerns, Americans tend to believe that many things are troubled, that governments are corrupt, that democracy is largely a failed concept, that hunger stalks tribal groups, that local civil wars threaten and children are kidnapped, and that diseases of all sorts sicken and kill thousands.[2] We will return to the problems that this image carries in later chapters.

Malaria flickered across my consciousness when I traveled, for, like any Westerner who has visited India or Southeast Asia, I took malaria prophylaxis—pills that I was warned needed to be taken daily, starting two days prior to my arrival and for a week after I returned. Most Americans could not have told you where the country of Burkina Faso or Mali was on a map of Africa. Malaria was on the list of diseases of the very poorest people in the world, intractable, inevitable. But as a bioethicist, what I did know a great deal about, however, were the ethical questions that surround the science of genetic engineering, both what was now possible and about the speculative future.

And that was why, in December 2015, I was invited to a small meeting of the British Royal Society and the US National Academy of Sciences to discuss some new projects in genetics and what is called "synthetic biology." I had been thinking and writing about the project of gene therapy—about stem cells, nanotechnology, and genetic testing—for the better part of three decades, and for the last several years, I have also been listening to scientists' narrative about the quest to apply principles of engineering circuitry to the study and manipulation of biological entities, which they called genetic engineering.

The meeting took place during an English early winter, in a Georgian country manor house shrouded by fog. There was a still, icy lake, a gravel, tree-lined walk, black, leafless trees in the wood at the end of the lane. We were a small group, and we fit into one small room with our computers and a screen for the PowerPoint presentations. The work presented, by design, was largely quite new, largely unpublished. At the end of the second day, Austin Burt, a quiet researcher from Imperial College London, put up his PowerPoint describing his idea to utilize what he called a "gene drive." Gene drives occur in nature, he explained, and described several ways that a genetic element "drives," or causes inheritance of genetic sequences in a biased manner, preferentially, so that it spreads a trait across an entire population. Gene drives use several different mechanisms, but all of them cause a selected trait to spread rapidly through a species via sexual reproduction over several generations by increasing the likelihood that a modified gene will be inherited by its offspring. Normally, genes have a 50:50 chance of being inherited, but gene drive systems could increase that chance to upward of 99 percent. This means that over the course of several generations, a selected trait could become increasingly common within a specific species.

This was the plan that Austin Burt proposed: to use one of these mechanisms, called a "driving Y," a homing endonuclease, inserted as the "trait" that could be driven in a mosquito population. I will describe this in greater detail in a later chapter, but briefly, a homing endonuclease is what is called a "selfish genetic element" that spreads by creating a break in a chromosome that does not contain that sequence, and that gets copied to the broken chromosome as a part of the repair process.[3] The plan was to use this capacity to place this element on the Y chromosome so that it would fragment the X chromosomes, during spermatogenesis, meaning that fewer female *A. gambiae* mosquitoes would be born than males and that this genetic element would be carried into each subsequent generation. This was important, he explained, because only female mosquitoes bite human beings, seeking a blood meal to mature their eggs. It is when they bite that they transfer the parasites that cause malaria into the bloodstream of the person they have bitten. If one could reduce the biting rate, then malaria would not be spread to as many people, and if fewer people were infected, the mosquito would be less able to act as a vector for disease. Fewer females would eventually mean that the mosquito population would be dramatically reduced and, theoretically, eliminated. There was a picture of how the gene drive worked, with little blue male mosquitoes replacing little red female mosquitoes in a population, then how fewer and fewer were born over time—a picture of nonexistence. Austin Burt then said a little about malaria, and one statistic was stunning: every two minutes, someone dies of malaria, usually a child below the age of five, usually an African child, and usually from the poorest part of the world, West Africa.

It was one of those rare times that I had heard someone talk about how genetic research could address a disease that was largely only a disease of the poor. I could count on one hand the number of times I had heard a research scientist focus entirely on a difficult problem that, if solved, would change the lives of the poorest, most marginalized people with whom we shared our world.[4] I told him so at breakfast the next day.

I explained that the usual concern of my field of bioethics was science at the most fantastic and rare. Can conjoined twins be parted? Are people who meet the medical criteria for death really dead? How should we protect astronauts? Is the neural tissue in the dish really conscious? If we reanimate the brains of animals, what is their moral status? Are designer babies allowable? Can we enhance ourselves and become transhuman or not?

When we thought about genetics, it was usually about interventions that would affect a handful of people or would be available only to the wealthiest and most privileged members of our society. Sometimes, we argued about obscure uses of human tissue or about artificially created balls of embryonic cells, called organoids, that resulted from human embryonic stem-cell research, and sometimes we argued about, say, face transplants.

I explained that I had not heard a paper in a long time that began with the question: What can we do for the poor of the world? I told him I would like to think about his project, what ethical issues it raised, and how a radical intervention in the natural world could be justified.

Austin Burt had been thinking about this for a long time, he told me, and he said that I should start by considering and understanding the science. He had written a book, he said, that explained the principle. A week later, the (very large) book arrived. *Genes in Conflict: The Biology of Selfish Genetic Elements*, by Burt and his co-author, molecular biologist Robert Trivers. This is a 602-page description of naturally occurring "selfish" genes, how they are driven across populations, and how they reoccur with frequency over time, acting as a "fifth force" in evolution, in addition to mutation, gene flow, genetic drift, and natural selection—when "the genes in an organism sometimes 'disagree' over what should happen."[5] Most of the time, genes in organisms contribute equally in reproduction, with each diploid individual contributing two copies of each gene with an equal likelihood—50:50—that it will be inherited. Each offspring has half of her genetic heritage from one parent and half, in most cases, from the other. However, Burt and Trivers go on to say, "As we shall see, selfish genetic elements are a universal feature of life, with pervasive effects on the genetic system and the larger phenotype, diversified into many forms, with adaptations and counter adaptations on both sides, a truly subterranean world of sociogenetic interactions, usually hidden completely from sight."[6] Most of these elements, they noted, had evolved to outwit the normal Mendelian genetic ratio of 50:50, and inserted themselves into 51 percent, 60 percent, or even 99 percent of the progeny. "Instead of being fair and transparent, the process of gene transmission in itself leads to an increase of gene frequencies. Genes inherited in a biased manner can spread in a population without doing anything good for the organism. Indeed they can spread even if they are harmful. Such a gene is said to 'drive.'" At the end of the book, Burt and Trivers speculate about how a naturally occurring phenomenon, such as, for example, killer gametes or homing endonuclease genes (HEGs), could shift inheritance patterns. The talk I had heard was the next step for this concept, looking for a genetic mechanism to alter inheritance patterns in the mosquitoes that were the most important vector for the deadliest sort of malaria in Africa.

Bioethicists have long been fascinated and worried by new genetic technology. This is, in part, because genetic manipulation, genetic testing, and, perhaps most importantly, the Nazi misuse of genetic data were the founding questions of our scholarly discipline. We count the Nuremberg Doctors' Trial, which traced the roots of the violent extermination of Jews and other "lessor races" of people back to the fatal gassing of disabled children, and then to the Nazi embrace of a euthanasia program prefigured by a genetic "race science" and an obsession with genetic inheritance. Understanding how genetic knowledge was used for such deadly purposes was one of the formative tasks of early bioethicists.

A second foundational narrative of bioethics was also about genetic knowledge and the possibility of its misuse without proper regulation. When scientists in the new field of molecular biology began work on the manipulation of genetic codes, first in single-cell organisms and then in animals, the question of fair limits on this sort of creation was raised. The discussions of recombinant DNA technology at a small meeting at the California State Park known as Asilomar are often cited as marking the emergence of bioethics as a multidisciplinary field with the power both to describe and to suggest normative constructs in science and medicine.

When considering a new technology, bioethicists had worked out methods for discernment. Since 1999, after a three-year project led by the American Association for the Advancement of Science (AAAS), and after a wide-ranging debate among scholars of religion, law, moral philosophy, molecular biology, and medicine, the AAAS released a method to assess germline genetic modification. I was a part of this debate and one of the authors of a book that it produced. Our methodology coalesced the questions about the many genetic technologies that were both permanent and unprecedented, and it became widely used as an assessment tool. Here is the list we thought important:

(1) Are there reasons in *principle* why using this technology should be impermissible?

(2) What contextual factors should be taken into account, and do any of these prevent development and use of the technology?

(3) What purposes, techniques or applications would be permissible and under what circumstances?

(4) What procedures, structures, involving what policies, should be used to decide on appropriate techniques and uses?[7]

This series of questions, I thought, would enable me to consider carefully the ethical issues in using gene drives to change the sex ratio or even perhaps risk the elimination of, the particular mosquito species that carried a terrible disease. I would be able to consider the usual issues: consent, privacy, regulation, safety, risks and benefits, and the problem of mastery and control of nature.

I was wrong. To understand a gene drive intended to address the problem of malaria, one needs to go far beyond the usual perimeters of bioethics. Why?

Bioethics is largely a field concerned with health-care intervention: how doctors treat patients, which assumes that patients can see a doctor; how treatment can be withdrawn, which assumes that elaborate treatment has been offered; how to distribute intensive care unit (ICU) hospital beds fairly, which assumes that there are ICUs and hospital beds; and, increasingly, how the most far-fetched and expensive technology should be developed and regulated. Issues of public health have historically been low on the list of priorities. All of these issues are important, and our field has contributed enormously to improving health care and improving the education of doctors, nurses, and health-care workers. Every large hospital in the USA—except for those depicted on television—has a process to consider ethical issues raised by the patients, families, and staff. Hospital accreditation is based, in part, on the existence of this process, on the documentation of informed consent to procedures, and on the use of advance directives for end-of-life care. Not only have genetic interventions, stem-cell projects, and all clinical trials sponsored by the National Institutes of Health (NIH) had Institutional Review Board (IRB) approval, but their studies are followed by a Data Safety Monitoring Board (DSMB). Bioethicists serve at all levels of this process. Genetic research that uses the recombinant DNA techniques was, until 2018, additionally reviewed by the national Recombinant DNA Advisory Committee (the RAC).[8]

However, the moral structure of bioethics oversight—again, largely because of the power of the Nuremberg trials and the horror of the Nazi treatment of Jewish prisoners—was created to foreground the individual's right to say no to the use of their body for experimental purposes. Against the power of a state, against the imperative of scientific progress, against the great goodness of the search for knowledge, one principle protects the vulnerable subject: autonomy, most often codified in the consent process. This encounter—powerful doctor or scientist, vulnerable patient or subject—is the core act of medicine. Bioethical analysis works to be certain that this moral gesture is transparent, fair, and nonexploitative. All of these principles, decades of steady research and implementation, have been valuable.

But when the subject is not an individual but rather a population or a region of the world, we do not have a secure linguistic framework. Public health experts, when considering how to make population-wide decisions, largely use a straightforward utilitarian framework to make policy. If an intervention—a vaccine or a new public water purification system, for example—will offer benefit to the greatest number of people, then it is, by this logic ethical and can be supported. This is the case, even if some will be harmed. In rare instances, some children will have a terrible reaction to a measles vaccine and become paralyzed. But since far more would suffer paralysis if measles sickened all children, it is ethical to administer the vaccine, goes the utilitarian reasoning. Every large public health infrastructure project will displace and displease someone. Here, autonomy cannot really play a role, for if too many families decline to vaccinate their children, the "herd immunity" is disrupted, and if a person cannot abrogate some property rights, the water purification plant cannot be built.

In classic liberal theory, utilitarians argue that individual rights can be abrogated when the social good of the group is at stake. An action that allows for greater human flourishing for the greatest number *must* be undertaken. This argument has been valuable, for it has allowed state action to protect the health of communities. However, the debate about this problem, in the case of COVID-19, shows how unstable our language can be, and thus we return again and again to thinking about how to obtain consent within communities.

But the questions raised by using a gene drive for malaria are of a different nature—something that I began to understand as I read about the problem over the next six months. First, while gene drives releases will of course be subject to complex and earnest risk assessments which will have to factor in pathways that could lead to harm, a risk assessment is not prophecy. Moreover, the entire point and the real promise of a gene drive is in its very capacity to spread widely and once established in the wild, continue to spread outside of human control, making consent difficult, where exactly are the borders of "the community" or "the population"? Second, while a gene drive as a control strategy is new, the story of strategies to combat malaria in which there are many subjects of research, not just one, and not just in one local area, is not—there is a long history of malaria and communities with which to contend.

And so, I began to understand that a book about gene drives needed to take a great many complex narratives into account. Good bioethics, it has long been said, begins with good facts. This means that I will bring into this analysis many stories: a long and complex history of malaria control; an intricate story about the mosquitoes, the malaria-causing parasite, and the human interactions; a long and competitive search for the cause of disease; and the science of parasitology. There is a dark narrative about the forces of colonialism and something called "the scramble for Africa"; and there are stories about the relationship between malaria and the act of war, the use of malaria as a weapon, and the near collapse of the Allied forces to malaria in 1943. There are many things still not understood about malaria: how the parasite shifts forms in the human body; how the gametocytes or sexual forms of the parasite are formed; why resistance to both insecticide and parasiticide has historically developed so swiftly; and why scientists in the past have thought that resistant mutations begin in the same region—the Thai–Myanmar and Thai–Cambodia borderlands. There is a story about native plants and the Jesuits, and another one about the Chinese Cultural Revolution. The price of grain in the Punjab region of India and the chaos of ongoing war both play a part. There is the story of malaria in the American South, in Russia, in Italy, all across the temperate zones of the East Coast and Midwest of the USA. Malaria was not eradicated in the USA until 1951, and we need to think about why.

There is a story about how malaria was used to treat mental illness and how research on malaria treatment was done on prisoners, including a famous prisoner: Loeb of the ill-famed Leopold and Loeb case. Malaria and its eradication cannot be understood without first understanding how the USA came to control the Panama Canal, and how Sunnis and Shi'as and Christians live together in West Africa, where the burden of malaria is so very high and where most of the deaths from malaria occur. I came to believe that I could not answer the question of ethics—what the right act is and what makes it so—without understanding all of the surrounding narratives, the history that feels so vivid in the community of health-care workers and policy makers that cope with malaria. All these stories need to be explored, reader, to work out our problem.

One of the points that Burt had made in his talk was about what is called "the last mile problem." This refers to the fact that many of malaria's victims live in villages far from cities, clinics, or hospitals, on dirt roads that are impossible to navigate in the rains and floods and this makes the final eradication of many diseases of the poor very difficult. People in these villages are desperately poor, and their poverty means that they live in huts exposed to mosquitoes, that health care of any sort is miles and miles of unpaved road away, and that the interventions—insecticide-treated bed nets, drugs to combat malaria, crews to spray insecticide, on river, streams, and culverts to kill mosquito larvae—all of which has to be done in person, one intervention at a time—have a very difficult time simply reaching them. Only the mosquitoes reach into their lives, only the parasites carried by the mosquitoes reach into their blood, and that, noted Burt, is why changing the mosquitoes is the only way to change the disease's deadly pattern. Malaria is a disease of poverty and of upheaval: newly turned soil, deforestation, changing the way water flows over the land.[9] There is also the upheaval of colonial extraction, and of war, which means that wherever there is chaos, in all the "last miles" of rural poverty, now in Africa and Asia and Latin America, in the first half of the twenty-first century, on every continent but Antarctica, malaria is with us. In the USA and Europe, malaria is our recent neighbor.

It may be so again. When I met Austin Burt, and first heard the story of gene drives and malaria, the world was on a record trajectory: malaria cases and malaria deaths had been falling dramatically, year after year. The last mile was difficult, and there was still that horrible death rate—one child every two minutes—but the progress was steady. Not so now. By the fall of 2017, during which I first wrote this introduction, the curve of progress had leveled off. But on World Malaria Day, held annually to discuss progress on malaria (originally World Mosquito Day, an annual meeting begun in the nineteenth century by the British discoverer of the mosquito transmission of malaria) and in the World Health Organization (WHO) Malaria Report for 2018, the news was grim. Malaria was now back up to levels not seen since 2012.[10]

> The global response to malaria is at a crossroads. After an unprecedented period of success in malaria control, progress has stalled. The current pace is insufficient to achieve the 2020 milestones of the WHO Global Technical Strategy for Malaria 2016–2030—specifically, targets calling for a 40% reduction in malaria case incidence and death rates. Countries with ongoing transmission are increasingly falling into one of 2 categories: those moving towards elimination and those with a high burden of the disease that have reported significant increases in malaria cases. In 2016, there were 216 million cases of malaria in 91 countries, 5 million more than the 211 million cases reported in 2015. This marks a return to 2012 levels.[11]

And of course, by 2023, when I finished this book, the one you now have, COVID-19 had made the situation far worse. Something written two years earlier was now out of date. By 2022, malaria deaths were up to 619,000 and cases were at 247 million. In 2023, cases continued to rise.[12]

Malaria has begun to reassert itself more quickly than the WHO can write the reports. This is due in part to drug and insecticide resistance and in part to an increase in conflicts in some of the ninety-one countries referenced in the WHO report. To some extent, it is due to population growth, and in large part, it is due to the strain on health-care systems that had to cope with a new pandemic. However, the most pressing indicator is climate change. The range of mosquitoes is larger because of climate change, as the world is wetter and hotter. Parasites spin through their life span faster, reproduce more, and can infect more people in warmer climates, and the disease can become constant, not seasonal. When I first wrote this introduction, the United Nations (UN) Intergovernmental Panel on Climate Change (UNIPCC) released yet another report about global warming—about the speed at which the climate is changing, with temperatures rising toward 1.5°C above preindustrial levels. The UNIPCC notes: "B5.2. Any increase in global warming is projected to affect human health, with primarily negative consequences (high confidence). Lower risks are projected at 1.5°C than at 2°C for heat-related morbidity and mortality (very high confidence) and for ozone related mortality if emissions needed for ozone formation remain high (high confidence.) Urban heat islands often amplify the impacts of heatwaves in cities (high confidence). Risks from some vector borne diseases, such as malaria and dengue fever, are projected to increase with warming from 1.5°C to 2°C, including potential shifts in their geographic range (high confidence)."[13] About malaria specifically, the UNIPCC states:

> Recent projections of the potential impacts of climate change on malaria globally and for Asia, Africa, and South America (Annex 3.1 Table S9) confirm that weather and climate are among the drivers of the geographic range, intensity of transmission, and seasonality of malaria, and that the relationships are not necessarily linear, resulting in complex patterns of changes in risk with additional warming (very high confidence) (Ren et al., 2016; Song et al., 2016; Semakula et al., 2017). Projections suggest the burden of malaria could increase with climate change because of a greater geographic range of the Anophel vector, longer season, and/or increase in the number of people at risk, with larger burdens with greater amounts of warming, with regionally variable patterns (high agreement, medium evidence). Vector populations are projected to shift with climate change, with expansions and reductions depending on the degree of local warming, the ecology of the mosquito vector, and other factors (Ren et al., 2016).[14]

And now, of course, every indicator is worse. Yearly, we release more carbon per capita, temperatures increase, and rainfall becomes more frequent. We face a world in critical danger, and with malaria, not only a disease of the Other, but one that could again reach into the lives of some of the most vulnerable people in the USA. It would not take much, for the lives of the poor are, by many measures, worsening. In 2016, directly after the election of President Trump, the US government invited the UN Commission on Poverty to submit a report on the poor of the USA. The results were startling, considering that this was written prior to the SARS-CoV-2 pandemic. Highlights included:

> By most indicators, the US is one of the world's wealthiest countries. It spends more on national defense than China, Saudi Arabia, Russia, United Kingdom, India, France, and Japan combined. US health care expenditures per capita are double the OECD average and much higher than in all other countries. But there are many fewer doctors and hospital beds per person than the OECD average. US infant mortality rates in 2013 were the highest in the developed world. Neglected tropical diseases, including Zika, are increasingly common in the USA. It has been estimated that 12 million Americans live with a neglected parasitic infection, largely hookworm. In terms of access to water and sanitation the US ranks 36th in the world. The youth poverty rate in the United States is the highest across the OECD with one quarter of youth living in poverty compared to less than 14% across the OECD. US child poverty rates are the highest amongst the six richest countries—Canada, the United Kingdom, Ireland, Sweden and Norway. In the OECD the US ranks 35th out of 37 in terms of poverty and inequality. According to the World Income Inequality Database, the US has the highest Gini rate (measuring inequality) of all Western Countries.[15]

It was this constellation of issues—how climate change affects human health, how malaria is both a cause and an outcome of extreme poverty, and how a radical new idea, a gene drive, could affect the disease—that interested me. I had long been concerned about the need to turn the attention of bioethics to the ordinary and persistent problems of the poor. In 2003, calling for a "Just Bioethics," I argued that although bioethicists are drawn to new technology and its remarkable power, we need to understand that the duty of the philosopher is to interrogate.

All of these technologies, I have argued, raise significant issues of justice and access as each remarkable gadget is released into a wider context. How do we address the issue of justice in a world of persistent health-care injustice? Reflecting on these issues will require an insistent tenacity as well as a discerning curiosity. It will require a shift from justification based on the mesmerizing ends of science to the constancy of, and practice toward, the daily moral appeals of community.[16]

This book aims to do several things. First, I will describe how malaria has been a part of human history, how the disease both shapes and is shaped by human activity, and why we are now at a particularly fraught moment in what has been a centuries-long struggle, since the disease was first understood in modern terms, a millennial-long struggle, in terms of our collective genetic heritage to defeat what is nearly always called "Man's Greatest Enemy." I will turn to the story of how malaria is closely linked to situations of war or social chaos, and how it cannot be fully understood without paying attention to race and class historical dynamics. I will describe how malaria—once the most important disease in the USA and Europe became a "tropical disease." I will describe how, in 1955, the world thought it had mastered the problem of malaria at last, and how that project failed, and how, now, well into the twenty-first century, we see again the patterns of resistance to nearly all our malaria-control strategies. That will set the stage for the rationale for new technologies, although everyone who engages with malaria agrees that every single strategy—drugs to fight the parasite in human bodies; clinics and health systems that can treat severe cases; preventative, community-wide dosing of pregnant women and children; larvae destruction, insecticide, bed nets, sugar traps, bacterial control, drainage, and case reporting—will all need to continue in a coordinated effort, even if new technologies are successful.

Then, I will turn to the science of gene drives, describe how Burt's laboratory at Imperial College London and then others have developed the consortium known as Target Malaria (where I served on the external international ethics advisory committee). I will describe the opposition to the project and explore, with care, the arguments of its leaders. After that, I will turn to consider the growing body of reports that suggest ways to regulate gene drive technology and that suggest "paths forward" to make the project safe, accessible, and ethically accomplished. Since one of the things that such reports universally agree upon is the need for community engagement and the delineation of the community, I will next reflect on the political and economic situation at the sites where permission for the use of gene drives might be first considered and sought: Burkina Faso, Mali, and Uganda. I will describe why these reports are useful—and indeed, how Target Malaria is already enacting them—but then I will tell you why the reports are limited. I will attend to the concerns raised by groups that fiercely oppose gene drives, and I will consider how the calls for "stakeholder engagement" are being understood and enacted in the project. Finally, I will think about the ethical issues, both the ones that have been encountered over and over in malaria research and the ones that are engendered by new technologies.

The New Vaccine

By now, alert readers will be wondering about the news that the WHO proclaimed as historic in the fall of 2021: the approval of the first vaccine for malaria. This vaccine announcement, which was made a week before I finished my manuscript, had been long anticipated. It is one of a series of hopeful interventions that offer a solution to a single piece of the complex puzzle that represents the landscape of malaria. Of course, every person who cares about malaria, and its impact, and everyone who champions scientific responses to human disease should celebrate this advance.

It is important to remember that the vaccine, Mosquirix™, is a complementary prevention intervention for children, but it needs to be paired with other interventions in order for it to work, such as indoor spraying (IRS), insecticide-treated nets (ITNs), and, at times, mass drug administration (MDA)—all were used to support the vaccine, when it was in trials, Mosquirix still is only 40–60 percent effective, cannot be used in infants, and loses its potency completely after four years. It requires multiple doses, which means going back to the clinic every month for three months, and then again a year or so later, which may prove difficult for families. It is a first-generation vaccine—there will be more development and its developers are optimistic about their capacity to improve it in later iterations.

You will see in this book how complex and dynamic a disease malaria has been historically. It changes its nature. The parasite has changed its vector. It mutates to resist interventions. It evokes up compensatory human biological and social responses. The vaccine reduces illness and death when used with the other interventions, but it does not eliminate malaria, not even locally. To make our world free of malaria is a larger project, and it is this project that is of interest to me, in addition to the goal of reducing the vast human suffering malaria causes at the individual level. Thus, despite the personal joy with which one can greet the vaccine—however imperfect—I will argue that gene drives for malaria could become one of the most important, durable, sustainable, and coherent preventive strategies for malaria and, of course, may offer proof of principle in the control of other deadly vector-borne diseases that sicken humans, animals, and plants.

This is what this book is about. Here is what it is not about. It is not a hagiography of one particular person or one particular project, although you will learn a great deal about one such project, Target Malaria. It is not a "how to" book or a handbook of regulations, although I consider regulations and their implications. It is a book that is, in a sense, a moment of thinking, it is a meditation on the complexity of the issues: nature, our power, research science, malaria, gene drives—midstream in the work, an unfinished discourse, for the work in the genetics of gene drives began more than five decades ago, and the work on the stakeholder engagement more than a decade ago, and gene drives will not be ready for deployment for a decade to come, even if all goes perfectly well. The idea may, indeed, fail in the field, or it may take decades to succeed, or history itself may turn in other directions entirely. Much literature about the ethics of gene therapy were written in the early 1970s for a medical promise that would go unfulfilled for the next thirty years and can only now be considered possible, finally come of age, at least for some who can afford its prohibitive cost.

Because I have been a bioethicist for nearly three decades, like all my colleagues, I have written—and written with cautious but very sincere optimism—about other projects that seemed to be on the brink of success— always ten years from clinical trials, I was told, a phenomenon that I began to think of as "decenniumophilia." First, it was gene therapy, then stem cells, then nanotechnology, then synthetic biology, then advances in neuroscience, then oncofertility, just ten years from the clinic, and here I am carefully considering gene drives. None of the previous projects have (yet) changed the world in the ways that their inventors imagined, although all are, of course, still possible. But nor has the grim descent into genetic reductionism, "designer babies," or any of the other sad fates that critics of the technology imagined, happened either. One reviewer of this book was quite concerned about this problem. "What are the odds this will *work*?" he asked. "Tell us about the odds of success," he asked again. But I cannot tell him that, nor could the scientists, not really. Rather, I will tell him, and you, reader, what the research is now showing, why it might succeed and why it might fail, and I can tell you how carefully the investigators are planning the next step. I am arguing, then, not for certainty but rather for thinking.

Let me add some important personal history at this juncture. After that 2015 meeting, and from 2016 to the present, I have served as one of the ethicists on what became the external International Ethics Advisory Committee to Target Malaria, the academic consortium of researchers where Burt was one of the two principal investigators (PIs). This is a group of scholars with training in various fields affected by the research. I am a bioethics scholar of religion and moral philosophy, but others come from conservation research, nongovernmental organization (NGO) leadership, global public health, or infectious disease practices, from Europe and the USA, from Canada, Africa, and India. This gave me an insider's view of this work. It also raised the very real problem of what bioethics calls "regulatory capture" and unfair bias, and this was raised by reviewers of earlier drafts. Of course, some of this is understandable. Why would I serve on a committee for a project I believed was ill intended, or review the work of a scientist I thought was mendacious? I am interested in Target Malaria, of course, but I am very aware of both its limitations and that it is not alone in gene drive research. I chose to focus on this one project in some detail not only because it was the first gene drive project and the one farthest along in the process, and not only because it is the one that I know the most about, given my proximity as a member of the Ethics Advisory Committee. but because the project was attempting to create a new way of doing science. First, it was a not-for-profit consortium, for the members had to first agree to share their work without patent restriction or unfair profits, should any technology be licensed. The goal was to ensure that cost would not be a barrier to the use of gene drives, and this is, in itself, remarkable in the competitive world of modern science. Additionally, the project was not to be entirely Western led, but rather built as a collaboration between and among Western and non-Western scientists. Our committee reflected that principle. Also, as I will explore in the chapter on community engagement, I was interested in seeing how the sort of fully "community engaged" science that bioethicists argue for in principle would work in practice. So, the project intended several experiments in its process—in ethics oversight, in collaboration, in stakeholder engagement, and in distributive justice—in addition to genetic innovations.

Let me also give you a reader's guide, or road map, to the argument of the book. I began my work in bioethics working in clinical medicine, where my colleague Susan Rubin and I developed a method for hearing and judging cases with local ethics committees. We always began with the scientific and medical facts of the case. Then, we reviewed the other sources of facts and critical narratives from the family, staff, and community that surrounded the patient faced with an ethical dilemma. Only then did we create a list of options and moral arguments and evaluate them.

I found this useful when I began to turn my attention to the ethical issues in emerging technology. We will begin in chapter 1 with a long (very long) history about malaria and the human encounter with the disease. In it, I will retell some of what I think are the most important narratives that still drive our evaluation of the ethical issues today. I will explain here some of the biology and etiology of the disease and of the long struggle to figure out its complexities. This is "thick description" that bioethicists need about the players in the case. Although I enjoyed learning about malaria's history, if you know a great deal about public health, you can go right to chapter 2. In chapter 2, I will describe the Imperial laboratories, which is one place among several globally where gene drives are being investigated. I chose Imperial because I had that front-row seat as a member of an independent ethics committee, but also because it is the first of the laboratories in the field with gene drive technology. In this chapter, I will give very much a layperson's description of the science of gene drives. It will focus on the two laboratories at Imperial, the Burt and Crisanti laboratories but also make brief mention of other gene drive projects, including ones at the University of California in Irvine and San Diego. Here, too, if you know the science, you can go to chapter 3. In chapter 3, I will give an account of three of the many regulatory plans that have been erected to create norms for gene drives in advance of the development of the technology. I will also give a brief history of the regulation of genetic research. In chapter 4, I will give you the final set of descriptions and observations that you will need to make evaluative judgments about gene drives. Here, I will describe the tangible realities of African stakeholder engagement and discuss how the history of colonial rule in Africa has shaped our perceptions of disease, and of the justification for intervention. You will find that I tell some historical narratives here as well, using the story of the first leader of the Royal Society, Humphrey Davy, as an example of how science has listened to the needs of citizens. These four chapters are like the investigative part of an ethics case consult. And you will note, reader, that I have made you my ethics committee, listening to the facts of the case first.

In the last three chapters, I will change register and walk you through the ethical arguments about gene drives and their implications. In chapter 5, I will allow the critics of gene drive to speak first, and we will listen to them, as one does in a consultative process, as they make their case. Then, I will address their concerns. In chapter 6, I will explore what I believe are the ethical issues we need to consider. First, we will explore the ethical issues that exist in all malaria research and treatment. Next, we will consider the ethical issues that exist in all genetic engineering. Finally, we will see what we make of the use of genes drives for malaria, given all these issues—sorting out the arguments to see them clearly and to reason our way to a conclusion and justification. In chapter 7, the conclusion of the book, I will consider the problem of uncertainty, and you will see how I justify the research and ways I suggest for going forward after careful thinking.

For to think carefully about the deeper moral justifications and implications of this project will mean far harder intellectual work. Why can "we" intervene in the lives of others? What does it mean to do so? How are we—the whole of humanity—going to address the very old problem of disease in a physical world that is now being changed in unprecedented ways? What language best articulates our duty to act in a world where, during the time it took you to read this introduction, two children lie dead? I am going to suggest that the discourse we will need will not be about insect cages, error reports, or even surveillance, although these are all critical of course. What is needed for the project to be ethical, I will argue, are not only the usual calls for autonomy, justice, and beneficence—the demands of human rights—but also the demands of duty—constancy, fidelity, and integrity—and I will explore how attention to these demands, their sources, and their meaning creates a more demanding but necessary framework for reflection on genes, diseases, humans, the natural world, and our shared, created, environment.

1   The World as We Know It: Malaria and Its History

1.1   The History of Malaria: The Nature of a Disease

There has always been malaria. Long before there was any human inquiry into why children sickened and swiftly died of malaria, before there was any human child at all, there was *Plasmodium*, the parasite that causes malaria. More accurately, there was a single-celled organism, likely plantlike in origin[1] because its genome still contains traces of proteins needed for photosynthesis, floating in small, warm tropical streams, near the banks of the slow, silty rivers of Africa, and near other single-celled organisms, perhaps near the tiny eggs of other aquatic creatures. By then, there were mosquitoes on Earth, for the delicate lacewing traces left in the fossil evidence shows how little they have changed, and they laid their eggs in these wetlands too. Scientists speculate that the *Plasmodium* somehow drifted into the eggs, hitched onto their larvae's bodies when they hatched, and then began living in the intestinal tract of the newly born mosquitoes. It is then thought that these single cells, living in the gut and parts of the mouth of the mosquitoes—largely the salivary glands—adapted into what we now know as the species *Plasmodium*. It had slipped inside mosquitoes and found a home in their gut, reproducing sexually, as it still does inside certain mosquito species.[2]

Malaria parasites are microorganisms that belong to the genus *Plasmodium*. There are more than 100 species of *Plasmodium*, which can infect many animal species such as reptiles, birds, and various mammals. Four species of *Plasmodium* have long been recognized to infect humans in nature. In addition, there is one species that naturally infects macaques, which has recently been recognized to be a cause of zoonotic malaria in humans. (There are some additional species that can, exceptionally or under experimental conditions, infect humans.)[3]

The mosquito species evolved along with the *Plasmodium* species, and they evolved to need blood—from reptiles, birds, or mammals—to mature the females' fertilized eggs prior to laying them. Mosquitoes fly randomly, taken by the air, following the currents of the wind, and they have evolved to sense something: the increased CO_2 in the air, the exhaled breath perhaps or the odor (it is not clear). They then alight on the skin of the creature to suck its blood. Scientists speculating about the odd, complicated dynamics of malaria theorize that the *Plasmodium* must have been dropped from the proboscis of the mosquito, onto the bitten creature, and found in its blood a second fortuitously hospitable place, dividing asexually and multiplying. *Plasmodium* flourished there, in the pierced capillary, living in the blood of the animal, evolving over centuries, amassing in huge numbers, filling the cells of the liver, returning to the blood until once again, another mosquito bit that particular animal and sucked that particular blood up again, invested now with the *Plasmodium*, which traveled into the gut of the insect, where it divided again, into female and male forms, which reproduced inside the mosquito, just as it had before it had stumbled into the animal blood. Over millions of years, this chancy, jerry-rigged, unlikely series of evolutionary events created an ecological niche for the *Plasmodium*, here, in these capricious animal bodies, and there, inside the small bodies of the mosquito.

Randall Packard speculates that the *Plasmodia* must have flourished in the bloodstream of many animals in this way, in birds and rodents, safe from predation, long before humans evolved from nonhuman primates also to become hosts. The *Plasmodium* that causes malaria changes shape, form, and function inside another creature. After the mosquito bites, the first form is the "sporozoite," and in this form—likened to clear, thin needles—the parasite goes immediately from the site of the bite to the liver of the animal. There, it "hides" or rather evades the body's immune defense systems, as each sporozoite enters a liver cell and slowly invades it, reproducing asexually, until the liver cell bursts, and the new form of the parasite, the "merozoite," spills back into the bloodstream. The merozoite form has evolved to pierce the sides of red blood cells, again evading the immune system by hiding within the cell, circling inside, sucking out its protein, and growing and dividing again and again. The white blood cells, "phagocytes," the body's defense mechanism, try, as the name implies, to "eat" as many merozoites as possible, especially in the brief moment they escape from the liver, but there are so very many merozoites in every infection, and most go from freely swimming in the bloodstream to quickly entering the red blood cells themselves. As each cell is depleted, the merozoites enter (the usual word here is "invade") other cells, reproducing, bursting, over and over, until the person, wracked by cycles of alternating chills and fevers, becomes anemic. Some of the merozoites change form again and, in smaller numbers, become "gametocytes," which are the cellular forms capable of sexual reproduction only in the gut of the vector, the mosquito. So, remarkably, and oddly enough, the human person who has become the host for the parasite has to be bitten again, so that a mosquito can suck up the blood that contains gametocytes, which travel to the mosquito's gut. There, the *Plasmodium* combines to make new a new form. This is the wriggling, mating, wormlike form that was one of the first indications of their presence to early researchers. It a form that moves through the inside of the gut to the outside to wait on the outside surface of the stomach of the mosquito as small, glistening, cyst-like orbs. These orbs then burst to release tens of thousands of the clear, glistening "needles" into the abdominal cavity of the mosquito. From there, they are swept into the mosquito's salivary glands—long, white ribbons that hold enormous numbers of parasites, which, when the mosquito thrusts its mouth into the skin of its victim, are squeezed out, along with an anesthetizing element, and a decoagulant. This allows the mosquito to bite and to fed on freely flowing blood as the sporozoites are pumped into the small wound. It is such an efficient and swift process that the animal, usually sleeping (since then the mosquito can find them easily), is barely aware it happened until the next morning.

It is a process so unlikely, so chancy, that it is extraordinary that it works at all. First, a mosquito must bite a huge creature, many times larger than itself. It needs to bite an animal that has gametocytes, which apparently are found most easily in the peripheral vascular system. It must take a blood meal and then fly, awkwardly swollen with blood, to find a safe place to rest before expelling the water from the blood solids. It needs the blood not for food but rather to use the proteins in the blood to mature the fertilized eggs in its body. The female—and only the female of the species—is driven to bite by powerful reproductive instincts. Males apparently exist only to drink nectar from flowing plants and for mating. What makes the odd, shape-shifting process work at all—there are seven separate body designs for this one parasite—is abundance, sheer numbers. At each stage, the parasite makes copies, at some stages, tens of thousands of copies of itself (often called "armies of progeny" in yet another military metaphor),[4] which overwhelm the immune responses of both mosquitoes and human beings—a formidable task, notes Sonia Shah.

As evolution filled the Earth with many species of mosquitoes, *Plasmodia*, and mammals, the mosquitoes began to prefer to bite certain animals over others. One of the favorites for some *Anopheles* mosquitoes were the hairless humanoids, our ancestors, and eventually, modern *Homo sapiens*, who liked to live and liked to sleep around one another in groups, who collect water that they left uncovered overnight, and who liked to climb trees—all very convenient as for a flying, biting insect. Historian Gordon Harrison writes, "Indeed, it is reasonable to suppose that our primate ancestors were recognizably malarious before they were recognizably human, that the parasite that causes the fever and the mosquito that transfers it from one person to another have accompanied us throughout the Darwinian evolution."[5] Many books about malaria start with this sort of long description of the biology of the mosquito for three reasons, I would argue: first, because of the terrible beauty of the life cycle of the organism, its otherworldly capacities and permutations and forms; second, because of the oddity and the unlikely chanciness of the entire operation; and third, because our story of gene drives begins in the prehistory of the Earth itself. Learning the natural history of the disease makes the long, difficult relationship between humans and vectors central to our understanding of our own present. We live, as this sort of long history makes clear, in a world not entirely under our control—a world in which the small, sticklike insect we can kill with a swat of our hand, the mosquito, delivers the parasite of deadly malaria, which makes it the single most deadly organism on the planet, as Sonia Shah notes in her extraordinary work, "*The Fever.*"[6] Here, she describes this, something that Bill Gates has also noted in his characterization of the mosquito as "the world's deadliest creature." As Shah notes: Such are the ironies of survival on this protean planet. A creature at the very bottom of the zoological scale, a humble being beneficently converting sunlight into living tissue (and thereby providing the basis for the planet's entire food chain) turns into one of the most ruthlessly successful parasites ever known, commanding two separate spheres of the living world, human and entomological.[7,8]

For malaria to flourish, it needs three organisms in perfect alignment—the parasite, the mosquito vector, and humans—all of which must be linked in an elegant, delicate relationship: *Plasmodium*, insect, person, and enough of both mosquitoes and people to keep the *Plasmodium* species alive. Reduce the number of *Plasmodia* or the concentration of mosquitoes or their biting rate or the number of people who carry the *Plasmodium*—any of this would disrupt the disease of malaria, which is why it has been successfully locally eradicated in many regions of the world.

And, yet here we are, with our cell phones and our Large Hadron Collider and our complicated apps, and we cannot—or have not—been able to eliminate either the mosquito or the parasite globally, or use any of our extraordinary power—vaccines, insecticides, drugs—to cure the disease permanently and for all. Consider this: there is not one place on Earth where humans do not know mosquitoes. They are there in the most intimate of spaces, where we sleep and eat, touching and softly penetrating our nakedness, leaving the round red mark of their presence, their sign, on our bodies. Every human everywhere knows to swipe at them, knows their high keening sound. And we know that they leave far more than the red itchy sign; they leave, especially in the small bodies of children, dreadful disease.

The gravity of our situation is the beginning of our evaluation of gene drives, and without these details, it is impossible to assess the ethical questions in the debates about their use. This is a book about the ethics of gene drives, but it is specifically about the ethics of gene drives for the elimination of malaria, and that—the human problem of preventing a devasting disease—is central to our thinking about the technology.

It is thought that the malaria caused by the *Plasmodia* species called *Plasmodium vivax* was the first one that humans encountered in Africa, when humans lived only in Africa, and this encounter was long into the evolutionary history of the mosquito–*Plasmodium*–animal relationship. It must have been a deadly, devasting disease, argues Shah.[9] Shah continues that disease outbreaks must have happened only rarely, for the first Africans were hunter-gatherers and lived in small bands that rarely encountered one another or an infected mosquito. But when the band was found and bitten by such a creature, having picked up the parasite from some other wandering hunter, the catastrophe of illness exerted intense selective pressure. Only a few people, Shah reasons, must have survived the first epidemic sweeps. The individuals with the capacity to resist infection might have done so because of a random mutation that made their red blood cells smooth instead of knobby, and this survival advantage spread this gene throughout the tribes then living on the African continent. Because the mosquito that carried the *P. vivax* parasite preferred the blood of humans to other animals, the parasite adapted to be exquisitely sensitive to the precise shape of human red blood cells. It could not penetrate the cells without the little protrusions—called Duffy bodies—that cover normal red blood cells. People who are Duffy negative, which includes virtually all people of African ancestry, are resistant to infection by *P. vivax*—a trait that both perplexed eighteenth- and nineteenth-century scientists and enabled racist explanations to take hold within the science of malaria itself. *P. vivax* parasites could not successfully persist in Africa. Thus, over time, mosquitoes that carried *P. vivax* found humans to bite farther north, toward the Mediterranean, where the population was slower to develop genetic adaptations.

Thus started new chains of malarial transmission around the Mediterranean, up to Italy, toward the land around Marmore, as we know, and finally, north to the Fens of England, carried in the blood of Roman armies. Malaria was not only a tropical disease. Diminished to the point of vanishing in Africa some 10,000 years ago, *P. vivax* reemerged some 5,000 years later in ancient Egypt, Greece, India, the Middle East, Europe, and China, and persisted. The *Plasmodium* only needed humans in dense enough concentration, the vector host species, *Anopheles* mosquitoes, in large enough numbers, and they were everywhere. In colder climates, mosquitoes wintered in the warm houses, emerging in great clouds in the medieval spring air.

However, into the niche in Africa that was abandoned when mosquitoes that carried *P. vivax* moved their territory, came both a new type of parasite and a new type of mosquito to carry it. Both had existed previously, but as hunter-gatherers gave way to Bantu tribes, who began small-scale agriculture, the forest environment began to change, giving a different mosquito species and a different parasite selective advantages. Several factors changed at once. First, the Bantu people, arriving from the north and sweeping across West and Central Africa, began to slash and burn and cut and clear the vast forest that once stretched across the continent.[10] Sunlight suddenly began to reach streams and pools, which favored the eggs of *A. gambiae*, a species that likes bright, clear water in which to lay their eggs.[11] *Gambiae* are what are known as "super-transmitters," because after the females emerge from their larvae stage, they are quickly fertilized by emerging male mosquitoes and do not need to mate again. Then, once matured on the nectar of plants, the females begin to bite humans—and prefer humans—with fierce frequency, laying several rounds of eggs in a lifetime. "There are three major species of "super transmitters": *An. gambiae sensu stricto, An arabiensis, An.funestus* . . . one or more were present across all African ecological zones, from desert-edge to dense rainforest, from the lowlands to the moderate highlands, in virtually all ecological niches. They were not alone. Other anlopheline mosquitoes, such as *An.nili, An moucheti, An melas, An. Mascariensisi* and *An. Paludi* were highly significant regional vectors with narrower ranges."[12] Second, the landscape was newly changed—plowed, with the earth turned up, streams dammed and diverted for irrigation, and young plants growing in soft depressions that filled with rainwater. And because the Bantu farmers did not leave their land like hunter-gatherers, settlements grew and attracted more people, who began farming, exchanging, and building small huts to sleep in safe from the rain that they gathered in pots near their homes. But the huts were not safe from mosquitoes that found it fortuitous to bite sleeping humans clustered in groups, humans who barely noticed the bites, as the mosquito vectors evolved to inject an anesthetic agent along with an anticlotting factor into the bite wounds as they fed, seeking a capillary, but not disturbing their host.

In the end, not only was the *A. gambiae* mosquito more aggressive but the parasite *Plasmodium falciparum* was far more deadly than *P. vivax*, causing more fatal disease, penetrating the red blood cells more efficiently, regardless of the lack of Duffy knobs, and making these cells so sticky that they clotted, blocking veins and tissues. Malaria parasites create crystallized hemoglobin that is ingested by the macrophages—and the white blood cells, which mobilize to respond to foreign parasitic cells, are unable to respond properly. Nor do they die, however. So the body does not create more macrophages, crippling the immune system.[13] Shah argues, "Blood cells infected with *falciparum* parasites become sticky and get clogged in the small blood vessels. This is likely a survival tactic for the parasite. Stuck inside the vessels, it avoids being washed into the bloodstream and neutralized by the pathogen-killing spleen. There it can grow undisturbed. But the clogged vessels deprive the victim's tissues of oxygen and clogged micro vessels in the brain can starve the brain and bring on coma."[14] Scientists had historically inferred that *P. falciparum* is the youngest evolutionary form of *Plasmodium*, but that is only a hunch because it is so deadly.[15] This one parasite accounts for 90 percent of all deaths from malaria. *P. falciparum* also attacks red blood cells at all of their life stages, not just young or old cells.[16] Gordon Harrison argued for this concept in 1978: "Since successful parasitism evolves toward accommodation, perhaps ideally, toward a fully cooperative commensalism in which the interests of both animals are served, the reckless behavior of

P. falciparum suggests that it is new to its host. Perhaps we have not had evolutionary time to develop effective controls over its fecundity, and it has not had time to oust the killers from its main genetic line."[17] Shah, too, continues that theory, claiming "Most pathogens mellow as they age. It's enlightened self-interest, as the theory goes. Diminishing virulence is a superior strategy for survival (but *falciparum*) remains essentially wild and untamed despite its great antiquity."[18] Of course, there is controversy on this point as well, for as we now realize from COVID-19, pathogens evolve largely to be more transmissible, which may or may not be less lethal to their hosts. But that is not the only argument at play. *P. falciparum* is also thought to be a more recent pathogen by because of the way that human hosts have genetically reacted to it, even under great selective pressure.[19] Scientists speculate the time when the parasite entered human history by the rate of mutations and of evolutionary changes left in the human genomic record. "Malaria has placed the strongest known selective pressure on the human genome since the origin of agriculture within the past 10,000 years. *Plasmodium falciparum* was probably not able to gain a foothold among African populations until larger sedentary communities emerged in association with the evolution of domestic agriculture in Africa (the agricultural revolution). Several inherited variants in red blood cells have become common in parts of the world where malaria is frequent as a result of selection exerted by this parasite."[20] Mutations in the red blood cells—the site of the attack, especially of the sticky, deadly cells infected with the *P. falciparum* parasite—give an advantage to the host if the cell could change shape or if their surface proteins changed. Thus, survival pressure from *P. falciparum* favored another random human mutation. This one was linked to red-cell protein production. But unlike the direct success of the Duffy mutation, this was only partly effective in avoiding the disease, and it came with fatal risks. The mutation changed the shape of the blood cells from spherical to crescent.[21]

This strategy proved to be costly. The mutation causes sickle cell disease when a child inherits copies of the mutation from both parents. A carrier of two these mutations has the capacity for their cells to "sickle" or change from a round to a rigid curved shape, and this keeps the *P. falciparum* parasite from entering the cell efficiently. Sickle cell anemia, the double mutation, which can be horribly painful and eventually fatal, and surely would have been in antiquity—was the high cost of avoiding malaria in some children, and it spread within African populations. Some 44 million people have sickle cell anemia, the most common form of the disease. Eighty percent of cases occur in sub-Saharan Africa.

Other blood dyscrasias, or thalassemias, akin to sickle cell, spread behind the infection of *P. vivax* and then *P. falciparum* as it swept into the Mediterranean basin. The mutation traveled across the Middle East, leaving a trail of people, some with overt sickle cell illness, others only with a glucose-6-phosphate dehydrogenase (G6PD) deficiency, which renders them unable to eat fava beans, a Mediterranean staple, or, as it later turned out, unable to take an important drug for malaria—primaquine.

Over the years, and after many repeated *P. falciparum* infections, the Bantu who survived developed what was initially thought to be an acquired immunity to the most severe form of the disease. But the inner landscapes of Africa were impenetrable to Westerners, who had no previous exposure to *P. falciparum* forms of the disease. When nonimmune people moved to the area, they immediately succumbed—a fate that would foil many later invaders of Central Africa. And even when people who had been immune moved away or were taken by war, they would lose their immunity. By 900 CE, *P. falciparum* malaria swept across all of Africa, and would, with rare exceptions, remain only there until the 1500s. But malaria was only in its early stages of explosion. The expansion of empires, the trade in humans, and new global travel would greatly extend its range.

Because the life cycle of the parasite was so complex and so very odd, and because so many diseases caused fevers and sudden childhood death, the history I have just recounted remained obscure. Humans did not guess the unlikely story of the life cycle of the parasite, half inside a mosquito gut and half inside human liver and blood, until nearly the twentieth century. "At every stage of *Plasmodium*'s remarkable travels the odds against its continuance are overwhelming. If a mosquito manages to pick up the parasite from an infected person—not a likely event to begin with—she must stay alive for the ten to twelve days that the sporozoites need to develop and lodge in her head . . . Malaria, is, in short, a most improbable disease. Yet it has demonstrated a durability and a resistance to attack second to none."[22] Because the etiology of the disease was so strange, and unlikely, other theories arose to explain the persistence of the deadly fever. Swamps were suspected in some way. By the time of the Rome Empire, citizens knew to avoid the deadly, swampy Campagna, and built houses on stilts on the highest places possible. Of course, the landscape of hill towns throughout Italy still offers mute testimony of this strategy. The existence of the Marmore Falls, built with such astounding effort, also testifies to this.

The medical literature in antiquity described what is clearly malaria: waning and waxing fevers that were predictable, both *P. vivax* and the deadly *P. falciparum*, and references to malaria in 4,000-year-old Sumerian and Egyptian texts record the disease as it swept over the Nile and then the Mediterranean basin. Antigens to *Plasmodium* in 5,000-year-old Egyptian and Nubian mummies have been found. By the fifth century, the school we know as the Hippocratic School had texts that described it as a disease "common around swamps." Homer is thought to have referred to malaria when he decried Sirius as an "evil star" that was the "harbinger of fever." Hebrew Scripture warns of the fevers that come at night, and Deuteronomy 28:22 says, "The Lord will strike you with consumption; and with fever, and with inflammation; and with fiery heat, and with the sword, and with blight, and with mildew, and they shall pursue you until you perish." This anxiety around going out at night would be codified centuries later by rabbinic law. Texts from the Qin dynasty (221–206 BCE) in China called malaria the "mother of fevers." Vedic texts from India 3,500 years ago describe the reoccurring fevers as the "king of all diseases," personified by the fever demon Takman. The Vedic sages accurately described malaria's signature chills and fever. "To the cold Takman," they wrote, "to the shaking one, and to the deliriously hot, the glowing, do I render homage. To him that returns on the morrow, to him that returns for two successive days, to the Takman that returns on the third day, shall homage be."[23]

By the time of the Roman imperial conquests, *P. vivax* had swept over Western Europe, for the Roman legions brought both the new religion, Christianity, and the new parasites on their long, slow marches. This was despite the cold winters, for there, the mosquitoes entered the houses and the newly created urban centers and wintered over. Records describe the disease's entry into Northern Europe during the early medieval period.[24] Malaria surrounded the birth and growth of religion and culture, a part of the human experience itself, as predictable as birth, unavoidable.

Hippocratic texts and Vedas alike described the peculiar "fever rhythm" of the illness, with wildly high fevers of 104–106°F, and debilitating headaches, which crested at the time when the parasites burst out of destroyed red blood cells, in synchrony with the hemolysis. In *P. vivax*, *P. falciparum*, and *P. ovale* malaria, there was fever every forty-eight hours on the first and third days, and thus it began to be called "tertian fever." Malaria caused by the *Plasmodium malariae* parasite peaks every seventy-two hours, or "quartan," on the first and fourth days. The fevers can be "benign tertian," usually *P. vivax*, or "severe tertian" or "malignant" tertian, usually *P. falciparum*. The incubation period between bite and illness varies. For *P. falciparum*, it is twelve days, and for *P. ovale*, it is seventeen days. For *P. malariae*, it can vary between eighteen and forty days, and for *P. vivax*, it can be as quick as fifteen days, but it can also be delayed by six to twelve months as the parasite waits in the liver.

The disease remained a mysterious, seemingly inevitable, part of the cost of human exploration itself. By the fifteenth century, *P. vivax* was well established in Europe and Asia, and the regnant of *P. falciparum* dominated the African continent. Wherever humans traveled, malaria was part of the human exchange. As people traded along the Silk Road and pushed into what is now Russia, malaria came as well. Ivory was traded for spices, Venetian glass for tea, fine woven silk for intricate embossed weapons, and everywhere, the disease passed between travelers as well. The mosquito that carried *P. vivax* proved quite adaptable—and the *Plasmodium* could live inside local mosquitoes that evolved to hide in warm cracks in houses when it was cold. The *Plasmodium*, which needs it to be 68°F inside the mosquito in order to reproduce, adapted to stay for long months in the liver of the human host, returning to the human's peripheral bloodstream, where it was then sequestered in the gametocytes form, until the mosquitoes, newly hatched, began to bite. *P. vivax* did not need a tropical zone. It just needed a mosquito—but not all mosquitoes. There are 3,200 species of mosquito, and far fewer are deadly vectors for malaria. Although *Aedes aegypti* carries many diseases, including dengue fever, Zika, yellow fever, chikungunya, and Mayaro fever, the complex cycle needed by the *Plasmodium* of malaria is only carried by a single genus, the *Anopeles*, and of the 430 known species of *Anopeles*, there only seem to be seventy that have ever been known to have carried malaria. But there were—and of course, there are—*Anopeles* on every continent, and as the patterns of commercial and cultural exchange quickened in early modernity, there was now malaria, too.

The fever, or marsh fever, shaped life in Europe. The huge, windy, wet marshes, the Fens of England, ridden with malarial mosquitoes carrying *P. vivax* parasites, were well known to Shakespeare, the marshland in *Macbeth* standing in for uncontrolled evil, the place of plots, darkness, and sorcery. The fever was on the margins of every life—a disease that was serious but

not as deadly as the plague, smallpox, or typhoid. However, when Westerners began to encounter the African settlements just inland from the coasts,
to take slaves, and to seek to explore the river valleys, something critical
changed. The act of exploration, extraction, and colonialization also created
an imaginary, in which the New World had a different kind of fever, far more
fatal than *P. vivax* that had taken up residence in European marshes. It was
P. falciparum, and indeed, for the disease-naive Western Europeans, it was swiftly
deadly.

As the fifteenth century began, Portuguese traders edged along the African
coastal harbors, encountering *P. falciparum* for the first time. Turning back
from deadly forays into the interior, they began to write of the fatal "fevers
of the rivers" that lead away into the forests. The death rate was appalling.
Thus, colonization and stable trading posts, which were a feature of earlier
conquests, were impossible to establish. Yet, the Portuguese were creating an
imperial system, seeking the goods—and the human slaves—they desired to
build and consolidate their economy.

The Portuguese developed another system, in which inland traders
brought the resources and the slaves to the coast—slaves who carried the
deadly form of *P. falciparum* in their blood, forced captive and exhausted
onto Europe's ships, bound for the New World. As the Portuguese and the
Spanish mounted their exploration voyages, taking with them slaves, and
went to South America, they brought malaria to the jungles, pampas, and
forests of the New World. From Britain, where malaria was endemic, British
colonists brought malaria to North America, both vivax, from Europe and
falciparum, from Africa, first to Jamestown, along with smallpox, dysentery,
measles, and typhus. Ships from Africa, carrying mosquitoes in the hold and
parasites in the blood of the slaves, traveled directly to Caribbean ports and
to the thin, snaking Panama region, where the parasites exploded into the
naive populations. Up and down the coasts and rivers of North America,
along the Mississippi, the Ohio, and the Illinois, mosquitoes carried malaria
deep into the riverbank settlements and to the newly growing port cities:
Philadelphia, Baltimore, and Boston.

The fever was everywhere—one of many diseases that were threatening the
entire project of colonial expansion. However, there was one intervention. It
was based on the close observation by early Jesuit priests and sent along with
the first soldiers, who quietly noticed that the native peoples in Brazil used the
powder from the bark of a tree to reduce fevers, even the fever of the new sort

of malaria. This bark came from the cinchona tree, native to Brazil and fussy
and difficult to grow when transplanted. The powder seemed remarkable. It
brought down the fever and eased the headaches, and the characteristic shaking chills of the disease ceased when it was given. It was known as "Jesuit powder," and it was brought back to Europe, where it was promptly denigrated as
mere "Indian medicine." But the Jesuits and then others continued to use it,
and over time, the powder's effectiveness meant it found its way into medical
practice. It was, of course, the drug we now know as quinine, and it was the
best treatment available for the next four centuries.

Italy, especially Rome, was so sickened that malaria was referred to as the
"Roman Fever." Large swathes of the Middle East, Turkey, and Palestine were
simply empty of people—it was not practical to live in a place with such a
high death rate. In any of the colonies where African slaves labored, largely
immune because of their Duffy mutation to *P. vivax*, they died in high numbers from *P. falciparum*. Sonia Shah argues that malaria has "killed half of the
world's population," having killed 50 billion people, 300 million in the nineteenth century alone. It is malaria's ordinariness—unlike the Black Death
or cholera epidemics—and its persistence and endemicity that has shaped
human history. "Even in recent millennia, it has frequently lain silent in the
diverse record of our pasts, too common a disease to claim much notice. At
other times, epidemic malaria has careened violently across the landscapes of
world history, leaving death and suffering in its wake."[25] Even as an endemic
disease, it would take a terrible toll. But malaria, especially *P. falciparum*, was
a particular problem for regimes of conquest and control in the New World,
Africa, and Asia. As the British, French, Belgian, and German empires grew,
joining Spain, the Netherlands, and Portugal in the colonialization project,
the armies were sent across the globe to defend the territory they had conquered from the native peoples. Invariably, they found malaria there. It had
not existed in North and South America before the regnant of the Atlantic
exchange and the attendant slavery, but it established itself quickly, for the
tropical climate affects how fast the *Plasmodium* reproduce and speeds up
every factor in the malarial cycle of infection—the reproductive cycle, the
biting rate, and the tendency for humans to sleep outdoors at night. The
Europeans, who had grown accustomed to *P. vivax*, were stunned by the virulence of this deadlier form of the disease.

By the early 1600s, malaria and its terrible dangers was understood as part
of life in the new American colonies. *The Tempest* is thought to have been

partially inspired by Shakespeare's reading of a real-life event: a public letter written by a William Strachey, detailing the experiences of a shipwreck
survivor. On July 24, 1609, a fleet of nine English vessels that were part of
"The Virginia Company" were nearing the end of a supply voyage to the
new colony in the Bermudas when they ran into "a cruel tempest." The
vessels in the fleet couldn't keep together, and two fared particularly badly.
One of them, *The Sea Venture*, carrying the fleet's admiral, who was to be
the new governor of the colony of Virginia, ran ashore, and the passengers
and crew were stranded for months on a deserted island in the Bermudas,
during which time they were believed to be lost at sea before they were able
to sail to Virginia a year later.[26] For Shakespeare, the mysterious and terrible
fevers of Africa, the *P. falciparum* with its neurological effects and its madness, and the newly discovered wild Americas were seen as allies of barba-
rism. This barbarous energy coalesced in one figure, Caliban, and the whole
drama of native anger, uncertainty, and strange powerful magic is portrayed
by this character. Read *The Tempest* after knowing this story, and you will
newly understand the figure of Caliban: dark, enslaved, dangerous, always
present, always at the margins of the action, until he calls down "fevers" as a
curse on his captors. Shah argues that the slave trade depicted in the play via
Caliban created another growing anxiety, for slaves seemed in the European
imaginary to be always about to erupt, burst out of confines, carrying Africa
with them, and carrying the diseases of Africa as well. Yet, slaves were always
needed the fulcrum in the project to keep the entire enterprise of the imperial
enterprise—the extraction, the construction, the agriculture, and ultimately,
the trade—intact.

The Atlantic slave trade meant that between 1500 and 1800, millions of
Africans would be bound to ships and sent off to American colonies. But the
colonists had no way to understand the particular vehemence of African's *P.
falciparum*, and they wrote about it as if it were simply a part of the wilderness
they had encountered. "Sixteenth century Westerners did not have a specific
definition for the disease of malaria . . . so they thought of it primarily as a
disease of the landscape itself . . . Malaria took a terrible toll on the new colonies—86% of European American babies in South Carolina died before they
reached the age of twenty. In one parish, a third of European American infants
died before their fifth birthday, with most dying in their first year between
August and November, when the malarial mosquitoes were biting."[27] Life in
these colonies was chaotic and uncertain. One Scottish endeavor, to Darien

on the Panama peninsula, in what would become known as "the Mosquito Coast," became a symbol of all the lost hopes, the word "Darien" itself continuing as a linguistic sign of folly. After spending an enormous sum, largely on inappropriate objects for a life they would never live to create, and nearly bankrupting hundreds of families, the project to establish a Scottish territory on the Caribbean coast ended with more than 300 deaths, almost every single one of them the optimistic colonists.

But since conditions in Europe for the poor were often just bad enough, the plight of second sons just chancy enough, the uneasy European conflicts just dreadful enough, and the promise of riches and resources of the Americas, Africa, and Asia just powerful enough to keep men and women coming, the enterprise continued in other places. European powers understood that trade dominance depended on the natural resources of newly acquired territory and that holding it was key. Thus, permanent settlement was also critical to their empires. The colonies were not just for trade and agriculture, but also were military outposts, and the governance of many of them, and the land around them, was performed as a military endeavor. The colonialists, for their part, counted on large garrisons of soldiers to defend them against native peoples.

Malaria raged in the new colonies in the Americas, but not only there. In Europe, even though it was endemic and by then well characterized, it remained a significant problem in the Balkans, including Sweden and Russia, where it would flare into fierce local epidemics. Malaria even reached the Arctic Circle. Malaria wasn't recorded in Finland until the seventeenth century, probably brought by migrant workers, and it gained traction among people gathered for summer infrastructure projects in southern Finland in the eighteenth century. Death records and physician reports indicate that during mid-nineteenth-century epidemics, the mortality rate reached as high as 3 percent of the population, with 7–20 percent infected. The worst epidemic occurred in 1862. It haunts the work of Dickens, in *Great Expectations*. The malarial barrens lie between the city and the village, always the place of liminality, darkness, and danger the fens and marshes playing the same role as they had in Shakespeare. The Romantic poets, holidaying in Greece and Italy, were beset by malaria, with Lord Byron dying of it in 1824.

The colonization and expansion continued around the globe, pushing farther into regions that had long been thought uninhabitable, too fever-ridden for settlement. As the Americas and then Asia were explored, claimed, and began to be settled, countries turned to Africa itself. Shah writes: "Beginning in 1879, European political authorities, whose national economies were locked in savage industrial competition with one another and suffering from a regional economic depression, launched campaigns in tropical Africa to stake out national territorial claims. . . . The "Scramble for Africa" called forth a new map of tropical Africa, with the boundaries of Portuguese, Spanish, German, Italian, Belgian, French, and British colonies inscribed upon it."[28] To build an empire and create colonies there meant conquest of the land: it meant cutting down trees, clearing forests, and placing humans in convenient tasty groups for mosquitoes to bite. It meant plowing up the exquisite, untouched New World landscapes, changing the ecology of each place, the relationships between animals, insects, and human beings. It also meant the housing, feeding, and care of large armies. For that, the armies sent doctors along with troops, newly trained in the science of the late eighteenth century.

It was these Army doctors, ambitious men sent to far-flung places in the empire, alone with primitive microscopes and hundreds and hundreds of sick, feverish, quaking patients, who both solved the mystery of causality and created the language that would frame malariology for the next 300 years—it was the language of conquest, the language of war. The world as they knew it was about to change. Let me now turn to the next part of our story and give you an account of how humans began to understand malaria and, in many ways, to understand the natural world as an adversary to be conquered, in large part because of malaria's virulence. It is a central part of my argument that to understand our contemporary ethical position, it is critical to understand this fundamental historical perspective.

1.2 The History of Malaria: The Language of Conquest

Alphonse Laveran was a French military doctor, son of a French military doctor, with the curious habit of careful and intense, even obsessive, observation. By age of thirty-four, he was already the author of a "Treatise on Military Diseases and Epidemics" and sixty-two other scientific communications. In 1878, he was posted in French colonial Algeria, in the military hospital in Constantine. It was one of the many colonial outposts, requiring large armies to be in places to which they were unaccustomed. Malaria was by then a

serious problem in the Army, and Laveran was surrounded by sickened, feverish, and dying patients—young men suddenly overcome with shaking chills,
dying of high fevers and with blinding headaches—and he was determined
to understand why. His work was untiring, meticulous in describing the disease's shifting clinical aspects and its anatomic pathology—providing, for
example, an excellent histological description of cerebral malaria. But he was
most interested in identifying the causal agent of the disease.[29]

It was the age of the microscope and of a dense, miniature world suddenly
alive with pathogens. In 1862, Louis Pasteur, curious about how beer was
fermented and milk spoiled, began to look for answers with the new Dutch
microscopes, the lenses ground with new precision, and reasoned that the
small objects he could see swimming about—what he called "germs"—were
the cause of fermentation and later of disease, thus "germ theory." At the
time, the current medical science favored "miasmas" or bad air for illness,
especially for malaria. Hence, the name for malaria was derived from the
Italian for "bad air": malaria. It was Pasteur who disproved this theory conclusively by showing that the germs could infect clean culture and that they
never emerged spontaneously. For this discovery, Pasteur won the Alhum-
bert Prize. He concluded, "Never will the doctrine of spontaneous generation
recover from the mortal blow of this simple experiment. There is no known
circumstance in which it can be confirmed that microscopic beings came
into the world without germs, without parents similar to themselves."

Illness was not "in the air." Medical science was moving quickly to understand a new sort of epistemic framing, now seeking microbial causes for diseases everywhere. By the time Alphonse Laveran has been shipped to his post
in Algeria,[30] bacteriologist Robert Koch, from Germany, found the microbes
responsible for tuberculosis in 1882 and for cholera in 1884. Quickly, new
discoveries occurred: syphilis, typhoid, tetanus, and the plague all had bacterial causative agents. All of the long-standing historical diseases suddenly
began to be understood as bacterial. Surely malaria would have a bacterial
cause as well?[31] Koch's method, called his "postulates," specified his criteria
for how to prove disease causation. First, a microorganism must be collected
from diseased individuals but not found in people who are healthy (Koch did
not anticipate asymptomatic occurrence). Second, it must be cultured from
the diseased individual. Third, a healthy individual has to be inoculated with
the cultured microorganism, and they then must acquire the disease (he also

did not understand genetic resistance factors). Finally, the microorganism must be re-isolated from the inoculated, diseased individual and it must be the same as the original microorganism.

And it was the Italians who came up with such a cause. Surely, they reasoned, marsh fever's cause must lie in the swampy marshes outside of Rome—in the Campagna. Surely the bacteria would be found there. It was there, in the steaming marshes, that Roman pathologists collected samples, from the air, the water, and the mud, and repeated the steps of Koch's postulates. Using their crude microscopes, they found what they described as long rods, and these seemed to them to be the organism they sought. Indeed, when they injected rabbits in the laboratory with them, the rabbits seemed to develop malaria, or what looked like malaria, with high fevers and trembling and they believed they had found the organisms when they dissected the animals. In 1879, they announced that they had named the microbe— *Bacillus malariae* and declared it the cause of malaria, even though the organism had been found in the mud and not in an animal or human. It was immediately hailed and accepted.[32]

But the careful, closely watching French Army surgeon, Laveran, surrounded by the sick soldiers, alone in the long, warm nights of North Africa, noticed something else. In the blood and tissue of patients with malaria, where one would expect to find the causative agents, as one did for syphilis and tetanus, he saw only tiny black dots. He took sample after sample of blood from his patients, and yet, as he looked carefully under his microscope, he did not see the Italian *Bacillus*. One day, instead of looking at the blood right after he drew it, he left the slide on the microscope for fifteen minutes (the standard narrative is that he left to get a coffee, being French). Feeling the drop in temperature, the parasite reacted as if it were outside the warm human bloodstream and inside the relatively cooler mosquito intestinal tract. The male gametes whipped out their long flagella and began moving about. Laveran, when he returned, could see this on his slide. He found it again and again: the black dots in blood, when cooled, had tails and, moreover, seemed to change into what he guessed were male and female forms. He tried putting drops of quinine on the slide, and he watched them vanish from the blood after quinine was given. Looking more closely now, he saw and then excitedly drew in his notes just the red blood cells themselves— filled with parasites, then bursting, and then forming the male and female forms he had first seen.

But no one believed him.

Meanwhile, stationed in China, on the other side of the world, another Army doctor was searching in the blood of patients who had a strange, horrible disease never seen in Europe: Filariasis, or "elephantiasis," so named because something caused a patient's legs or groin or testicle sack to swell to huge proportions. Looking in the blood, Patrick Manson saw the "tiny worms" that other scientists had seen in such cases of the illness—but the worms only appeared briefly. How did the worms get from one patient to another if they were not in the blood all the time, he wondered? Manson, who detested his tropical posting, was certain that the clouds of insects that swarmed at night must surely play a different role from the one they had in England, something unlike fleas, lice, or leeches did there, where filariasis was unknown.[33]

Manson tested his theory by making one of his filariasis patients sleep in a contained area. He knew a little about mosquitoes. He knew at least that after the mosquitoes bit a person and had a blood meal, they were too heavy to fly far, and so they rested on the next vertical surface while their body absorbed the blood. So, in the morning, he had a servant collect the blood-filled mosquitoes resting on the wall of the sleeping area, after their meal, and when he cut them open, he found the "worms." Manson was Scottish and thought himself living in "an out of the way place, away from libraries."[34] He did not understand insects, could not tell the difference between species, and could not figure out how the "worms," once inside the mosquito, could get back into humans. His theory was that mosquitoes laid their eggs in water, died, and contaminated the water. Then, when humans drank the water, they became sick. And he held to this theory, even while he returned to London, to libraries, and promoted this theory to great prestige and power. Moreover, he then decided that this must be the way that all mosquito-borne disease was transmitted, and he began to lecture about this theory widely and lucratively.

Meanwhile, Laveran's research had finally been accepted by then, in France, and it cohered with what the Italians, by far the most skilled entomologists, had at that time seen. It was the Italians Amico Bignami and Giovanni Grassi, working in Rome, the site of the long legacy of the "Roman Fever," who understood that there had to be a link between malaria, swamps, and mosquitoes. They had spent decades studying insect behavior, and they also understood that Manson had to be mistaken. The Italians, and Laveran, ever the naturalists, understood that the parasite could not survive in water and swim about. It needed to live inside the insect gut or the human blood-stream. Manson dismissed "the French and Italians" and simply insisted that British science was far more advanced. But he was unwilling to leave the salons of London again to do the research to prove this claim. And thus, Manson found someone who would: a young man, another military doctor, whose temperament, utter lack of training in entomology or in malaria, and nationalist convictions matched his own. It was someone who was as eager as Manson was not to go out into the field to test the theory.

This man was Richard Ross, who, having barely passed his medical exams, had been sent to India, to Madras, the farthest reaches of the empire. India had two things that interested him: sports and lots of free time to write the poetry that was his real passion, for he was considered quite the failure at studying medicine. Ross set about organizing sports leagues and poetry readings for the wives of officers, for he rather disliked sick people. But, like Laveran, he was surrounded by hundreds of malarial soldiers, and even a not very enthusiastic doctor could see there was an enormous problem. His superiors, alarmed by the disease outbreaks, sent him to take a course in the new science of bacteriology, and there he found something he did like about medicine—he loved the beauty of the world safely tucked under the microscope. He set about trying to understand and replicate Manson's work. But he was as hopeless a scientist as he was a physician. He could not tell the mosquitoes apart; he struggled to breed them, and they died before they laid eggs. In his writings, he is increasingly frustrated and somewhat bewildered. He did not use their proper scientific names, instead calling insects by their colors and spots ("the stripy ones").

His rapport with human research subjects was no better, but then, he was forcing them to drink mosquito-ridden water to please his mentor, Mason, so it is difficult to tell. It is recorded that natives fled when he came toward them, lest he used them as subjects for his research. His letters are full of anger: at the Indians, who he thought dirty, at Hindu customs, which he despised, at mosquitoes ("they are as obstinate as a mule"), and most of all at the Italians, the careful scientists who had studied malaria in other species and were aware of the rules of evolutionary biology—Amico Bignami and Giovanni Grassi. By 1896, Bignami had published the first paper on how malaria was transmitted to animals by the bites of mosquitoes of the genus *Anopheles* or *Culex*.

Ross and Manson began a bitter epistolary battle to "defeat the Italians," even though their own theory about water made no sense. Ross did not know which mosquitoes carried the disease ("There are so many kinds!" he complained in his letters). Finally, when Ross was guided by his servants, gently, out of pity, to see the correct mosquitoes—*Anopheles*—and dissected them, he too found what Laveran had seen and what Bignami and Grassi had just published. The salivary gland in the probiscis of the creature—the very place where the creature touched the human body and breached it—was filled with the parasites that Laveran had seen.

Because Ross could not get humans to work with him, he had worked largely with birds, which could not refuse. Ross began a grueling, exhaustive, obsessive project: capturing the stripy mosquitoes in the hundreds (actually, ordering his servants to capture them), dissecting their tiny mouth parts, carefully looking over and over for the silver rods. He saw, and drew, over and over, the complex life cycle of the *Plasmodium*, finding the parasite at each stage in its different forms—an extraordinarily difficult task. What he lacked in insight or entomology, he made up for with a level of persistence that was staggering. He learned at last how to breed the insects. Then, he set up trials in which the birds were kept in cages with and without mosquito netting. He watched the course of their illness, hatched new young mosquitoes, had them bite the sick birds, and then transferred the blood-filled mosquitoes to the cages of healthy birds, which became sick with malaria from the bites of the infected mosquitoes. This was a version of what Pasteur had done, a version of the Koch postulates, the definitive proof of transmission.

Then, he wrote a (rather bad) poem to celebrate. He had found "the murderer."

Meanwhile, the Italians followed out their theory as well and did the same work, but in humans not in birds, and were the first to infect a human with malaria. Not to be left out, Robert Koch claimed he had known all along, and that *he* had discovered the vector and the route of transmission.

Then, Manson made the audacious claim to the British Medical Association that it was he and Ross who had discovered the mosquito's true role in human malaria and not the Italians after all. A bitter, terrible academic fight ensued, and it ended with Ross receiving the Nobel Prize, to enormous acclaim, along with the uneasy, persistent, reputation of its theft.

While the Europeans were wrapped up in this battle for credit, the Americans, who had themselves quickly disproven both the earlier bacterial theories and Manson's woebegone theory of "mosquito tainted water," understood and embraced the science behind the Italian and French work. Malaria, as we have seen, stalked the colonies since the 1600s, and as the country coalesced and expanded, so did the range of the disease. According to Shah, by 1901, malaria was the leading cause of death in America.[35] Entire geographic areas lay under its grip—along the swampy Ohio River, down many parts of the Mississippi basin, near the salt swamps on both coasts. Malaria and mosquitoes were seen as a stubborn barrier to progress. If the Europeans did not want just to kill all mosquitoes, the Americans would. Thus began a new way to understand malaria—as a military battle, discovered by Army surgeons, campaigns led by Army officers, under the new discipline of modern armies enforcing the police power of the state.

Read any account of malaria, any report on eradication, and to this day, the print of war is still linguistically apparent. The language of war permeates the literature: the parasite "invades," humans "lose the battle," malaria takes "casualties," we need a new "weapon," malaria is a formidable "enemy" who takes "territory" and has to be "beaten back," the doctors "waged" a "war" on the vector. In my first account of the disease and its discover, that you just have read, I attempted not to use this language, for it is my argument that seeing the "battle against malaria" as a battle shapes our capacity to understand fully our relationship to the disease and to the people who suffer from it and, not tangentially, to our natural world. However, from the beginning, it was as a war that malaria was understood. Consider how Gordon Harrison, a military historian, writing in the mid-twentieth century, reflects on this period:

> It was mankind's first war against another species. . . . the early fighters referred modestly to their campaigns, yet for most control always meant defending people chiefly by killing mosquitos. Most of the doctors in the field saw themselves at war; the language of battle came easily to their minds and pens . . . then as now it was predominantly an affliction of warm climates and particularly lethal to White agents of empire. The doctors who first fought malaria in the tropics went out explicitly to challenge the mosquito for possession of the rich lands that she and her supercargo of disease organisms dominated.[36]

Once mosquitoes had been identified, the tactic of destroying their habitat was the first act in this war. Oddly, defensive measures, such as providing screens on every house, would not occur for years later—window screens were not invented until 1861 and were not in wide use, even in the USA, until early in the 1900s. (In fact, even today, screens on windows in clinics, universities, hospitals, dormitories, and prayer rooms in most of the world are still rare.[37]) At first, the "assault" went well. For some species, draining swamps and putting a coat of petroleum oil over every ditch and stream killed larvae and reduced breeding sites. This strategy was carried out in what Harrison called the "high noon of the White man's empire," the end of the nineteenth-century and the dominance of European powers. It was, at first, successful. "Success produced an ecstasy of self-congratulation."[38]

However, the mosquito proved a difficult creature to kill. As Harrison noted: "Any attempt to banish disease is by definition an attempt to alter evolved relationships among living things . . . to try to banish disease by killing its insect vectors carries the process of intervention in the natural order a step further. Finally, to attack disease vectors as in the war against mosquitoes by making the world less fit for their habitation is to engage on a grand scale in the kind of environmental manipulation that has been characteristic of man's approach to his inexplicably flawed by perfectible world."[39] Malaria is formidable because not only does the parasite change shape and change vulnerabilities seven different times in one life span, but the parasite also overcomes the bodys defenses by reproducing in sheer numbers that overwhelm the immune system. And it is formidable because the mosquitoes that carry the parasite also reproduce in enormous numbers, overwhelming human efforts to contain them. British, French, and German officers would spray insecticide, spread oil, and drain swamps, with huge numbers of soldiers involved in the effort. But leaving even one breeding pair of mosquitoes would make the entire project useless. Consider the mathematics:

> One female mosquito, depending on her species and environment may lay a little less than 50 to about 500 eggs in her first brood, slightly fewer in each subsequent delivery, of which there may be eight or nine before she dies. Taking 200 eggs as an average clutch and assuming half of these will hatch out females, then the theoretical progeny from a single female insect in five generations would be twenty million . . . each life cycle from egg to egg takes, under good conditions, two weeks . . . In some tropical locations where reproduction goes on all year round, one female could theoretically be ancestor to mosquitoes numbering twice ten to the twenty-sixth power . . . in practical terms the calculus means simply that were one to wipe out 99% of a given mosquito population, the survivors could quickly make good the loss.[40]

Mosquitoes are tiny. They hide in tree holes and lay their eggs there. They only need enough water to breed—for example, the water left in a bottle cap from the ubiquitous bitter and tonic that the British used to swallow their quinine is enough for a brood. They bite without causing pain. Their life span is quite short. Usually, depending on the breed, females can live from forty-two to fifty-six days, although most only live around 14–21 days, males only ten days (their major accomplishment is completed when they mate, usually on day 1). This means that life spans are quick. A female is able to breed quickly as well. In many species, she will usually only mate once, typically right after emergence. Then, she will store the male's sperm in her *spermatheca*, releasing it with each ovulation cycle. Males swarm at night when females feed, it is thought, to attempt another chance at mating to ensure species fecundity.[41]

It is the enormous prolificacy that gives the mosquitoes another advantage that in disease vector is even more daunting that mere numbers: adaptability. Because their breeding time is short, mutations can quickly arise, and if these mutations give even a very small fitness margin, the species can adapt. This is why resistance arises so quickly in mosquitoes and why every single drug, and every single insecticide, has given rise to resistance. Where bed nets are used, mosquitoes adapt to bite before bedtime. When swamps are drained, the mosquito with the mutation that gives her the capacity to lay her eggs in temporary puddles, allowing them to wait for rain to achieve maturity, passes on these genes, and the species shifts.[42] They have adapted to salt water in this way, and they would adapt to quinine, a drug that, it could be said, made the entire colonial enterprise possible. (Not tangentially, as we will see later in the story, they will adapt to dichlorodiphenyltrichloroethane [DDT] and to artemisinin, and they will of course adapt around vaccines and even gene drives if they are not carefully designed and effectively implemented.)

But the war continued. Quinine was taken ubiquitously by European settlers in large quantities, now added casually to certain tonics and aperitifs. A new disease emerged from quinine overdosing—blackwater fever—always fatal after an agony of fever and black diarrheal stools and urine as red blood cells burst directly into the bloodstream and traveled to the organs, causing kidney failure, usually as a result of the interaction of quinine with the parasites. Quinine, despite its complications, was used through Europe—it was called the "European Way." The longer that Europeans stayed in tropical Africa, the more prone they seemed to be to blackwater fever.[43]

The "American way" was largely funded by the Rockefeller Foundation and was based on a more aggressive strategy: kill all the mosquitoes, drain all their habitats, and insist on the mass spraying of Paris Green or petroleum on every body of still water to eliminate malarial mosquito breeding grounds.

Malaria had begun a slow, imperfect retreat in the USA. This was due not only to the campaigns against mosquitoes but also to the slowly changing agricultural practices, the use of machines to plant and harvest, which took people out of the fields in the early mornings, the slowly improving economic situation, which meant that people could afford to build houses with closed doors and windows, the capacity to isolate a sick person in a room, away from mosquitoes, and being able to afford better food, all of which make humans able to resist malaria parasites. As the industrial economy strengthened and more people moved into cities, working in factories, as more land was settled and plowed and crops were planted and rivers were diverted, malaria waned. This process was replicated slowly all over the Northern Hemisphere. Malaria was becoming largely a disease of the rural areas and of the poor. This meant that in the American South, desperately poor and rural since the mid-nineteenth century and physically torn by the American Civil War, malaria was still a primary cause of death, especially pediatric death, but it no longer haunted northern cities or farms.

By the fall of 1923, the directors of the Rockefeller Foundation decided that the USA's malaria problem weighed too heavily on the country's economic potential: malaria had to be eradicated. The foundation's secretary-general called malaria "probably the heaviest handicap on the welfare and economic efficiency of the human race."[44] In particular, they were aware that the burden fell on the American South. The Foundation was particularly concerned that malaria stunted the growth of an entire quadrant of North America—it was unacceptable. It funded the largest scientific and sanitation campaign yet, aiming to learn about the species, their habitats, and their habits and to find new methods to eliminate them. It trained the scientists of the entire next generation of American malariologists, bringing expertise and, importantly, funding.

Sanitation campaigns took on a moral fervor both in America and Europe. Ross, writing in 1923, said, "they were the most important task" of modernity. "Great is Sanitation. The greatest work, except discovery, I think, that man can do. . . . What is the use of preaching high moralities, philosophies, policies, and arts to people who dwell in. . . . Appalling slums . . . ? We shall reach the higher civilization not by . . . methods of government, manners of voting, liberty, self-determination and the rest, all of which have failed—but first by the scientific ordering of cities until they are fit for men of the higher civilization to dwell in. We must begin by being Cleansers."[45] The poorest region in the USA was the Southeast, but in Italy, it was the countryside outside of Rome. In Italy, the Campagna di Roma remained a terrible problem, essentially unchanged in the transmission of disease from the medieval period, despite Italy having long been a center of scientific study for malaria. Now, Italians began to use the tools of social science in their war. The Italian hygienist and sometime socialist politician, Angelo Celli, was the director of the Department of Hygiene at La Sapienza University in Rome, and he was deeply concerned by the impact of economic and social factors on health. He noted that the mild form of malaria in the north of Italy did not prevent industrial and agricultural development there, whereas the more severe cases in the south impeded both economic and social development. In collaboration with physicians, engineers, farmers, and teachers, Celli proposed a variety of public health interventions, including the usual interventions against mosquito habitat—adequate drainage and water management interventions. But he added full local employment, local health clinics, and public education. He argued for combined efforts, not only against the direct causes of malaria (the parasite and mosquitoes), but also against the concomitant causes of the disease—the environmental and living conditions of the affected populations. It was his insight that a good stable job was an important as drainage when thinking about the health of a family. In particular, he was concerned about railway workers.

By the summer of 1900, Celli began a new pilot research project to assess the effectiveness of a set of new ways to prevent malaria by preventing mosquito bites. He began by recording the numbers of malaria cases in the local railway workers and their families living near five of the most malarious railway routes. Then, he began a controlled experiment in some of the workers' houses. He screened the porches, doors, and chimneys with wire mesh and covered the windows with thick muslin. The inside walls of these homes were whitewashed, as mosquitoes were thought to be repelled by reflective surfaces and also could be better seen and subsequently killed. To prevent bites at night in houses in which mosquitoes were noticed, families were told to burn special powders (probably pyrethrum, an effective insecticide). Railway workers from these homes who were working on night shifts were equipped with veiled hats similar to those used by beekeepers and given large leather gloves to prevent mosquitoes biting them. Quinine was only administered to some of these workers. In short, Celli used every single intervention known at the time. But none were used in the families he used as a control group. By the end of the year, the results were dramatic: ninety-two percent of the control group became malarious, and only four percent of the intervention group did (largely people who had resisted some of the advice to cover themselves up in the sweltering heat).[46]

Frustrated by the reluctance of his superiors to see how critical were the social and economic issues of malaria, the resistance to what seemed suspiciously "communist," and by the apathy of some of the workers, Celli noted that attempts to implement these public health interventions sometimes met with "apathy, ignorance, and prejudice." He would finally come to use quinine for everyone. In fact, the reforms he had proven effective were only able to be instituted when a military dictatorship took over the country, forcing people to comply with strict public health measures by using the Army to organize the programs on a wide and universal scale. In a campaign waged by Benito Mussolini, taking power initially as a national socialist, new workers' houses were built, massive drainage projects completed, spraying and larvicide applied using the newly discovered and powerful Paris Green, which was cheaper and more effective as a larvicide than oil, and screens placed on all public building. He called this effort the "Bonifacio Integral" or "Integrated Improvements." There were three steps to the plan. First, the Italians constructed an elaborate, detailed engineering project that dug ditches, built dikes, and constructed a vast system of pumps that moved swampy water into the sea. As a part of this step, Paris Green was sprayed everywhere that mosquitoes laid eggs, which meant the entire Pontine Marshes and roadsides along the Appian Way, so famously malarious that they were cited as dangerous in Byron and Goethe, a synecdoche for impenetrable and deadly.

The second step in the Bonifacio was to construct new housing, schools, health centers, and extensive roadways for some 60,000 formerly landless settlers brought in to reclaim and farm the land. Although Mussolini claimed credit for this effort, in fact he had good advice from a number of Italian malaria experts such as Grassi and Celli, fresh from his study of railway workers. Previous experience had shown that simple drainage was not enough; it was also necessary to maintain the drainage system and develop the new settlement by reclaiming the land for agriculture and by enacting consistent measures until the parasites was eradicated and both poverty and disease addressed in Italy's poorest people, the *paisanos*. It was wildly successful—this area is still the most productive agricultural area in Italy, for example, and it created a devoted base of support for Mussolini. The third step was medical treatment of malaria infections, using the new clinics and mass administration of quinine.[47]

It would take an Army. It would always, it seemed, take an Army to enforce the public health rules to eradicate malaria because mandated and maintained social practices for public health was often resisted. The military approach was also critical in other geographies. For example, the US Army marched into the Caribbean and began the clearing of occupied Cuba after the Spanish–American War. Lessons learned there to eliminate *Aedes* mosquitoes that carried yellow fever were used against malarial mosquitoes as well. This particular effort was led by a young US army captain and surgeon, William Gorgas, who was selected for leadership, initially only because he had nearly died from yellow fever and thus was immune, but who turned out, somewhat surprisingly, to be a genius in military management.

As soon as the Spanish–American War ended in 1898, Gorgas was sent to Havana, where yellow fever had been endemic for centuries, often flaring into epidemics that swept the island. Gorgas plunged in: he sent soldiers to overturn potted plants, marching them in formation through villages and towns to look for any water stored overnight, to smash fountains, and to pour Paris Green on every open sewer, irrigation ditch, stream, and marsh and puddle. After three months, he had mapped the entire island and destroyed every mosquito breeding area he could find. Yellow fever was eradicated. Malaria, too, dropped dramatically. Gorgas, with his grid maps and his zeal for military campaigns was eager to continue. And he found an ideal place to try his methods: the Isthmus of Panama. Gorgas immediately understood the potential for trade if a canal could be built across the peninsula, and he also understood the magnitude of the problem. When the French abandoned their efforts, and the US government decide to build the Panama Canal, he immediately asked for a transfer.

The French left Panama after their own disastrous attempts to build the canal, having been defeated by massive malarial fevers despite their pretty hospitals, lovely courtyards with decorative fountains, and best of plans. What was needed, Gorgas believed, was to use the Army to clean everything up, eliminating mosquitoes as much as possible, just as he had done in Cuba. Gorgas was enthusiastic, imagining that the tropics would be more productive than the temperate zones. He enthused to Theodore Roosevelt, "White man could take over and produce many times the amount of food now produced in the temperate zone."[48] This entire activity was known as "cleaning the tropics," a slogan proudly displayed on pharmaceutical company ads of the period. They picture a tall white guy in tropical military gear, pith helmet on head, map in hand, gun on hip, leading a little band of soldiers with rifles, and trailing along beside him, small, dressed in rags, barefoot, are his Black slaves, carrying his scientific equipment in large, wooden chests.

It was an enormous task, for yellow fever and malaria sickened and killed his soldiers as it had done the French, and it was accomplished against passionate opposition from officials convinced that yellow fever was caused by filthy habits and environmental degradation, not mosquitoes.[49] President Theodore Roosevelt supported Gorgas' efforts, and the Canal Zone was "free of yellow fever by 1906, followed by eradication of malaria a few years later."[50]

It was not, however, entirely free. Gorgas cleared a five-mile zone on either bank of the Canal, aggressively ditching and draining, slashing against the jungle underbrush, applying larvicide, carefully screening the hospital the French has left behind, and taking out the lovely courtyard gardens with their pools and palms that that French had so loved.

The end of the nineteenth century also marked mass migrations of peoples as the new conflicts of modernity pushed them into marginal areas where it had long been impossible to settle. Pogroms and riots in Kishinev, Russia, in 1882 convinced many Jews that they would be better off living anywhere else. Jews had for centuries yearned for a return to Palestine, and as anti-Semitic pogroms swept the Pale of Settlement, it looked more likely as a future. Thus began what was called the First Aliyah—a movement of Jewish immigration that lasted from 1882 to 1904. Jews came to Palestine prepared to buy property for collective farms, and the Arabs in the region were happy enough to sell land they considered uninhabitable. So, the land the Jews found for sale was largely the barren, empty coastal plain, swampy and malarial, which they did not know was a problem initially—in fact, they thought it was rather pretty, with water everywhere. The settlers came with few skills as land assessors or as farmers, for that matter, for land ownership by Jews had been prohibited in most areas of Russia from which they had come. Hundreds died nearly immediately, sickened by the clouds of malaria-bearing mosquitoes. By the Second Aliyah, from 1904 to 1920, new settlers were prepared to buy better land, supported by their benefactors, the Rothschild family, for the Second Aliyah's largely socialist, idealist, vision.[51] Yet again, the land they were sold had been largely abandoned as impossible to work, because it, too, was highly malarious. Settlements, largely early kibbutzim, were built near lakes, as they were in Europe, which was a disaster, for in the rainy season, the lakes were marshy, hot, and mosquito ridden. The death toll was again terrible. Desperate, digging grave after grave, settlers planted eucalyptus trees, imported from Australia in huge numbers, for they were told that their roots would soak up the wet soil and reduce the number of mosquitoes. It did not work. Entire kibbutz communities were stricken and had to abandon the newly purchased land. Malaria killed thousands of people each year, and 20 percent of the population suffered from the disease. Entire regions were abandoned due to malaria. Some people in the Zionist movement believed the disease would entirely wipe out the Jewish community in Palestine.

It was not only the Zionist kibbutz members who were dying. During World War I, malaria was a bitter enemy of General Allenby's Egyptian Expeditionary Force (EEF) in Palestine. "This is one the most malaria-afflicted countries in the world," wrote Allenby's chief medical officer. [52] In 1918 alone, more than 28,000 cases of malaria were reported among British soldiers in the EEF.

One visitor in 1902 remarked that the Turkish soldiers at one border garrison had to be replaced monthly because all would contract malaria in little over a week and simply die. A report from 1917, the year the British arrived, noted that Palestine was "notoriously malarious" and that an estimated 90 percent of British soldiers at the town of Beisan—today's Beit She'an, in the Jordan Valley—were ill within ten days. [53]

For the British, whose doctors, such as Ross of the Indian Medical Service, had led the charge against malaria, the level of malaria in their colony of Palestine was intolerable, and they were determined to act. Moving to eradicate malaria, they found a partner in the odd little socialist colonies of Russian Jewish settlers who had narrowly survived and were eager to farm in the impossible marshes they had rather naively bought. Meanwhile, newly arrived in Palestine was a diminutive, Rockefeller Institute–trained scientist, Israel Jacob Kligler, who had just been commissioned to write a report on malaria in Palestine by US Supreme Court Justice Louis Brandeis and to see if he could do anything about the terrible toll it was taking. Brandeis, committed to settlement in Palestine, gave him $20,000 of his own money so that Kligler could begin the campaign to eradicate the disease. He came prepared with the newest research on malaria and, understanding that he would need a way to enforce the public health program he needed, sought out British military support to implement his ideas.

Kligler, ever an optimist, found a land devastated by malaria, far bleaker than he had imagined. The illness was, a British report said in 1921, "by far the most important disease in Palestine." Much of the territory the Jews had purchased for settlement "was in lowlands impossibly infested with malaria," he wrote, because of course that was one of the main reasons it was available. Some settlements had been abandoned altogether as a result. "The once famous city of Beth Shan, standing in the midst of an intensively irrigated plan, was in the course of time completely surrounded by water-logged marshes, became one of the most malarious points in a highly malarious area, and dwindled to a small village," he wrote. Describing the coastal plain, he wrote, "One sees large stretches of richly watered, potentially cultivable land inhabited only by a few Bedouin tribes, all infected with malaria, and eking out a precarious existence from the proceeds of baskets made of marsh reeds, and from the milk of buffaloes which wallow in the marshes."[54]

He began by organizing Jewish settlers, Bedouins, and Arab villagers for a systematic and prolonged fight against the mosquito, finding each marsh, wadi, and water storage area, draining and treating it, and teaching the techniques of oiling the water to kill larvae. Working with the British Mandate officers, they established a grid, as had been done in Cuba, with a systematic screening network of inspectors. At its peak, there were hundreds of people taking part in the campaign. Most of the budget came from Zionist movement members in America and Europe, but Arab villagers participated and offered resources too. The anti-malaria network was one of the few services that continued to operate even during periods of violence between Jewish and Arab communities, which flared up as the Zionists entered in larger numbers. When Mufti Amin al-Husseini tried to prevent anti-malaria workers from entering Arab villages, the workers, both Jews and Arabs, returned, this time accompanied by British soldiers.[55]

The eucalyptus trees that were thought to assist in warding off the disease by drying swamps did not impress the British or Kliger, who knew that the trees could actually cause damage, since their roots sometimes blocked drainage channels. Instead, Kliger imported *Gambusia* or mosquito fish, native to the American Midwest, to eat the mosquito eggs in the swampy marshes. Quinine was distributed as well, but since Kliger was an American, he concentrated on killing the vector.

Kligler set about creating the Malaria Research Institute to develop new techniques to improve the work. With the help of the Army, he found new ways to drain marshes and began spraying areas where hidden concentrations of larvae were found. He developed new ways of dealing with the different species of mosquitoes and, by periodically changing the direction of water flow in an irrigation canal, disrupted the breeding sites. Combined with a general improvement in public health under the British Mandate, the results were striking. In Jerusalem, for example, according to British statistics, 633 people were treated for the disease in 1923. The following year, the number had dropped to 347. Four years after that, in 1928, the number was 16.[56]

The British Army was pleased, if surprised. The small Jewish scientist and his crews of Russian Jews, Bedouins, and Arabs had begun to make a difference. One officer noted in his report: "An interesting recent feature has been noticed. In a number of areas where intense endemic malaria had resulted in NO population for generations, recent schemes (of malaria control) have created large tracts of cultivatable land."[57] The British continued to wage anti-malaria campaigns run by the military in every one of their tropical colonies. In India, malaria proved far harder to eliminate. Ross's call for cleaning up was harder to enact, especially in North India. Here, the industrious British had dug a vast network of new irrigation canals where newly abundant, sluggish water was intended to help grow crops, and railway lines the building of which created upturned soil, poor drainage, and disruption of local, fast-flowing rivers that had previously tumbled seasonally from the Himalaya. All of these inadvertently made the mosquitoes more abundant.

It was also hard to develop a local source for quinine. While quinine could be locally produced, it was found to be of poor quality. The colonial enterprise, which instituted farming practices for cotton, indigo, and rice at far larger scales than sustenance agriculture, required the amassing of large armies of workers, often from different areas of the country, some with malaria, some with no immunity to malaria and they lived in huge camps with poor sanitation, open toilets, and only basic shelter, exchanging malaria between one another. When the harvest, bridge or dam, or railway or other British project was done, the workers dispersed home, often taking malaria with them to new areas.[58]

In general, North India and Punjab were too dry for the main malaria vector, *Anopheles culicifacies*, which barely managed to sustain itself in sufficient numbers to keep the parasite circulating. But monsoon rains now filled the new ditches and flooded every pothole and work site, and the mosquito population exploded, rapidly colonizing the temporary waters that appeared suddenly in the oversaturated lands.[59]

Interestingly enough, some years, following rain, there were no epidemics of malaria, and in others, the disease swept terribly across the plains. Colonial agriculture was based on aggregation—cash crops such as cotton were planted, and when the crop failed or the prices of cotton dropped or a drought occurred, famines then took their terrible toll. Army surgeon Samuel Rickard Christophers, another British army doctor fascinated by malaria and a methodical keeper of detailed statistics, noticed a trend: when it rained after a prolonged drought, the epidemics began; when it rained after a normal cycle of wet and dry weather, they did not. He carefully charted the pattern, going back to Army records kept over decades.

Why? Christophers thought that perhaps drought causing crop failure weakened the resistance of people by malnutrition. He tried out a correlation between the price of grain (a surrogate for scarcity), rain, and fever and found that it could account for four fifths of the epidemics. Rainfall made the mosquitoes more abundant; famine made the people more susceptible (and made grain prices rise). "There seems little doubt," Christophers concluded, "that the two factors, rainfall and scarcity are the determining causes of the epidemic malaria seem in the Punjab."[60] He had noticed what Celli would see half a world away in Italy: the disease was driven not only by a vector, a parasite, and a human host, but also by the social and economic conditions in which the human host lived.

This critical insight—that the disease was driven by economic factors, by poverty, rather than just the parasite itself—was always in tension with the new scientists of the late nineteenth century, who saw the direct cause of illness unfolding under the microscope. Pasteur was convinced that all that needed to be done to eradicate disease was to find the bacteria and describe the etiology and kill it—pasteurize it. Social conditions and the environment had nothing to do with illness, he said confidently. "Whatever the poverty, it will never breed disease," he wrote. This view of scientific hygiene developed in Germany at the end of the nineteenth century and was subsequently transported to the USA. It also permeated the work of the new international health organizations that arose at the end of World War I, whose goal was translating concerns into the universal language of science. This led, during the 1920s, to a series of narrowly defined technical responses.[61]

The alert reader will see that this essential debate—ethical in nature—would persist, lacing through the narrative from Christophers's charts to our own discourse. Thus, despite the Italian insight that malaria could not be eliminated without attention to the social and economic conditions of a population, and despite the evidence of the waning of the disease in the Northern Hemisphere as economic and social conditions improved and basic nutrition and public health became more accessible, the military model of single disease eradication—of a war against the mosquito foe—was still seen as the imperative. I will return to this issue in more detail in chapter 6.

In part, this was because of the logic of colonialism. The people seen most at risk were the non-native Westerners, who built hill towns above mosquito ranges and who had access to quinine in reasonable concentrations and Army doctors for their health care. What Westerners with no immunity needed was eradication; what villagers and native workers needed was housing, food, and clinics—and these were not usually provided.

As the twentieth century proceeded, the world began to turn from this debate to think about another sort of war: World War I, whose chaos threw the British, French, German, Italian, and American Armies and all their colonies into confusion. Research that had been undertaken in virtually every European medical school was stopped. After the war, famine, disease, and political unrest was widespread, and malaria resurfaced, even in areas where it had been eradicated:

> The First World War and the political and sanitary chaos which followed in its wake in Eastern Europe and the Balkans resulted in a new state of affairs. The medical strategies designed before the war, which were based primarily on the widespread use of quinine, had certainly proven effective in controlling malaria outbreaks locally. However, despite this knowledge and experience, the number of malaria cases still rose after the war, reaching a peak in 1922–1924. Malaria had re-emerged in areas where it had ceased to be endemic, and appeared with greater frequency and severity everywhere else, including in Italy, where the death toll climbed from 1 per 10,000 inhabitants in 1910 to 3.2 at the end of WWI (Celli, 1933).[62]

Not only was the malaria widespread, but *P. falciparum* also emerged in areas where it had rarely been seen before. In Russia, the revolution of 1917 and then the counter revolution meant that the new Soviet governments could pay little attention to malaria. A terrible famine drove populations south to seek food to areas in the Balkans and southern Russia where malaria had been endemic and the population relatively immune. Not so the refugees, who died in great numbers and then fled back to areas across the north of Russia, carrying malaria as far as the Arctic Circle.

In 1913, malaria was occurring at a rate of 500 cases per 10,000 people, but by 1923, it had reached about 5,000 cases per 10,000 in the Volga German

Republic, with an estimated death rate of at least 3 percent. It is estimated that in 1923, 18 million people suffered from malaria in Russia, and that 60,000 deaths occurred out of a total population of about 110 million.[63]

Throughout the Ottoman Empire and southern Europe, the war meant that malaria again became a leading cause of death. Similar observations were made throughout the whole of Eastern and Southeastern Europe and the former Ottoman Empire. Alarmed by the postwar collapse, the new League of Nations had established not only a special health office but also, within it, a special Malaria Commission. In 1931, after a decade of epidemics and despite growing information about its causes, the political turmoil had increased the death rate from malaria. The situation was well summarized in a 1931 report by Émile Marchoux on the activity of the Malaria Commission of the League of Nations between 1924 and 1930.[64] The report noted that the war had introduced new, large-scale changes to mosquito and *Plasmodium* distribution, including the forced migration of large numbers of people from infected areas, the sudden exposure of populations to *Plasmodium* species that were new to them, the collapse of health systems due to war, and the unavailability of quinine in most countries, all in the context of the worst poverty seen in years. The "sanitary landscape" of Eastern Europe was rendered even less palatable by epidemics of typhus cholera and relapsing fever, on top of hunger and even famine in European Russia and Ukraine.[65]

War continued to be the operative language. One reason why the history of malaria is so tied to war is that the conceit that it was a war, and the logic of war, and the language of war shapes the response but, more importantly, the response was shaped by the officers that were assigned to wage what they understood as the battle. In war, you need to kill the enemy, not build a health-care infrastructure. Thus, of the two "paths" toward control, only one could really be waged by an Army officer. It was frontal assault, the foe defeated, disease by disease. Armies were not really equipped to set up long-term basic health-care systems or address poverty. Thus, the war metaphor became the official language and thus a battle successfully waged became the official role of the Malaria Commission. Economic and social reform were seen as the task not of international experts but rather of individual economies and, finally, as no one's task at all.

Ironically, it is war itself that potentiates malaria rates. War offers a perfect opportunity for the mosquitoes and the parasite. War first brings horses, then marching troops, and then tanks—all of which drive their prints into the muddy ground. Shells and trenches pockmarked Europe, and natural predators—fish—were eaten in the first months of postwar famine. There was always a torn-up landscape, always people living outdoors, and always a lack of available medical supplies, and this all contributed to the death toll. War destroyed public health systems and civil societies and focused attention on the immediate crisis and on attacks on specific problems to address immediate crises.

The military historian Harrison noted that malaria upsurges have been associated with nearly every major armed conflict of the nineteenth and twentieth centuries. "War has enhanced the spread of malaria in a number of ways. It has weakened and destroyed existing health systems, making it difficult for people infected with malaria to obtain treatment. . . . warfare prevented the effective operation of malaria control."[66]

And of course, the first scientists who unraveled the secrets of the etiology of malaria were serving in remote posts in colonial armies, thinking like soldiers. The discoveries of Laveran, Ross, and Grassi occurred at a time when the practice of public health as a whole was becoming increasingly focused on the identification and elimination of microparasites and when this project was linked to the establishment of Western settlements in regions seen as new and uncharted, needing to "be cleansed." It is thus not surprising that these discoveries led to similar concentrations of malaria control efforts to be focused on eliminating the proximate cause of the disease—parasites and mosquitoes—and the neglect of the broader social and economic conditions that played an important role in the epidemiology of the disease.[67]

By 1924, the Malaria Commission had traveled throughout Europe and the Middle East, stopping to admire the efforts in Palestine as the first colony to eradicate malaria there, but they did not visit Latin America or Africa—a problem that would characterize the response well into the twentieth century. The world then went about rebuilding, only to be beset by the Depression and the growing tensions that would lead to World War II. It was this structure of anti-malaria attention—on the Middle East and Europe—that came to haunt the combatants in World War II. It was a war that was waged not only in the trenches of Belgium and northern France, but also in Northern and Western Africa, Southeast Asia, and the South Pacific, where malaria was endemic. It would begin "the greatest war on malaria" yet, as we will see.

Meanwhile, as in Italy, social reformers such as Celli made the case that improving living conditions and eradicating disease needed to be addressed in one campaign. In America, first the Progressive Era and then the New Deal marked a change in the attention paid to malaria in the American South. The Tennessee Valley Authority began to build hydroelectric dams on the malarial rivers to bring electricity to the South. After initially ignoring the problems that changing water courses and digging roads in a malarial habitat created, thus giving the North American *Anopheles* new habitat, the Roosevelt administration and the Rockefeller Foundation sent entomologists and malariologists to organize a sanitation and larvicide campaign, spraying insecticide on regional Army barracks and Works Progress Administration camps. But most of the improvement in disease prevalence was due largely to a change in the economic conditions. M. A. Barber, the US Public Health Service officer who had first developed Paris Green and who was also the president of the American Society of Tropical Medicine, noted in 1940:

> Apparently, the amelioration in malaria prevalence in *Anopheles* infected regions occurs only where improved agriculture or other social factor has brought about a general economic improvement in the condition of people . . . It would seem that with even a moderate betterment of social conditions, malaria in the United States tends to disappear or become relatively inconsiderable provided such improvement is general. Or, to state the proposition in another way, the maintenance of high endemic malaria requires a permanent reservoir of infection such as is furnished by a considerable body of people lacking proper housing, proper food and adequate medical treatment.[68]

Sent to China in the 1930s, American doctors saw that here too, even in the midst of Asian poor, rural communities, small improvements in standards of living made significant differences. Many scientists in the public health services began to press for such reforms. Stampar, the new head of a US Public Health mission to China, wrote: "After working nearly three years in China, I am especially impressed by one fact, Successful health work is not possible where the standards of living falls below the level of tolerable existence. Public health policy must be intimately connected with a programme for general social improvement."

1.3   The History of Malaria: Modernity and Mortality

Then, the world went to war again. Social improvement would have to wait because the scientists and the public health officers had all been recruited to the American military.

World War II would be a global crisis for malaria control, and it would transform, as the apotheosis of the war against the disease, the way that malaria would be fought because of two powerful new interventions. It was the Rockefeller-trained scientists, skilled in eradication and entomology, who led the anti-malaria campaign, but it was once again organized and implemented by the US Armed Forces. America at war had several enemies. The war took millions of men and women into malarial countryside regions right across the globe, in North and West Africa, in Southern Europe, and throughout Asia. Malaria took a shocking toll on the Allied troops in the Pacific theater in particular, sickening a third of the invasion forces at Guadalcanal and nearly half of the troops in New Guinea and the Pacific Islands, and sickening British and Australian troops as they surrendered, exhausted, in Burma and Bataan and throughout the Philippines, to the Japanese. Of the 75,000 American and Filipino soldiers involved in the desperate campaign to stop Japan in the Philippines, 24,000 were sickened with malaria.

Quinine forests on Java, the sole source of the enormous Dutch quinine production farms, and storage centers for quinine in the Netherlands were all under Japanese or German control. Dutch quinine plantations produced 2,000 pounds of quinine a year by 1941. Germany took Amsterdam's stores, and Japan invaded Indonesia and took control of Java's cinchona plantations in 1942. The sole available drug once quinine was unavailable, Atabrine or Quinacrine, worked only sporadically, had to be taken precisely once a day, made men nauseous, paranoid, and wracked by vivid, violent dreams, and, moreover, turned their skin bright yellow. The soldiers hated it. Meanwhile, the filthy, desperate army camps, the trash, and the lack of supplies made other illnesses worse, and thousands of men and women kept sickening, unable to fight. Even when they could clean up the camps, periodically, the surrounding jungles were a reservoir of parasites—and as soldiers went to fight or to patrol, they would return infected. Infection rates were high across the entire Southwest Pacific Area, astronomically so in some localized hotspots. One of the hardest hit areas was the Allied base at Milne Bay, Papua, which provided support for the campaign against Buna and Gona in late 1942 through January 1943.

During the campaign, malaria was rampant. According to the US Army Center of Military History, the incidence of the disease reached an astounding 4,000 cases per 1,000 soldiers per annum. On average, this was the equivalent of every single soldier at Milne Bay coming down with the disease at least four times throughout the course of the year. This had a devastating effect on the efficiency of the units based there, where it was estimated that they lost around 12,000 man-days a month in work due to the disease.

Infection rates for the rest of the area of operations were not much better. Shah writes: "In Papua New Guinea, malaria laid claim to four times more casualties than the ferocious battles themselves, with more than 70 percent of Australian soldiers down with malaria. Every single soldier of the American Division, sent to Guadalcanal in the Solomon Islands in late 1942 came down with malaria, some more than once. Overall, malaria sickened more than 60 percent of the Allied troops in Southeast Asia. Most notorious was the island of Bataan—85% of the men lay sick."[69]

By the winter of 1942, the Army sent out "mosquito brigades" led by the Rockefeller-trained scientists to study, map, and treat anopheline breeding sites, and a "year later, more than two hundred malaria units were in every theatre of the war."[70] They used Atabrine and something they called "bug bombs"—repurposed air conditioning units full of African chrysanthemums—which were used as insecticides. The head of the unit reported directly to General MacArthur—malaria had become a central issue of the war. Winning Guadalcanal was one thing, but if no troops could live there without becoming sick with malaria, it could not be held. On average 5,332 men were on the sick list a day. By the fall of 1943, the Pacific saw ten hospital admissions for every one battle casualty, and the majority of the Allied division were now incapable of effective military duty. Major General Norman T. Kirk wrote in desperation to his superiors:

> The malaria situation in the South and Southwest Pacific is bad, as I originally mentioned. The attached report, which is authentic, shows that some six divisions have already been incapacitated because of malaria infection. Thus malaria handicaps the war effort in that area. The same thing will happen in North Africa if troops occupy any of the island in the Mediterranean, or southern Italy itself . . . Malaria control is a command function and the protection of troops from mosquito bite is essential. The war effort in these areas can be badly crippled, if not lost, by malaria infection alone.[71]

The medical department estimated that casualties due to this disease for this period outnumbered combat casualties on an order of seven to ten times. Lieutenant General Robert L. Eichelberger, commander of the US forces bogged down at Buna, noted that "disease was a surer and more deadly peril to us than enemy marksmanship. We had to whip the Japanese before the malarial mosquito whipped us."

The South Pacific was not the only place where malaria threatened to derail the entire Allied offensive. Indeed, in Libya, Liberia, and the Gold Coast of Africa, where thousands of soldiers were shipped, *A. gambiae* mosquitoes were everywhere. By July 1943, malaria was the number 1 problem of the war in nearly every theater of the conflict.[72]

The Army launched a massive propaganda campaign, illustrated by a young Ted Geisel, who would later be known as Dr. Suess, to convince the troops that basic nineteenth-century hygiene, swamp clearing, larvicidal oil, Paris Green, nets, and rigorous use of Atabrine would stop the deadly epidemic. Giesel leads a group of illustrators to create leaflets and pamphlets to convince the troops to take the hated Atabrine. In them, the anopheline mosquito was portrayed as a lethal, female sexual predator. Always with large breasts, always scantily clad, drinking blood from a wine glass, she appears to us now, looking at these pictures, as a wildly erotized but oddly Suess-like creature. In the Army anti-malaria literature, the female mosquito seductresses look Asian. They are always flagrantly sexual. They are out at night, slinking into one's bed, sharing fluids, sickening the victim, who is unsuspecting, careless, or naive. The unstated subtext was "Don't go out of your bed net at night to Asian prostitutes." Using all the tropes of racism and misogyny, completed by linking sexual seduction (as a kind of death) and the actual risk of malaria, the campaign used a teasing innuendo to convince the troops that they were always at risk of death from the dark and dangerous world. (There is no mention of the half a million women serving or any pictorial account of the women in the propaganda—women were not your colleagues, they were the dangerous, whoring mosquitoes.)

Geisel, to be sure, was faced with a difficult problem. Atabrine turned the person who took it bright yellow and caused nausea and disturbing neurological symptoms—mental instability, terrible headaches, and terrifying, hallucinogenic nightmares. The Army grew desperate, posting human skulls around their bases, with threatening signs: "This man did not take his Atabrine." Hollywood got involved. Disney made a version of *Snow White*, in which the seven dwarfs were enlisted to clean cheerily not only the house but also the surrounding forest. Small birds and bunnies poured Paris Green on the forest ponds, all the while singing happily about the virtues of cleanliness. In another Hollywood film, a soldier comes home with malaria, and sickens his fiancée and entire family, who die horrible deaths. In another, a swarthy farmer fails to put screens on his cabin windows, gets malaria, and cannot care for his family, resulting in his farm falling into darkness and despair. All seems lost until the swamp is drained, Paris Green is applied, and he changes his ways. His farm is restored, and he, now cleaner and oddly whiter, sits happily on his rebuilt porch. In another film, an old, vaguely Italian prostitute, "Annie," sits in a bar with three young Asian prostitutes. All are wearing bright red lipstick and outrageous outfits—black lace, fishnet stockings, nine-inch heels. She is telling them about the good old days before the Army's anti-malaria campaigns and gives a little account of colonialism while a series of night-clubs in Asia, Latin America, and North Africa flash on the screen, in which she appears, happily drinking blood with unsuspecting soldiers. "But we have been driven out, hunted, killed," she complains, against a montage of images of bulldozers, men with spraying gear, and canisters of Paris Green. "But don't worry," she tells the young hustlers, "there are always one or two. . . ." Don't let that be you, warns the film, as Annie is locked out of a tent and squished. "Don't go to bed with a malaria mosquito . . . be sure no mosquito is waiting for you!" warned the posters.

Meanwhile, scientists conscripted into the war effort, including the scientists who had been instrumental in combating malaria in the American South, worked frantically to replace Atabrine and find some drug that would work against mosquitoes. Here, too, the language of war, of total victory and bombs and defeats began to work its way into the scientific projects. Called the Malaria Project, its main task was to try to find a drug to replace quinine without the side effects of Atabrine.

In the last year of the war, two new—one can, by now, only call them—"weapons" were developed that finally proved effective against malaria. They were the first new weapons of the twentieth century. The first was DDT, and the second was hydroxychloroquine.[73]

DDT was called "Gerasol" by its German inventors, chemists of the J. R. Geigy company of Switzerland.[74] It was a powder that killed by insinuating itself into the tissues of the organisms, who died later. The residue, if left on surfaces, would kill for six months in most cases. Since mosquitoes rested on vertical surfaces right after they ate, waiting until they could excrete excess fluid from the blood out of their bodies, it was highly effective to spray DDT on the walls of houses, where the mosquitoes would touch the residue, so highly lethal that it killed them nearly immediately. Its first important use came at a critical moment in the Italian campaign, when Allied troops were poised to advance on the Campagna di Roma and the Pontine Marshes. As the Nazis withdrew their troops, they opened the floodgates and reversed the pumps, knowing that the area would flood, that the heat of the oncoming spring would hasten the laying of eggs, and that in a month, the mosquitoes would again spread parasites—a very primitive but effective germ warfare plan. But knowing this, the Allies sent in troops to spray the area with DDT, giving them time to fix the pumps, drain the marsh, and neutralize the threat.[75] DDT was then used in massive amounts in the Pacific theater, with entire bases sprayed repeatedly with DDT. Aerial spraying was done ahead of invasions, eliminating the threat of malaria and, to be sure, dengue fever, elephantiasis, and any other vector-borne disease almost entirely.

DDT was not the only radical new weapon in the war. The troops that marched into Rome had come from North Africa, and in the fierce fighting there, they had come across a terrified but clever Swiss scientist, who had run a small clinical trial with a new drug he had acquired from Germany called sontochin. In its composition, sontochin, or hydroxychloroquine, was found to be very similar to a drug tried and rejected earlier by the Malaria Project scientists—but perhaps that was a mistake? Clearly, the drug had to be tested to be certain it was not a Nazi trick.

Thus began one of the largest clinical trials held during World War II.

To understand how it was tested, I need to reverse the arc of our malaria history timeline to go back to the nineteenth century in Europe to the State "Lunatic" Hospital in Graz, Austria. It is 1883, and psychiatrist Dr. Julius Wagner-Jauregg is worried about a syphilitic stage actor, a gentleman of his class, who seemed to have lost his mind entirely.

Shah describes the problem. Syphilitics filled the asylums in the late nineteenth and early twentieth centuries, occupying an estimated 10–20 percent of hospital beds. Syphilis is first noted in medical records as a new disease, part of the Atlantic exchange, perhaps because it had been unknown before, or perhaps it was a mutation of a skin disease called yaws, which is caused by the same bacterium. In any case, it swept across European before it attenuated, and then, in the late 1800s, it changed again, developing the ability to infect the brain, causing a measurable increase in dementia in relatively young people. The mutation from skin disease to venereal disease occurred just as Europe's population had exploded, when there were houses of prostitution, more sexual freedoms, and, of course, more warfare—with mass movements of arms and refugees to spread the disease. Syphilis was a feature of life in many intellectual circles, making appearances in literature and plays. Philosopher Hannah Arendt remembers her father dying of the disease and remembers how delirium and rage took over his personality. Beethoven, Shubert, Nietzsche, Manet, and others died of the disease. "This new type of psychosis caused a somewhat sudden personality change that brought on wild mood swings, followed by profanities, inappropriate sexual behavior and muscle paralysis. . . . it burned through the middle classes at infection rates as high as 20 percent in Europe."[76]

Julius Wagner-Jauregg, frustrated but always attentive, noticed that when one of his patients with syphilis also had a very high fever, that seemed to moderate the symptoms. What causes the highest and most recurrent of fevers? Malaria! Perhaps if one could be deliberately given a fever, it might somehow clean the blood of the syphilis bacteria, he reasoned. He tried *Streptococcus*, then tuberculosis, both of which were too dangerous. Patients were cured of syphilis but died of the other illness. Then, he tried the blood of patients with malaria, injecting it directly into the veins of patients with late-stage syphilis. The immune response, marked by fever, seemed to kill both the malaria parasite and the syphilis bacteria. One had to be careful, using only *P. vivax* and not *P. falciparum*—but it was the first hope of a cure, albeit a very arduous one, for a tragic disease, and for it, he was awarded the Nobel Prize in Medicine.

By 1942, the treatment, while rare in America, was still being used. (After penicillin became widely available, five years later, it was abandoned entirely.) This presented an interesting opportunity. The only way to test the new Swiss doctor's drug for malaria was to do a full-scale clinical trial with a control group, using a technique called the challenge trial. In a human challenge trial, the research subjects are deliberately given the disease to be studied, allowed to sicken, and then the intervention of choice, or a placebo, is given.[77]

Thus, in the middle of WWII, The University of Chicago was not only the site of the development of nuclear weapons, a biological Manhattan Project was also carried out there. Two University of Chicago physician scientists—Lowell Coggeshall, a veteran of anti-malaria campaigns in the South and member of the Malaria Project, and Alf Alving, a professor of medicine—were enlisted to run the trial to test sontochin at the nearby Stateville Penitentiary. They would use the institutionalized patients who had been given malaria to cure their syphilitic madness.[78]

A strain of malaria (*vivax*) was maintained in the psychotic patients at Manteno State Hospital, Maneno, Illinois by blood inoculations. University of Chicago researchers had conducted initial clinical trials of anti-malarial drugs involving mentally ill patients before establishing the malaria research facility at Statesville prison. Mosquitoes were fed on some of the malaria infected mentally ill patients prior to being transported to Statesville for inducing malaria in volunteers at the prison.[79]

By all accounts, the trial was conducted within the ethical boundaries of the time. It was thought that using prisoners was more acceptable than using mentally ill patients, for example. There were many such experiments, and after all, the patients were receiving the malaria treatment for which the Nobel Prize had been won. If the "fever therapy" was given incorrectly or to the wrong patients, or if it was a bad idea in general, the researchers would not have known this in 1942. By every account, including one by the most infamous of the prisoners who volunteered to be both a participant and a laboratory technician, Leopold Loeb (of the Chicago "Leopold and Loeb" case, in which he and his friend had brutally killed a young boy just to see how it would feel), the prisoners thought it was fairly done. Dr. Alving, also by all accounts, was the model of kindness, compassion, and ethical veracity. He told the prisoners how it would feel to be sick with malaria, promised to stand by them, and spoke of the nobility of such volunteerism. He offered no inducements and made no promises about reduction of sentences. The prisoners were offered $100 to participate, and many chose not to take part. And despite retrospective alarm in my field of bioethics, and new rules in the 1970s that prohibited prisoners being used as research subjects for fear of unjust coercion, firsthand reports at the time did not reflect any undue coercion. Yet, not everyone saw the project as benign or even morally justified. The experiment, when portrayed in *Life* magazine, featuring, of course, Loeb and showing mosquitoes biting prisoners, was used by the defense in the Nuremberg Doctors' Trial. How is this different, the defense tried to argue, from using imprisoned Jews as research subjects? Of course, the idea that terrified, tortured, and fatally trapped Jews in the Dachau and Auschwitz concentration camp could be compared to prisoners at Statesville was not persuasive. The argument quickly fell apart as scientists anxious to protect the project testified to its difference.[80] The science itself was a war effort, it was argued, and it was the eagerness to be a "part of the war" in some way that was the most persuasive argument for prisoners volunteering to be research subjects. After all, men their age were stationed in malarial areas, wrote Loeb in later accounts, so they would endure the same disease in the hopes of "winning the war" on malaria.

The drug worked extremely well. And now, in addition to the powerful DDT, the armed forces finally had another weapon: the anti-malaria drug they called chloroquine. It would be this combination that would be used all over the globe, and it would quickly end the threat of malaria in the US Army.

When the Army doctors emerged from the war, after seeing this enormous success, they turned their full attention to the eradication of malaria in general, convinced it was possible. They were certain that it would also be possible to eliminate all vector-borne diseases and liberate agriculture—they just had to kill all the mosquitoes.

DDT was remarkable, powerful, and shockingly effective—it was universally malignant, especially to insects. It did not seem to affect mammals or birds, it was thought, and could be easily sprayed by hand or by plane. It seemed to last long after it had been applied, poisoning the environment and the mosquitoes for months. And even if sprinkled on human skin or inhaled, it seemed to have no discernable effect on people. It also meant that it could persist in the environment, exerting its poisonous effects for months, which, at the time, seemed entirely like a good idea.[81]

By the end of the war, DDT was made available for domestic use, and farmers and gardeners around the world used it indiscriminately (as did my family), excited and thrilled by its immediate effects on pests. Crop yields skyrocketed. "Never in the history of entomology," enthused Sievert Rohwer from the United States Department of Agriculture (USDA), "has a chemical been discovered that offers such promise to mankind for relief from his insect problems as DDT."[82]

And the popular press loved it. "Our next world war," *Popular Mechanics* called it, "a long and bitter battle to crush the creeping, wriggling, flying, burrowing billions."[83] The political community, too, was convinced, and the new agency, the UN, organized a UN Relief and Rehabilitation Administration (UNRRA) endowed with billions. Campaigns led by former Allied officers on islands on which they had been stationed—Sardinia, Sri Lanka—sprayed millions of gallons of DDT everywhere. It could blanket the countryside. It was easily applied by semi-skilled workers with minimal training, wearing cheap backpacks with spray canisters and spray guns. It worked on all mosquitoes (and, indeed, all annoying insects), and there was no need to establish clinics, train medical personnel, or distribute chloroquine.

By 1956, convinced that "malaria could be eradicated in just a few years" with the use of massive DDT spray campaigns, the newly formed UN WHO announced plans to support the effort, along with its campaign to eradicate smallpox. Thus began the tale, central to every malaria effort since, of the "two campaigns." Vaccination for smallpox, however, turned out to be far simpler, despite its enormity, than the malaria campaign. It is important to stop for a moment to consider this, for its failure created a fatalistic tone in all further malaria projects, and it still plays a role in how gene drives are understood and in the structure of the opposition to them. There are several reasons why.

First, the 1956 campaign (as will be a theme is all modern malaria elimination efforts since) was dramatically underfunded. Second, the WHO decided that the malarial forests and plains of Africa were too "difficult" to cope with. They left Africa out of their campaign, limiting efforts there to "demonstration projects," not eradication efforts, leaving, of course, a huge reservoir of potential infection, not to mention abandoning communities beset by the worst form of the parasite, *P. falciparum*, and the most aggressive vector, *A gambaie.*

Third, the WHO did not plan for failure, which meant that they did not have a solution for a problem that had been worrisome since at least 1939, when the husband and wife team—identified always as "Dr. and Mrs. Wilson"—began to notice that when soldiers from East Africa were deployed away from the villages where they were born and where malaria was endemic, they lost their acquired immunity in six months.[84] Describing why so many had what he thought was immunity but which we now understand to be low-level chronic malaria in a world prior to DDT, Dr. Wilson said:

> There were always infected anopheles present in houses . . . at a very rough estimate it might be said that an individual was likely to receive an infective bite every twelfth night, or thirty times a year. Anopheline control under such circumstances in tropical Africa is impossible, or perhaps I should say that I have not yet seen a village having this type and degree of endemicity in which control would be possible. These villages, it is true, have been protected during the dry season, when breeding places are reduced to a few wells, the pools in a half-dried stream and some other almost permanent pools. But with the rains and after every heavy storm innumerable natural hollows fill with rain water or formed swamps; in addition old pig holes, hoof marks, and the multitude of manmade evacuations which surround every African village and are constantly renewed—all contributed to a breeding area

so large that the available methods of anopheline control (this was prior to DDT) are utterly beyond the resources of such people.[85]

Not only was the situation bleak, he thought, but interfering might actually make it worse, argued Miller.[86] Miller noted: "The main object which I have in mind has been to arouse discussion on what, in my opinion, a question of increasingly pressing importance, namely, the relevance of what has been called 'natural immunity' to malaria in deciding on an anti-malaria policy; and secondly to draw attention to some of the lacunae in our knowledge of hyperendemic malaria."[87] But the Wilsons were wrong. There is no acquired immunity to malaria. What was supposed to be full immunity would quickly disappear when the person left for war, for work, or for migration. When they returned to a malarial area, they would have lost their capacity to resist malaria and would quickly sicken again—something called the "rebound effect." This phenomenon changes the disease. Unless it is eradicated, even people who thought they were immune are at risk. Even seemingly immune Africans would lose the capacity to resist the organism, and returning soldiers, newly infected, could spark a new epidemic. Additionally, because they present to the vector as malaria naive, they are far sicker that they were with their first infection. What looked like immunity was likely a persistent low-grade infection—one that prevented a second, more severe case.

By 1955, the WHO was aware of this problem, and WHO officials were also aware of the unsteadiness of health-care funding. By the time they were scheduled to start, WHO only had about 50 percent of the money that they need would need to complete the anti-malaria campaign in the countries it had already begun. Would beginning a campaign in Africa and then stopping end up doing more harm than good?

> Nobody disputed that DDT would depress malaria to begin with. But freed from chronic exposure, local people would quickly shed their acquired immunities. And then, if for any reason—lack of funds, lack of roads, lack of popular support— malaria returned, they'd be especially vulnerable. More people would die.[88]

A less-than-perfect eradication campaign, in other words, would end up being much deadlier than no eradication, changing a disease from one that kills infants to one that can kill the now-unimmune adults—causing more deaths.[89] In part, this fear represented a confusion in what immunity really was. Researchers distinguish between three types of this acquired or adaptive immunity: (1) anti-disease immunity, (2) anti-parasite immunity, and

(3) premunition, which maintains a low-grade and generally asymptomatic parasitemia and thereby protects against the clinical manifestations of new infections.[90]

1.4   The History of Malaria: The Global Campaign

The WHO campaign did in fact exclude Africa from anything but a few pilot projects. We will return to this problem when I carefully focus on the ethical issues in malaria treatment in Africa in a subsequent chapter.

The WHO campaign began in earnest, and by 1960, it was succeeding as promised: ten countries had eliminated all traces of malaria, and fourteen had seen enormous declines in infection and death rates. By 1956, malaria was eradicated in the USA, with the last cases in Louisiana. Cases across Central America, where the hard-fought battle for Panama had been so difficult, began to decline, and in the villages of Papua New Guinea, where Marines had sickened in enormous numbers, malaria receded, and even in malarial India, despite unrelenting social and economic struggles, an annual caseload of 75 million dropped to fewer than 100,000.[91] Across the world, new agricultural land long abandoned to disease was reclaimed, and as children began to survive in larger numbers, the population rates and life expectancy rose dramatically—raising concerns among some, who then began to worry, ironically enough, about "population bombs." Of course, killing mosquitoes also eliminated other vectors, and the WHO campaign was carried out at the same time at a vast, successful vaccination program for smallpox, all of which played a role in changing death rates dramatically.

A rise in population in the formerly most stricken and poorest areas of the world was not the only consequence of the extensive spraying. There were also unexpected negative aspects that vexed the project, little of which had been foreseen. All insects, including beneficial ones, were caught up in the killing. The plan called for spraying twice a year, but because the mud walls of primitive houses in the developing world absorbed the poison, this was less effective than planned. This meant that teams had to return often to remote, sometimes bewildered, sometimes hostile villages and demand that the villages empty their houses entirely and put the furniture, decorations, bedding, cooking pots, clothes, utensils, and food outside until the spray dried. When harvesting season came, in some countries, villagers moved to the fields and slept in open huts, leaving their homes locked so that the spray teams could not go inside. Some pretended not to be home to avoid moving out and back in again. In one story (which might be apocryphal but is widely told by people who participated[92] in the Borneo campaign), the DDT killed the mosquitoes, and then the geckos that ate them became contaminated by massive doses of DDT, and when the cats ate the geckos, they died (other accounts credit the DDT directly for killing cats), and then rats began to take over villages because the cats were dead. In a desperate response, the WHO opened "cat distribution centers," and in remote areas, the British Royal Air Force dropped healthy new cats in specially devised baskets along with seeds and "4 cartons of stout for a recuperating chieftain."[93] Moreover, in village after village, thatched roofs collapsed—as the bugs that ate the eggs of caterpillar species died, the caterpillars overgrew, eating the thatch until the roofs fell in. To enforce the rules about spraying, of course, the army was needed again. Soldiers began accompanying spray teams and medical surveillance researchers who were tasked with taking blood from sprayed villagers to check for parasites—a task so difficult that some resorted to using fake samples rather than going into hostile territory twice weekly to draw the blood. Although it was easy to skip a hard-to-find random house, sometimes, whole areas were missed. Shah notes:

> On the fortnightly rounds, it was not likely to be serious, but there was evidence in India, for instance, that some teams routinely avoid remote villages and concealed their delinquency by taking an excess of blood samples from families more easily reached. . . . In one hospital, they forget to reorder slides. In many, there were too many slides to process . . . A two or three month back up for slides was common . . . as usual, the system was designed to press against the limits of human capacity . . . no one wanted to put more money or manpower into it than was absolutely necessary.[94]

There were more problems in the Global South—cultural clashes, more difficult terrain, the more challenging weather—than in the Global North. Thus, most of the real progress was made in the Northern Hemisphere, where there were far more resources and armies (always armies) that could be deployed. Of the ten countries where eradication had been achieved, noted the WHO, four were in Europe. The other six were in the Americas, and they were Chile and five Caribbean Islands.[95]

For the plan to work, it needed to work rapidly. Instead, it stalled, and a new problem, which had been emerging since the first few years of the eradication campaign, began to become terribly clear. The DDT no longer seemed to work as effectively. It had been ignored at first but could be no longer: the mosquitoes were becoming resistant to DDT.

The plan for global eradication should have worked. A mathematical model, developed by MacDonald as early as 1947, showed that everything came down to how an epidemic spreads: if there was a slight increase in longevity in the female mosquito population, if the biting rate was higher per insect, or if slightly more humans were available—slight changes where the numerator affected the denominator—then you would have malaria epidemicity. And slight permutations should have also changed the disease dynamics. Reducing the mosquitoes with DDT and reducing the parasite in the blood with chloroquine should have been enough to end malaria. But it was not. Resistance, probably because of mass agricultural spraying, grew so rapidly that the rates of malaria began to climb once again.[96] Slowly, sporadically, not only the mosquito, but the parasite too, developed resistance.

For many communities, the DDT project promised so much reward. It replaced the serious issues of land reform, health-care accessibility, income redistribution, and fair labor practices, long advocated by the Italians as fundamental to creating a durable response to malaria. DDT was a solution that did not fundamentally change the structure of countries or empower communities. Everything would be just the same—only without mosquitoes, and eventually without the *Plasmodium*.

Politics and logistics had created hurdles, and that work "turned out not too satisfactory." An interviewed Peruvian official saw DDT and SN7618 (plasmochin) as a cheap alternative to expensive land reforms. Public health officials all over Lima now eyed these wartime technologies as miracle weapons against malaria. "Everyone tended to seek an easy way out of the malaria control problem . . . (not realizing) their uses might prevent the development of permanent means of control."[97]

There was one more serious problem: scientists and lay observers began to notice a decline in some bird species, and it was discovered that birds with high levels of DDT, from eating insecticide-treated insects, could no longer lay eggs with solid shells. Instead, the shells cracked, and the eggs were destroyed. Human DDT levels, once tested, showed the ubiquitous nature of DDT, which accumulated in the fat cells of mammals, including, of course, people. Rachel Carson's bestseller *Silent Spring* documented these facts and added a grim prognosis: without insects, and without their capacity to pollinate crops, and without the birds that ate them, silenced by DDT, and without the predators that ate birds, our world would begin to unravel completely. The book was a wild success—and DDT sales plummeted. (My father began to turn to organic gardening.) DDT was swiftly banned in many cities. In the tropics, funding by Westerners for spraying DDT stopped, and there was already little money to continue from within the countries that were most at risk. Meanwhile, what many thought were the root causes of malaria—things that allowed the vector to flourish such as poverty and instability—had been left unchanged.

At the same time, the political calculus that had enabled the funding stream changed. In the USA, enthusiasm for bold chemical attacks on insects started to give way to fear of poisoning and a more political, most troubling concern about overpopulation, especially in the Global South. Poor children were surviving, and for some, who echoed the same fairly racist concerns of the British politicians who first raised them after Ross's discoveries, this was worrisome. By the 1960s, several prominent public health experts had reached a consensus that the most serious problem facing humanity was not excess death from disease but just the opposite: overpopulation.[98]

The idea of "preparation, attack, consolidation, and maintenance" of the disease, which was the optimistic plan, stalled at the attack phase. A final terrible resurgence in Sri Lanka discouraged many, and the five-year funding promises ended completely. The country had nearly eradicated the disease, with six cases reported, but when the USA withdrew funding, it took only five years before there were more than 1 million cases. Disenchantment with malaria control was only part of the problem. Since much of the funding was tied to Western efforts to win over countries defined as neutral in the great postwar struggles of the Cold War, political calculation was also a part of the structure of the eradication campaign. When a country made a choice to affiliate with the Soviet bloc, US funding and Western support often disappeared. That had been the case in Sri Lanka when its leadership began to embrace a socialist economy.[99]

Worse still, it could be argued that the situation had deteriorated. The mosquitoes were swiftly becoming resistant to DDT. The *Plasmodium* was becoming resistant to chloroquine and quinine, the only readily available and inexpensive ways to address the problem. *P. falciparum* was entrenched throughout Africa and Southeast Asia. However, as soon as it was no longer a problem for developed countries, malaria was marginalized as a tropical disease and was not a priority for health-care dollars. It is also worth noting that in many of these countries, malaria control programs had succeeded in eliminating malaria as a problem for the economically well off and politically powerful. Malaria, in effect, had settled in among the poor and the powerless.[100]

By 1974, the campaign for eradication was officially ended by the WHO. As new nations gained independence in the 1970s and coped with instability as the colonial order ended, endemic malaria in the poor countries of Africa and Asia became a fact of life, unchanged since it had arrived at the beginning of human history. Attention turned from Africa. The Cold War ended, and what money there had been for African health care needs went to cope with the aftermath of wars, droughts, and famines that called for attention instead. Shah sums up the WHO analysis:

> Between 1957 and 1967 the war against *Plasmodium* cost $1.4 billion or about $9 billion in 2009 dollars [and $10.5 billion in 2018]. To this day, malariologists and historians disagree over whether it was worth it. . . . In just over a dozen years, malaria had been lifted from the shoulders of 32 percent of the human population. . . . [But] others see [this] as "one of the greatest mistakes ever made in public health." Malaria had been eradicated from just 18 countries in the world, all of them either prosperous, socialist or island nations. That left some two billion souls still burdened with malaria.[101]

The neglect of Africa was another error in the WHO campaign. To some extent, the emerging nations began to address malaria themselves. The first African Malaria Conference had taken place in 1950 in Kampala, where the problem of rebound was discussed. Although adults did seem to be immune, at least to the deadliest aspects of *P. falciparum*, this fragile immunity was won at a high cost: 25 percent of all childhood deaths in Africa were due to malaria. Delegates understood that the WHO only committed to supporting pilot programs, and at first, they decided to try elimination themselves, but then they too settled on pilot programs for malaria control. But the rebound effects, even in the smaller pilot programs, were devastating. In the aftermath of the pilot project in the Kpain region of central Liberia, epidemic malaria struck adults as well as children in the once-protected communities.[102]

And in these communities, indeed across African nations, there were few laboratories, hospitals, or local clinics. So convinced were the scientists of the 1950s that spraying would work, they failed to create durable health-care structures—a problem in malaria control that still haunts Southeast Asia and Africa. New nations struggled to build schools, workplaces, and clinics. The malaria projects had not been designed to create a malaria service or any other type of public health infrastructure, and the institutional capacities for

medical surveillance in tropical Africa in the 1950s and early 1960s were rudi-
mentary at best. The lack of medical surveillance meant that not only were
public policies difficult to establish because of a lack of data, but also ethical
issues, including responsibility for the failures of the lapsed control projects,
were often ignored.[103]

Migration added another problem. As populations moved in response to
the political winds of nationalism and revolution, thousands shifted across
country lines. This had profound implications because new roads and new
railways meant that when drought or famine or war pushed populations out
of established regions, they could travel widely across the continent. New
malaria infections followed the railways and were borne in the blood of the
refugees, spread in the vast new camps, across the entirety of sub-Saharan
Africa. When a robust and successful anti-malaria campaign was waged
in one region, it was meaningless unless adjoining regions—now often in
adjoining independent nations—cooperated. In many countries, the newly
independent governments had little effective reach into large parts of their
state territories.[104]

For many, the global campaign had uncomfortable echoes of colonialism.
Little attention had been paid to community consent, much less to education. Webb notes that the failure did little to create trust in science or agreement with shared goals: "The aborted malaria eradication campaign had been
driven by the insights and assumptions of Western bioscience. Western perceptions of the seriousness of malaria were shaped by knowledge of the vulnerabilities of the non-immune settler in tropical Africa, economic arguments
about the loss of worker productivity, and growing evidence that malaria killed
many African children and wreaked havoc with the lives of some who survived. . . . For African adults, malaria was largely perceived as an annoyance,
an unpleasant reality, rather like the seasonal flu, rather than a vital problem
to be tackled with scarce resources."[105] The sense of failure after the optimism
of the early victories permeated the public health workers and the literature
describing the events. Because it had been constructed as a war, the failure
was not an event in a health-care narrative but rather a defeat by a fierce, evil
enemy. This sense of defeat was pervasive. Look at how the leading historians
write of this period. For Harrison, the war historian, "It is a failure—failure so
universal, so apparently ineluctable, must be trying to tell us something. The
lesson could be, of course, that we have proved incompetent warriors. It could
also be that we have misconstrued the problem."[106] For Packard, the scholar

of public health, it was a failure to understand the early lessons learned by Celli and Sopher about the need for economic reform and social changes that included land redistribution and health-care infrastructure. Commenting on a visit to a South American health administrator, Packard said, "The problem is worse in many parts of the globe over the last 30 years. The limited effectiveness of recent efforts to eliminate malaria as a public health problem stems in large measure from a failure to appreciate the importance of social and economic forces in driving the epidemiology of the disease. Or, put another way, it flows from a failure to appreciate the lessons of history."[107] For Webb, scholar of African history, "The failed pilot projects had produced untoward malarial dynamics in their wakes. Severe morbidity, and an increased incidence of mortality had been inflicted on those age cohorts whose acquired immunities had been lost during the era of malaria control. The extent and the ethical dimensions of this medical crisis for African adolescents, parents, and grandparents in the project zones went unexplored."[108] For Sonia Shah, "After the ignominious defeat of the 1950-era DDT blitz, malaria disappeared from the headline. Books on the topic went out of print. Scientists stopped studying the disease; educators stopped teaching it. So completely did malaria vanish from the public mind that many people in the West grew up thinking that there was, literally, not more malaria in the world."[109]

1.5   The History of Malaria: The Unstable Advance

Meanwhile, China, which had been largely ignored by the WHO because it was a newly communist country, was organizing itself after its successful revolution and decades of Western colonial adventures. The Chinese Communist Party (CCP) went to work reversing centuries of isolation from normative public health initiatives and the utter neglect of the poor. For decades, elite Chinese scholars had studied in Europe and were aware of the international public heath standard. In the first years after the revolution, public health measures focused on large sanitation and public hygiene campaigns. For generations, the Chinese used human waste, called "night soil," directly on crops, and the CCP taught a method for composting to reduce the concentration of intestinal parasites prior to application. The CCP began vaccination campaigns. Incredibly, between 1950 and 1952, more than 512 million of China's 600 million people were vaccinated against smallpox, massively reducing case numbers. The last outbreak of smallpox in China occurred in 1960—twenty years before smallpox was eradicated globally.

By 1957, more than two thirds of China's then 2,050 counties had an epidemic-prevention station or a more specialized clinical center for the control of specific diseases (such as malaria, plague, schistosomiasis, leishmaniasis, and brucellosis) modeled on those established in the Soviet Union earlier in the twentieth century. Their efforts included "patriotic health campaigns" focusing on ensuring a clean environment and safe drinking water, vector control, latrine construction, and human waste disposal. Each of these short-term interventions (on average twice a year, lasting for around a week) required the mass mobilization of peasants and so served to increase the "health literacy" of the rural population.[110]

Twelve years after the revolution, the CCP's new chairman, Mao Tse Tung, organized a massive campaign called "Away with all Pests!" The Four Pests campaign was aimed at eradicating those pests most responsible for the transmission of malaria, plague, and leishmaniasis: mosquitoes, rats, flies—and the non-native European sparrows, which ate grains and fruit needed to feed humans. (They relented on the sparrows after entomologists pointed out that they also ate flies and mosquitoes.) Killing the mosquitoes meant draining swamps, examining village water storage, and spraying Paris Green on waterways and DDT in every house—but the intensity of party discipline, held over from the revolutionary days, meant that it was carried out with far more zeal and persistence.

In 1970, a new program was begun to create a more enduring system of health care, beyond the Four Pests campaign. In every village, the CCP trained a "barefoot doctor"—literally a poor peasant who would be in charge of a village-wide cooperative medical plan, including a clinic, obstetric care, basic health services, ongoing education, and advice on child-rearing. Trained by physician volunteers from urban areas (and in a few cases from foreign supporters), the "barefoot doctor" movement, which grew to nearly 2 million trained medics spread across the rural countryside, transformed health care and created the foundation for a widespread network of accessible clinics and hospitals—exactly the opposite of what had been done in Africa. It was Celli's socialist ideas put into practice.

There were of course many complex aspects of the period known as the cultural revolution in China in the period after Mao's death, which are beyond the scope of even this extremely long historical chapter to address. However, one little known aspect of that period by Westerners is that Chinese scientists began to consider traditional epistemic categories as they thought about diseases such as malaria, reasoning that since their civilization had dealt with diseases over centuries, there must be textual traditions about how to treat them. Thus, the Chinese began to look to their own historical litera-ture for cures, especially since the Western drug of chloroquine had begun to fail as the parasite mounted its resistance. Determined to rely on their own medical history, scientists turned toward a renewal of acupuncture, herbal medicine, and a search for native medicinal plants. This led them to review old textual sources, including *The Handbook for Emergency Treatments*, writ-ten in 340 CE. One plant mentioned as a malaria preventative, *quinghaosu* or Chinese wormwood grown in the highlands, turned out to be a sturdy, weedy plant that, unlike the fussy quinine tree, took root almost everywhere. Shah describes this vividly:

> The scientists gathered at a Beijing restaurant in May 1967 and hatched their plan to comb through traditional medicines and ancient Chinese medical texts for leads. Tucked inside an ancient medical document called "52 prescriptions," dating from 168 BC[E] they found descriptions of the medicinal properties of *Artemisia annua* or sweet wormwood tree, an unpretentious little shrub related to sagebrush and tarragon that will grow like a weed, in any kind of disturbed environment. Inside *Artemisia* flows a fragile compound called artemisinin, which can kill malaria para-sites the way that bleach kills microbes by exerting oxidative stress on their cell membrane. The ancients knew it too. Ge Hong described how a bitter tea of *Arteme-sia* provided relief from fever. By 1972 it was synthesized.[111]

They followed the 2,000-year-old instruction manual carefully. When it was soaked, purified, and analyzed, the active component was a compound called artemisinin. It turned out to be effective not only for every strain of *Plasmo-dium*, but also for treating *P. falciparum* cerebral malaria, even in advanced cases. China immediately began to use it in clinical trials and then in prac-tice, sharing it with allies in North Vietnam. But despite the fact that they also shared knowledge of the new drug with the WHO, Western officials were wary, and, locked into Cold War suspicions, it took twenty years for the enor-mous value of artemisinin to be recognized and approved by the WHO and for it to be used as treatment in chloroquine-resistant areas.[112]

Shah describes the problem:

> Western scientists frowned on the unorthodox method of extracting it . . . scientific commentators pointed out that Chinese scientists had used equipment that was "rudimentary" and "obsolete" by Western standards. WHO refused to approved the drug unless production facilities moved to the United States, a requirement with which the Chinese scientists refused to comply. A chasm of mistrust between Chinese and Western science sucked artemisinin into the vortex. Between 1980

and 1990, artemisinin drugs slashed China's caseload from two million to ninety thousand. But the Chinese developers of the drug couldn't interest a world-class drug maker in producing the world-class drug until 1994.[113]

That year, Novartis bought it—and priced it initially at $45 per course versus 25¢ for chloroquine.[114]

In Africa, meanwhile, malaria care languished. There were "no real health care system, no real labs—for many, there was barely electricity, and the labs were lit only by sunlight."[115] Reports from Nigeria, in one example, described a sub-Saharan Africa largely untouched by the aggressive anti-malaria and public health measure introduced in other locations. Consider this, from 1984: "Despite health delivery care, parasite [malaria] rates in Nigeria are the same as they were in 1934. Only 1 percent of the population is covered by vector control."[116]

The attention of the West had been captured by another health-care crisis: the sudden appearance of a what at first looked like fatal and rare form of cancer, and pneumonia, and a wasting illness among gay men. This—acquired immune deficiency syndrome (AIDS)—was caused by a virus, human immunodeficiency virus (HIV) which, after a brief initial infection, stayed in the body and depleted its t-cells until the immune system burned through its capacity to defend against any opportunistic infections, and these would overwhelm patients. By the middle of 1990, Africa was stricken with a full-blown AIDS epidemic among men, women and children, and worse yet, it soon became clear that people with AIDS had a significantly poorer prognosis if they were coinfected with malaria.

Wars, both for national liberation and for land seizures and political power, swept over Africa, doing what war historically had done to potentiate the malaria epidemic outbreak. The war forced farmers from fields and marketplaces and into refugee camps. Harvest and planting time was disrupted, leading to years of recurrent famine. Impoverished, malnourished families struggled to combat the effects of malaria infection. The changing climate further exacerbated the problem. First, the chaos in agriculture meant that people had no crops to sell. Without income, families could not afford medication to treat malaria. States could not afford to intervene, as tax revenues fell. As always, terrible social and economic conditions deepened the crisis. Meanwhile, the conduct of the war itself destroyed natural ecologies.[117]

Meanwhile, a larger international monetary crisis meant that newly created African countries, which had been loaned millions of dollars by the West to build industries and infrastructure—with huge portions of the money going to corruption, private potentates, and graft—were pressed to repay loans. Western countries began to want repayment, with interest.

"There wasn't much interest on the part of international anti-malaria financiers. . . . The world's biggest funder of aggressive attacks against the disease, the United States, had all but written off the notion of helping African countries with anything," noted one commentator. According to Shah, "The global recession of the 1970's hit newly independent African economies hard, and by the mid 1980's, the World Bank and the IMF had taken over the $1.3 trillion in debt they and other developing countries had accrued."[118] Faced with massive continent-wide economic collapse, the World Bank stepped in to take over the loans. But the World Bank had but one theory of justice: libertarianism, where the free market would equalize demand and need. Coping with the AIDS crisis and with malaria proved difficult, and the free-market plan failed to address the issues. Next, the World Bank demanded reorganization of government agencies, including the beleaguered health-care services, along market-driven rules. Cuts were made, staff laid off, and services that had once been provided free of charge were no longer free. The World Bank believed that people would value things more if they had paid something for them. They encouraged privately run clinics, payment for services, and decentralized health care. Teachers were laid off, infant mortality rose by 25 percent, and, worst of all, malaria entered the cities.[119]

This was just at the point that many in the West noticed the crisis in Africa—the time of celebrities' and rock bands' interest in African charity. Massive amounts of money were raised for bed nets, which the World Bank had decided must then be sold. In line with a policy advocated by the World Bank, many African governments introduced new user fees for health services. Then, when citizens could not afford such services or the proper bed nets, a new malaria epidemic hit East Africa. As one policy maker noted:

> The government of Madagascar had borrowed heavily to finance a program of the nationalization of industry and by 1980, the IMF had imposed an austerity program and price reforms. When the epidemic struck, there was a dearth of anti-malaria drugs to treat the critically ill. Yet beneath the swirl of complex and countervailing forces that complicate the analysis of the epidemic lie two fundamental epidemiological facts. The first was that the colonial-era programs had transformed the mix of malaria parasites. Chloroquine is differentially more effective against *vivax* than *falciparum*, and the campaign of chloroquine prophylaxis had all but eliminated

vivax from the highlands. The second fact was that this chloroquinization program, in combination with the dramatic reduction in malaria transmission that had been achieved through vector control had created a population nakedly vulnerable to malaria.[120]

There continued to be successful campaigns in some areas, and it was discovered that using artemisinin in combination with other therapies kept rapid resistance from occurring. It became clear that pouring money into AIDS relief alone was insufficient—tuberculosis and malaria were far bigger killers. In the late 1990s, three important funds—the Global Fund, the President's Fund (PEPFAR) and the Bill & Melinda Gates Foundation (BMGF) fund—and numerous smaller NGOs were formed to address this issue. Some focused on drug development and distribution, others on bed nets. Not only were artemisinin-based combination therapies (ACT) important, so too was a new treatment modality: intermittent treatment. It was found that groups at highest risk—most notably pregnant women and infants—tended to be protected against the worst forms of malaria if regular doses of ACT were given, and the terrible mortality could be slightly altered if ACT was given seasonally to school-age children,

But the WHO did not approve and change the guidelines for the ACT until 2001, which was tragically late. Eventually, the price dropped to $2 for a course of treatment. But the US AID office did not approve the therapy. It said that it was "not ready for primetime" and so distributed bed nets instead. African children were still being given old drugs, funded by the Global Fund. Finally, after an outcry in 2004, the policy changed, and in 2006, the Global Fund gave money to the malaria efforts. It had taken three decades.[121]

Underground black markets developed as individuals heard of the drug and began to demand it. To stretch supplies, it was adulterated, and fake versions were sold at fake clinics and at corner shops. There was no oversight for dosing. And by 2007, resistance first emerged to artemisinin.[122]

In 1998, Roll Back Malaria, a new, joint international philanthropic effort, began a campaign for bed nets, combined artemisinin therapies (ACT) and insect-treated bed nets (ITNs.) Bed nets, an intervention that predated Laveran and Ross, proved to be effective when used faithfully, and treating them first with insecticide made them even more effective. But getting people to sleep every single night inside a white, shroud-like, hot sweep of fabric proved more difficult than expected. In general, only about 17–20 percent sleep inside the nets. Instead, many use them for privacy, for tying loads on to the top of cars, or for fishing (which might be more cost effective and rational in terms of assuring the survival of one's family).

Reasons for not using bed nets abound. One reason that sleeping under bed nets was resisted was that it was the white colonialist's habit. Another was that the long, thin, white nets did indeed look like burial shrouds and some cultures would not use them until health workers dyed them bright green or then bright blue. For some families, who had to pay for them to meet the World Bank standards, it made little sense to use such expensive items on tiny children, and they were saved for working adults. Some people did not like the smell of the nets, dyed and treated with insecticide, or the idea of ITNs inside their homes, close to their babies. Others, when the babies inevitably got the nets messy with urine or feces, were ashamed and would wash them, scrubbing off the insecticide. Others, feeling ashamed of the dirtiness of the nets, would not take them for the annual insecticide retreating and would hide them from aid workers. Many people reported that a net with small enough holes to keep out mosquitoes was horribly hot and stifling. The nets tore and were hard to repair, and the insecticide wore away in one or two years, not five as had been promised. Worst of all, sometimes the mosquitoes were caught inside or crept inside during the day. Hence, at night, they were trapped inside the net with the child and bit and bit until they were sated.

In some countries, behavioral resistance emerged: the mosquitoes began biting earlier, before people went to sleep under the nets. And by 1993, resistance to the insecticidal pyrethroids that soaked the nets, which came from the African chrysanthemum plant, had also already been noticed.[123]

But steadily, and despite all of this, progress against malaria continued. From 1998 to 2015, rates of infection dropped incrementally, first to a million and then further—a triumph. Still, more than a half a million people died annually, largely children under the age of five, almost all in Africa of *P. falciparum*, nearly all of cerebral malaria. Then, slowly, a little under half a million died, still unacceptable but clear progress. It seemed that the efforts were gaining ground.

Then, in 2016, progress stopped, and by 2017, the rates had plateaued and finally, in 2020, they began to rise. It seemed that a stalemate had been reached, and then, even the stalemate was threatened, first by COVID-19, then by a shaken economy. In part, this was because the critical health-care structures had never been built. People still lived hours, even days, away from clinics. And again, the political tension between public health strategies, with an afterlife long after the end of the Cold War, was still at play.

The history of malaria, as you have seen, reader, is a complicated interplay between all the forces that shape human societies: social relationships, biological realities, economic forces, and the constancy of environmental terrains. How these were organized, how they were understood, and the systems for addressing them shifted and realigned over vast historical horizons. This order has largely determined the locale of the disease, the populations it has affected, and its spread and expansion along with global imperial projects. The parasite is located in places that are understood as marginal—it seems like a tropical disease of the rural poor not because of the etiology of illness but because these are the last people to have the tools to eradicate it. But it is also marked by a history, since the late nineteenth century, of how medical science proceeds. Since Koch and since Ross, a targeted narrative emerged: malaria is not in the air, it is in the specific parasite, and all our efforts were targeted on specificity. One organism, one disease, one cure—this is the biological model, and it privileges the attack on the mosquito as a sort of war, as we have seen. But there have always also been scientists who worried about the condition, especially the social condition, of the human host. In that model, for malaria to be eliminated, poverty needs to be ameliorated, health care needs to be distributed, and the economic system needs to be at least marginally just. As Packard noted: "The tension between ecological approaches to disease prevention and control and narrower biomedical strategies is by no means limited to the problem of malaria. It is a fundamental dilemma of modern public health. Do we develop targeted strategies for attacking the immediate causes of disease or focus on the broader determinates of ill health?"[124] Because the immediate cause of disease was always the target—the mosquito, the *Plasmodium*—the underlying causes—the lack of clinics, the poverty—always lacked funding to address them. Like so many illnesses, the social and economic conditions that potentiate human transmission of disease, and malaria in particular, include patterns of labor and exploitation that place workers at risk of infection, warfare that disrupts local ecologies and health services, population displacement that has exposed millions to malaria, and poverty that prevents individuals and countries from achieving and sustaining adequate levels of malaria protection. All these factors need to be reduced or eliminated. Real economic development that leads to broad-based improvements in the quality of life, as opposed to growing disparities between haves and have nots, needs to be actively encouraged, argued Packard: "The history of malaria over the past 50 years is strewn with examples of control programs that have broken down, allowing a resurgence of the disease. . . . In the long run, addressing the ecological determinants of malaria will reduce and in some cases eliminates the need to continually protect populations at risk."[125]

In 1950, when the WHO decided to drop Africa from the planned eradication campaign, the WHO's Director-General for Tropical Africa said, "The most we may be able to do is to ensure that everyone that has an attack of malaria can go and pick up some tablets."[126] By 2018, even that goal had not been realized. In fact, rates were rising in both numbers and percentages because the population today is far larger. Packard notes:

> The momentum of human expansion of out of Africa into Eurasia and much later, the thickening of the webs of global intercommunication in the post-Columbian period that included the Americas, eventually created a global distribution of malaria in three great zones that was at its maximum extent during the nineteenth century. During the twentieth century, malaria was banished from approximately a quarter of the earth's surface, roughly half the domain of the nineteenth century. However, owing to massive population growth, particularly on the African continent, by the end of the twentieth century, the number of people expose to malaria had increased dramatically, by more than 300 percent. Early in the twenty first century, the malarial area remaining are mostly those of intense transmission, and *falciparum* infections constitute a far larger percentage of infections than a century earlier.[127]

In some areas, the problems were worsening. In 2019, the disease was still ravaging Africa and Southeast Asia. "After years in decline, malaria infection rates seem to be on the rise in northeastern Cambodia, where people are moving deeper into lush, mosquito-ridden territories in search of timber."[128]

Resistance to ACT, which had been reported since 2015, was growing. Researchers uncovered a "secret weapon" that parasites had gained against artemisinin: mutations in a gene called Kelch protein13 Pfk P553L mutation. One lineage of *P. falciparum* from Cambodia was found to contain both a powerful Kelch 13 mutation and a gene duplication that help it to survive treatment by the partner drug piperaquine. In October 2017, molecular biologists reported that this parasite had spread to Thailand, Laos, and Vietnam. Now, some members of that family also resist another partner drug, mefloquine.

The problem of under-resourced public health departments the problem getting treatment and prevention out to the "last mile," and the issue of persistent and asymptomatic spread all continued, as well as the constant problem of inadequate funding.

Beginning in 2014, local organizations in Thailand strengthened a network of 1,222 village malaria workers by training and paying them to treat and report any malaria cases they found. In addition, they analyzed blood samples across the state with PCR tests to find pockets of malaria. They then asked every healthy person in these pocket outbreaks—about 4 percent of Keren's population—to swallow ACTs once a month for three months. In surveys after the intervention, the researchers found that the incidence of malaria in the state had dropped by 90 percent. But it was too costly and difficult to continue this at the regional level. The researchers noted: "It takes a great deal of work to convince people who don't feel ill to take medicines that can cause fatigue and nausea."[129]

Notice that I have argued that most successful eradication projects called for massive state action. Usually, in the colonial period, that meant armies or, in democracies such as the USA, the National Guard or deputized public health officers, wearing military uniforms and bearing military rank. Colonies needed armies. Public health required armies. Thus, the military, often an occupying force, existed in a complex, ambivalent role, establishing social order, for both healing and discipline and punishment. This capacity, not only the language of war also but the entire apparatus of war, is also part of the history of malaria. Without the police powers of the state the leaders of the project of colonialization, winning the battle of eradication would falter both for the Western settlers and for the indigenous population all over the newly globally connected world. And as former colonies asserted their independence, and the British or French or German or Italian or America militaries left, that power and that expense had to be shouldered by new governments, often states facing debt, other new obligations, or other new external enemies and carrying the long legacies of colonial rule and in many cases, a long history of failed efforts to eradicate malaria, as well.

Why is this long history important? In this chapter of the book, I have asked you to consider the world as we find it and as we came to know it. It is my contention that we cannot understand gene drives without understanding the complexity of malaria, the elegant menace of the parasite, the intricacy of the disease dynamics, and the long history of attempts to eliminate it. We cannot afford to make the mistakes of the past. So, it is critical to know them. We cannot use arguments to think about gene drives or genetic modification that are simply factually improbable or historically invalid. Moreover, we are not merely "thrown in" to history without agency. We partake and benefit from the moral choices made, the chances taken, and the structures that benefited some and exploited others. When we scholars in the West critique, as we should, emerging new technologies, we also need to be aware that we are speaking and professing from our position of relative privilege within that history. Good ethical decisions need to begin with a firm grip on the actual world.

There is another reason why this history is important. Readers of the history of the human efforts to eliminate this disease, as is also true of the other epidemic diseases that have marked human life, will see that there were always conflicts about the social nature of disease. There has been an ongoing struggle about disease etiology and prevention since the early modern period. Was each disease particular to the individual person, and were the ailments of the rich and poor the same, or were some races and people uniquely subject to disease? It was the argument of physicians and democrats such as Locke and Sydenham that diseases were the same, no matter who bore them, but others, as we have seen in the history of malaria, thought certain races were "syphilitic" or "malarial" or, to the contrary, impervious to malaria.

A parallel struggle since the nineteenth-century discovery of germ theory was whether environmental remediation or a single biomedical technology—an antibacterial, a vaccine—was needed to end an epidemic or whether social and economic changes were also needed. In the nineteenth and twentieth centuries, advocates for what would become known as public health began to argue for restricting and managing the environment that allowed disease to flourish. Cholera could only be prevented by reimagining cities and restructuring water supplies for both the rich and the poor; rats needed to be prevented from spreading in the waterfront ports and in wealthy neighborhoods alike to prevent bubonic plague; waste needed to be cleaned from the streets in every neighborhood. These all required enormous public will and vast public resources.

In my city, Chicago, the nineteenth-century planners decided to remake the world. They reversed the course of the river that carried human waste into Lake Michigan, so that the drinking water would be pure. Huge pumps pounded the reversed river downstream, along with offal from the stockyards, human waste, and cholera bacilli—which promptly infected the people of St. Louis, who drank the water from the river downstream. For Koch and others in the germ theory camp, the problems needed to be addressed with medication, not public health remediation or the restructuring of cities. For Celli, malaria would be ended only when people had jobs, education, local clinics, and enough food.

Typhus was another example. In 1849, after investigating a devastating outbreak of typhus in what is now Poland, the physician Rudolf Virchow wrote: "The answer to the question as to how to prevent outbreaks . . . is quite simple: education, together with its daughters, freedom and welfare." Virchow was one of many nineteenth-century thinkers who correctly understood that epidemics were tied to poverty, overcrowding, squalor, and hazardous working conditions—conditions that inattentive civil servants and aristocrats had done nothing to address. These social problems influenced which communities got sick and which stayed healthy. Diseases exploit society's cracks, and so "medicine is a social science," Virchow famously said.[130]

 This "fundamental dilemma of modern public health," as Packard noted, was that Koch and Pasteur, and Ross understood the fundamental purpose of medicine as waging a war against an extremely tiny but deadly enemy—a microbe, a parasite, that could be slaughtered the way that the new weapons of the early twentieth century slaughtered unruly or rebellious native people. The solution was not to make the world, in this theory, it was to kill it. And each individual would need their own solution. Syphilis was addressed one fever at a time, not by changing the economics and the social repression that so drove prostitution. As Alan Wong wrote recently in *The Atlantic*: "Germ theory allowed people to collapse everything about disease into battles between pathogens and patients. Social matters such as inequality, housing, education, race, culture, psychology, and politics became irrelevancies. Ignoring them was noble; it made medicine and science more apolitical and objective. Ignoring them was also easier; instead of staring into the abyss of society's intractable ills, physicians could simply stare at a bug under a microscope and devise ways of killing it. Somehow, they even convinced themselves that improved health would 'ultimately reduce poverty and other social inequities,' wrote Allan Brandt and Martha Gardner in 2000."[131] Wong notes that this was just as much a political battle as a scientific one, and this is made clear by the history you have just read. I will return to this issue in my final chapter, but I note here that the history of combatting malaria is always linked to how the public understands disease itself: how inevitable, how preventable, how social, and how individual our fates.

By the 1990s, it had become clear that both approaches—public health and individualized responses—had faltered in the treatment of malaria. And as the rate of deaths plateaued, scientists looked for new answers to one of humanity's oldest problems. The older solutions had halted but not eliminating the persistent threat of disease.

And by 2015, when the WHO released its Global Technical Strategy for Malaria 2016–2030, they outlined the problem.[132] "Since 2000, eight countries have eliminated malaria and many others have reduced transmission and many others have reduced transmission to low levels," the report stated. But this was not nearly enough progress. Moreover, "The fight against malaria is being prolonged, and in some places slowed down, by several interconnected challenges. The greatest of these is the lack of robust, predictable and sustained international and domestic financing. This is compounded by the difficulty in maintaining political commitment and ensuring regional collaborations at the highest levels. The second important challenge is biological: the emergence of parasite resistance to antimalarial medicines and of mosquito resistance to insecticides."[133] Once again, the lack of funding was a core issue, despite the fact that molecular and genetic biology had vastly improved our collective understanding of the disease. To meet even the UN Sustainable Development Goals for 2030, the WHO noted, would mean dealing with a host of systemic and technical issues.

They include the inadequate performance of health systems, weak management of supply chains and the unregulated private health sector in many countries, which allows the use of ineffective antimalarial medications or vector control practices; weak systems for surveillance, monitoring and evaluation, which compromise the ability to track gaps in program coverage and changes in disease burden; the lack of adequate technical and human resource capacities to sustain and scale up efforts, the disproportionate risk of malaria among hard to reach populations, including high risk occupational groups, migrants, people in humanitarian crisis, and rural communities with poor access to health services, and the lack of adequate tools to diagnose and treat effective infections due to *P. vivax* and other non-*P. falciparum* parasites. Another challenge is that many people who are infected with malaria parasites remain asymptomatic or undiagnosed and are therefore invisible to the health system—(creating) an infectious parasite reservoir.[134]

In the language of the report, the WHO outlines the failure of three "pillars" that were needed if malaria was to be addressed competently and effectively. So far, they noted, progress had slowed, even stopped. First, the world would need to ensure universal access to malaria prevention, diagnosis, and treatment. To do this would require efficient vector control and the management of resistance driven by evidence, which would mean that mosquito ecologies would need to be continually monitored. They are not. Second, chemoprevention—subtherapeutic doses of antimalarial medication at regular intervals sufficient to prevent malaria would have to be administered to entire populations, when cases are discovered, especially to the most vulnerable, meaning intermittent preventative treatment for pregnant women and infants and seasonal preventive treatment for all children below the age of five in at-risk areas. Moreover, all nonimmune travelers and migrants would need to have prophylactic treatment. Third, the WHO restated the need for universal testing of all suspected malaria cases, giving treatment in all cases, and treating every severe case with intravenously administered artesunate or artemether followed by a full course of ACT, which is fourteen days of primaquine for *P. vivax* or *P. ovale*. This would mean radically scaling up community-based diagnostic testing and treatment, monitoring the safety and efficacy of antimalarial medicines that are sold so that fake ones cannot be used, and managing resistance to ACT as it occurred—which would mean more monitoring and some way of removing the fake antimalarials. Special attention would have to be given to eliminating *P. falciparum* from the Mekong region, so that it does not become multidrug resistant and completely untreatable, and more research is need on *P. vivax*, which is developing new resistance to chloroquine. And all of this is only the first pillar. The WHO called for the acceleration of efforts for the world to be malaria free, and to create an ongoing, hypervigilant surveillance as "a core intervention" within a robust health-care system.

By 2016, ninety-one countries reported a total of 216 million cases of malaria—an increase of 5 million cases over the previous year. There were a total of 445,000 million deaths, about the same as the previous three years. Fifteen countries, all but one in sub-Sahara Africa, carry 80 percent of the global malaria burden and 90 percent of all deaths. Just over half (54 percent) of people at risk for malaria in sub-Saharan Africa were sleeping under an ITN—the primary prevention method, after decades of distribution and public health messaging. It seemed, according to the WHO, that about 25 percent of all bed nets got "lost in transit." This was better, but it was still nowhere near what would be needed if this method was to work. And the health-care systems, clinics, and hospitals never materialized. There was no funding to build them or to staff them.

Two years later, in the WHO's World Malaria Report 2018, little had changed.

> For many years the global response to malaria was considered one of the world's great public health achievements. WHO reported time and again on the massive roll-out of effective disease cutting tools, and an impressive reduction in cases and death. Last December (2016) we noted a troubling shift in the trajectory of this disease. The data showed that less than half of the countries with ongoing transmission were on track to reach critical targets for reductions in the death and disease caused by malaria. Progress appeared to have stalled. The world malaria report 2017 shows that this worrying trend continues. Although there are some bright spots in the data, the overall decline in the global malaria burden has unquestionably leveled off. And in some countries and regions, we are beginning to see reversals in the gains achieved.[135]

The new report noted: "Access to the health care system remains far too low . . . only about one third (34%) of children with a fever are taken to a medical provider in the African region."[136] Member nations simply made inadequate investments. The WHO guessed that by 2020, a minimum of 6.5 billion would be needed to provide the basics of the 2030 WHO program, every single year. The US donates 2.7 billion, less than half, and since 2014, investments have on average declined. "Among the 41 high-burden countries, overall, funding per person at risk of malaria is below \$2.00. In 34 out of 41 high burden countries which rely mainly on external funding for malaria programs the average level of funding available per person at risk in the past three years was reduced when compared to 2011–2013."[137] Meanwhile, indoor spaying campaigns have faltered, protecting fewer people each year.

Among fifty-five countries where the burden of malaria was estimated, thirty-one have a malaria case reporting rate of less than 50 percent. This includes high-burden countries such as India. Although some of countries remained on track to achieve their elimination goals by the year 2020, eleven reported increases in indigenous malaria cases since 2015, and five countries reported an increase of more than 100 cases in 2016 compared to 2015. In

2015–2019, a slow and steady increase in cases continued. And the pandemic accelerated the pace and the magnitude of the problem, with case levels not seen in a decade. Meanwhile, it was becoming harder to track malaria, even in places with adequate testing regimes: In some settings increasing levels of histidine-rich protein (HRP2) deletions threaten the ability to diagnose and appropriately treat people infected with *falciparum* malaria. An absence of the HRP2 gene enables the parasite to evade detection by HRP2 based RDTs resulting in a false negative test result.[138]

Worse yet, new variants in *P. falciparum* have not only made testing more difficult, but also created a more deadly form of the disease, cerebral malaria—a swift and deadly form that can kill within hours. Pal and others in new research noted:

> Cerebral malaria (CM) is a disease of the vascular endothelium caused by *Plasmodium falciparum*. It is characterized by parasite sequestration, inflammatory cytokine production, and vascular leakage. A distinguishing feature of *P. falciparum* infection is parasite production and secretion of histidine-rich protein II (HRPII). Plasma HRPII is a diagnostic and prognostic marker for *falciparum* malaria. We demonstrate that disruption of a human cerebral microvascular endothelial barrier by *P. falciparum*-infected erythrocytes depends on expression of HRPII. Purified recombinant or native HRPII can recapitulate these effects. HRPII action occurs via activation of the inflammasome, resulting in decreased integrity of tight junctions and increased endothelial permeability. We propose that HRPII is a virulence factor that may contribute to cerebral malaria by compromising endothelial barrier integrity within the central nervous system.[139]

Other variants increased drug resistance. Of the seventy-six malaria-endemic countries that provided data for 2010–2016, resistance to at least one insecticide in one malaria vector for one collection site was detected in sixty-one countries. In fifty countries, resistance to two or more insecticide classes was reported. In 2016, resistance was present in all WHO regions. Resistance to pyrethroids, the only insecticide class used in ITNs, is widespread. The proportion of malaria-endemic countries that monitored and subsequently reported pyrethroid resistance increased from 71 percent in 2010 to 81 percent in 2016—highest in the WHO African and Eastern Mediterranean regions where it was detected in malaria vectors in more than two thirds of all sites monitored.[140]

But because the dramatic drops in infections and deaths slowed and plateaued, a new urgency was felt, a sense that new tools were needed, because the older ones were threatened. Rising resistance in vectors and parasites and the changing climate added to the sense that innovation on a grand scale had to be mounted. Thus, researchers turned to other ideas, and for the first time, scientists using the new tools of genetics were able to turn their attention to the endless and age-old problem of malaria. New ideas from researchers in developmental and evolutionary genetics and questions about how species changed, adapted, or became extinct began to have a practical application. The hermeneutics of genetic research became a part of the landscape of malaria eradication efforts.

As bleak as this picture seems, the SARS-CoV-2 pandemic, as it did for so many aspects of our shared life, made everything far, far worse. By 2021, after a year of the pandemic, cases of malaria and malaria-associated deaths were now no longer flat. They were rising for the first time in decades. All the crisis caused by COVID-19—the collapse of supply chains, the diversion of funding for COVID-19 needs, the death of essential health-care workers, the resistance in many cases to health-care interventions, and the social chaos—made every aspect of malaria prevention and care far more difficult. When borders closed and flights from the West were cancelled, so were critical deliveries. Moreover, when I began to write this manuscript, in the fall of 2018, writing that a person died of malaria every two minutes and that a half a million people died each year seemed impossibly catastrophic—too large a number to ignore. Now? After more than 1 million people have died in the USA alone in two years, with no real end in sight, and after each minute is now crowded with the death of COVID-19 patients in addition to malaria, my perspective has shifted somewhat. But the last WHO World Malaria Report in 2021 recorded 627,000 malaria deaths that year. In 2022, it was 644,000.[141]

Despite these terrible setbacks, 2021 also marked a remarkable moment in our long historical narrative: the development of the first vaccine for malaria. Let me conclude our historical overview with a brief account of this development.

1.6   The History of Malaria: Enter the Vaccine in the Fall of 2021—Mosquirix™ and the Ethics of Compromise

Vaccines for malaria are extraordinarily difficult to make because of several factors. First, there is no lasting immunity to malaria. Unlike many infectious diseases such as yellow fever or measles, a single infection with malaria does not confer immunity. In fact, the average child in high-incidence areas of

Africa catches malaria an average of six times before the age of eighteen. If
the child survives and stays in Africa, they will mount some defense against
new infections, but if they leave, even for a short period of a few months,
they will lose all immunity and, if reinfected, may have a violent case, which
may even be fatal. Second, there are many strains of malaria. There is extensive antigenic variation, and an effective vaccine would need to address all
of them. Third, the parasite changes shape, form, and function in a complex
life cycle that has a different relationship to the human immune system at
each stage. It impacts different cells, and it can lay dormant for months or
even years. These relationships are poorly understood and hard to characterize. There was no vaccine, in fact, for any disease caused by parasites. Yet, in
the 1980s, research began on a malaria vaccine that would be called RTS,S. It
contained a piece of a *P. falciparum* protein linked to a protein from the hepatitis B virus,[142] which was added as an adjacent to create a stronger immune
response. The intent was to block the virus from its first invasive stage, the
liver cells, as sporozoites, prior to entering the red blood cells.

RTS,S/AS01 was created in 1987 at GSK. In 2001, GSK and PATH began
working together to develop RTS,S for young children living in malaria-
endemic regions in sub-Saharan Africa. Over the past two years, the health
ministries of Ghana, Kenya, and Malawi, through a large-scale pilot program
coordinated by the WHO, administered more than 2 million vaccine doses
to 800,000 children below the age of five, despite the ongoing COVID-19
pandemic. This effort was achieved by working closely with GSK, PATH, the
London School of Hygiene and Tropical Medicine, and UNICEF, among other
partners. Financing for the pilot program has been mobilized through an
unprecedented collaboration among three key global health funding bodies:
Gavi, the Vaccine Alliance; the Global Fund to Fight AIDS, Tuberculosis and
Malaria; and Unitaid.[143]

Researchers from GSK struggled to make the vaccine work in Phase I clinical
trials, which began in 2003 after some promising results in animal studies.
Initial results were somewhat underwhelming. First, unlike the usual schedule of childhood vaccination, the vaccine did not protect well in babies younger than six months. Beginning vaccination at six months meant that the
four-dose schedule would stretch out over two years, which would require
repeated visits for each child, each on their own schedule, in various seasons, where travel is difficult and health care unevenly accessible. Even with

complete adherence, the vaccines were only 30–40 percent effective initially, which cut the risk of clinical malaria by 30 percent. Perhaps the most disturbing trends in early trials were a slight increase in mortality in females and an increased risk of developing cerebral malaria—the worst and more deadly form of the disease.[144]

But childhood mortality from malaria remained high, and the slow rise in death rates called for aggressive action. Catching malaria repeatedly in childhood, even if not fatal, still took a terrible toll. Many children suffered cognitive decline, exhaustion, and weakness—some temporary, some permanent. It was felt that even a vaccine that was 40 percent effective might save or improve some lives. In 2015, the European Medicines Agency approved the vaccine. This caused an immediate controversy. Many argued that the safety signals needed to be taken more seriously and studied in a larger clinical trial. Others argued that 40 or 50 percent efficacy was essentially no better than a coin toss and not nearly high enough for a disease with this level of morbidity and mortality. Still others doubted that the logistical hurdles—getting the vaccine into the arms of children in rural areas—could be overcome. Others objected to the use of African children to test a proof-of-concept parasite vaccine that may raise risks with a benefit that was not conclusive. Finally, many, including Doctors Without Borders (MSF), heavily involved in the distribution of bed nets, were concerned that families might abandon proven measures if they assumed that their children were vaccinated and thus safe from infection, as they would be with, for example, measles and polio vaccines. Citing the fact that only 30 percent of children with fevers get taken for medical care, critics of the vaccine argued that even fewer would be taken to a clinic if it was assumed that the fever was not malaria. Yet, it was the first encouraging vaccine yet conceived, others argued. Thus, a larger pilot was initiated in 2015, and the debate continued.[145] MSF, for example, opposed the pilot as wasteful of scarce resources, taking away attention from other modalities.[146] And finally, questions were raised about the informed consent process of the pilot study itself, for it was unclear if parents understood that the vaccine, which was given within the usual structure of pediatric vaccines at the well-baby clinic visits, was still unproven, calling the trial "a serious breach of international ethical standards" in the *BMJ*.[147] A petition in the *BMJ* article was offered as a part of the protest against the trial. The WHO contended that the study was a pilot introduction and not technically "research activity" that fell under the rules for research with vulnerable subjects, and that the consent was "implied" when the parents came for the rest of the approved vaccines. A WHO spokesperson said, "An implied consent process is one in which parents are informed of imminent vaccination through social mobilisation and communication, sometimes including letters directly addressed to parents. Subsequently, the physical presence of the child or adolescent, with or without an accompanying parent at the vaccination session, is considered to imply consent."[148] If the study was classified as research, several ethicists pointed out, then the careful rules would all apply. A separate IRB and ethics review process would have to approve the protocol and consent form, and, they argued, it is doubtful if any ethics committee would have waived the informed consent altogether.[149]

Yet, the project, which began in 2019, continued. As I was finishing this manuscript, the results of the pilot were presented at a Zoom meeting of the Malaria Policy Advisory Group. The pilot, which included more than 800,000 children, was launched in Ghana, Kenya, and Malawi, and it was approved by each state entity. Based on the results thus far, the WHO, acting on the advice of its scientific advisors, announced that it would recommend a broad rollout of the malaria vaccine, now called Mosquirix™ and sold for the reduced price, GSK said, of $5 a dose. First, let me review the positive features of this decision.

The safety signals of increased female mortality were not evident in the larger study and thus seem to have just been a coincidence, and likewise the incidence of cerebral malaria, which was no more likely to occur in the treatment group. The vaccine seems to be 50 percent effective when given only to children at aged between six and eighteen months. While far less than ideal, this puts the effectiveness rate at about what the influenza vaccine offers in some years, for example, and it is far better than bed nets for young children, where the prevention rate, given the uncertainty of use, is around 20 percent. It is clear that a vaccine, even a flawed one, has the potential to save thousands of the 279,000 children who die annually.

The WHO's Director-General, Tedros Adhanom Ghebreyesus, who has had an extraordinarily difficult tenure because of COVID-19, was happy to announce good news: "As some of you may know," he said, "I started my career as a malaria researcher, and I longed for the day that we would have an effective vaccine against this ancient and terrible disease," he concluded during a news conference from Geneva. "Today is that day, an historic day."[150] Interestingly enough, by 2021, only the results from the first three inoculations were known because the project had not gone on long enough for most of the children to receive the fourth dose. So, it is not fully known if parents will return when their children are older to get it, the rate at which immunity drops to zero, which happens by the time the child is four years old, or how to plan booster doses. And critics have pointed out that unlike other vaccines—polio, for example—which were created by using several different strains of the virus within one vaccine, to approximate real-world conditions of contagion better, the GSK vaccine used only one strain, and it was a laboratory-acquired strain. Thus, children who contracted a different strain would essentially be unprotected. Others pointed out that leaving babies younger than six months out of the project changed the data but did not change their vulnerability.

However, the scientific advisory board was clearly supportive of the vaccine. The most important reason for the advisor's decisions was not only the vaccine—it was that the vaccine, when given along with a widespread MDT program, with prophylactic antimalarials given to everyone just prior to the rainy season, became far more effective than either intervention alone.

A study *The New England Journal of Medicine*, found that when children were given an antimalarial drug along with the vaccine, the combination reduced hospitalization with severe malaria by 70.5 percent and death by 72.9 percent compared with just the antimalarial drug alone.[151] "A modeling study last year estimated that if the vaccine were rolled out to countries with the highest incidence of malaria, it could prevent 5.4 million cases and 23,000 deaths in children younger than 5 each year. A recent trial of the vaccine in combination with preventive drugs given to children during high-transmission seasons found that the dual approach was much more effective at preventing severe disease, hospitalization and death than either method alone."[152] Using the vaccine and drugs together was close to 70 percent effective in preventing infection. Meanwhile, R21, a variant of Mosquirix™ tested in Burkina Faso in 450 children, showed 77 percent effectiveness with the vaccine alone, and is both more potent and cheaper. A trial for this vaccine with 4,800 children began in the summer of 2021.

The vaccine proved to be easily delivered using the existing vaccine delivery systems established in the smallpox and then polio networks. In urban well-served areas or places with clinics, it was administered as part of the usual routine immunization systems. Even at a time of considerable stress on health-care systems—a global pandemic—the trial was able to proceed. More than 2.3 million doses of the vaccine were given. Reaching the unreached, RTS,S increases equity in access to malaria prevention.

Results were apparent, and they were especially vivid in children, who were not protected by other means, given that more than two-thirds of children were not sleeping under bed nets. There were few side effects, and the fear that parents would abandon the use of bed nets proved to be unfounded. Once people understood that both bed nets and the vaccine were needed, parents largely complied. The same was true for parents seeking medical care for fever. The intervention was considered "moderately cost effective," especially in areas with high malaria transmission. Most importantly, it reduced the worst of *P. falciparum*'s deadliest effects, with a 30 percent drop in in these cases, even in places with bed net use and good clinical treatment.

Critics have questioned whether African countries can afford and can mobilize vaccination for both COVID-19 and malaria at the same time and have also raised concerns about side effects that may not appear for more than two years. However, most researchers and clinicians have welcomed the vaccine, flaws and all, as an extremely important new tool to respond to malaria—the first one in the decades since artemisinin. Although it is imperfect, it is seen as a critical step toward understanding the dynamics of malaria. And the chance finally to save lives, after so many failures, was clearly a victory. Let me end my history here, not because the vaccine is the answer to the problem of the disease, but because we have what is needed to assemble enough history to understand why determining the next step in the story is so complex.

Now that you have read even a brief account of the complicated, fraught relationship between biology, medical research, and social policy, you have a sense of the many, many intricate narratives and the many factors at play all at once as we consider the ethical implications of a using new technology to, as we have historically spoken of it, "combat" malaria. In the next chapter, I will turn to a similarly abbreviated account of the scientific intervention itself.

The vaccine had taken two decades to come to fruition. At the same time, a new idea was being considered to respond to the cessation in the progress against malaria, humanity's old foe. This idea would use both a somewhat obscure capacity that occurred in the natural world and the radical new tools of molecular genetics and synthetic biology to search for a different way to address the problem of malaria. In the next chapter, we will turn to the beginning of the new idea: gene drives.

2   The World as It Is Imagined: Gene Drives for Malaria

2.1   The Fifth Force: Finding Gene Drives in Evolution

Austin Burt is looking down as he speaks behind the large podium of the dark auditorium at the National Academies of Science. It is a formal building, standing on the top of a wide, green lawn overlooking the Lincoln Memorial in Washington, DC. There are marble steps and marble floors, and the auditorium is tastefully done in shades of gray. There is a bright white light that shines on the stage.

He is wearing a plain white shirt, no tie, open at the neck, and a black suit jacket. He puts one hand in his jacket pocket and uses the other to point at PowerPoint slides on the huge screen behind him. He stands at a slant, which gives the talk an intimate, quiet tone. His voice is quiet too, with a soft lilt that raises at the end of sentences, and he has a faint Canadian accent. He thanks the organizers for "the task they have taken on," which is to write a formal report about the new technology: a "gene drive" that he has largely conceptualized. It is the reason that everyone is in the room. He does not draw attention to this, always using the "we" to describe his work—"we saw that" and "we discovered that," meaning his laboratory, his colleagues. This is rare in a scientific talk these days, in a time of patents, profits, and press. Austin Burt has discovered a way to understand and then use biology to, perhaps, just perhaps, solve one of humankind's most intractable and complex problems.

He apologizes to his audience for beginning with "what you already know": that a gene drive is a preferential inheritance of a certain trait from one generation to the next. In the simplest case, he explains, when "+" and "–" gametes come together to make a heterozygote embryo, and when that heterozygote grows up and makes its own gametes, they are made not in a

50:50 Mendelian ratio, with one gamete from each parent, as is normally the case, but in a 70:30 or 95:5 ratio. And that means there has been an increase in frequency in one allele, say, the "+" allele, just due to gene transmission. All things being equal, then, in the population as a whole, a gene could increase in frequency relatively rapidly, increasing to 95 percent in twenty generations that started with a 70:30 split. "The drive process can even lead to the spread of genes that are harmful to the organism, and it is that property that makes them such attractive tools for pest control," he says, and he pauses, looking up briefly at the watching scientists.

The National Academies of Sciences, Engineering, and Medicine (NASEM) report that followed their two-day meeting and months-long process begins like this: "Austin Burt had a question: Can an insect's genes be manipulated to stop it from spreading disease? " It was an acknowledgement of his central role in the field, his long, thoughtful search within complex biological processes of insects,[1] and of the singular importance of his research for human health. Burt had been thinking about how genes drive evolution for more than four decades. He was born in Winnipeg, which, it turns out, has a mosquito population so massive that it has its own interactive map and biting report. The report notes that Canada's mosquito population is so huge that "Roy Ellis, former chief entomologist for the city of Winnipeg, has estimated that during an horrendous year for mosquitoes on the Prairies, 10 million mosquitoes per square kilometre is possible."[2]

Burt received his undergraduate degree and PhD in biology at McGill University in Montreal in September 1990, but he had already published an article in 1987 with Graham Bell, who worked on adaption, extinction, and global change and was his advisor. The article, "Red Queen versus Tangled Bank Models" was published in *Nature* as a letter, explaining their research on how Red Queen models worked.[3] The "Red Queen" model is named of course after the imperious character in Lewis Carroll's *Alice in Wonderland*. The "Tangled Bank" is a reference to another Cambridge scholar's work: the last page in Charles Darwin's *Origin of Species*,[4] in which he describes his theory of evolution.

> It is interesting to contemplate an entangled bank, clothed with many plants of many kinds, with birds singing on the bushes, with various insects flitting about, and with worms crawling through the damp earth, and to reflect that these elaborately constructed forms, so different from each other, and dependent on each other in so complex a manner, have all been produced by laws acting around us.

These laws, taken in the largest sense, being Growth with Reproduction; Inheritance which is almost implied by reproduction; Variability from the indirect and direct action of the external conditions of life, and from use and disuse a Ratio of Increase so high as to lead to a Struggle for Life, and as a consequence to Natural Selection, entailing Divergence of Character and the Extinction of less-improved forms. Thus, from the war of nature, from famine and death, the most exalted object which we are capable of conceiving, namely, the production of the higher animals, directly follows. There is grandeur in this view of life, with its several powers, having been originally breathed into a few forms or into one; and that, whilst this planet has gone cycling on according to the fixed law of gravity, from so simple a beginning endless forms most beautiful and most wonderful have been, and are being, evolved.[5]

He then studied as a postdoctoral fellow in William Rice's laboratory at the University of California in Santa Cruz until December 1992, and then he went to the John Taylor laboratory at the University of California, Berkeley, in January 1993. He has been at Imperial College London since 1995.

The Red Queen theory explores how, as in Burt's seminal 1995 paper, "The Evolution of Fitness," organisms are in balance between adaptation and failure. "In every generation, the mean fitness of populations increases because of natural selection and decreases because of mutations and changes in the environment."[6] Organisms rely on adaptation to the niche that they occupy, constantly evolving and expanding in competition with other forces—other organisms, the climate, predators, parasites, and habitat changes. Burt noted that sexual reproduction confers an advantage to species, just as Darwin noted in 1889: "It is not the strongest of the species that survives, nor the most intelligent, but the one most responsive to change.[7]"

Evolution, by which species change their traits and adapt to their niche, occurs because they "must constantly adapt, evolve, and proliferate not merely to gain reproductive advantage, but also simply to survive while pitted against ever-evolving opposing organisms in a constantly changing environment. The hypothesis intends to explain two different phenomena: the constant extinction rates as observed in the paleontological record caused by co-evolution between competing species, and the advantage of sexual reproduction (as opposed to asexual reproduction) at the level of individuals."[8] The concept of the Red Queen is taken from a passage in *Alice in Wonderland*:

Alice never could quite make out, in thinking it over afterwards, how it was that they began: all she remembers is, that they were running hand in hand, and the Queen went so fast that it was all she could do to keep up with her: and still the

Queen kept crying "Faster! Faster!" but Alice felt she could not go faster, though she had not breath left to say so . . .

The most curious part of the thing was, that the trees and the other things round them never changed their places at all: however fast they went, they never seemed to pass anything. 'I wonder if all the things move along with us?' thought poor puzzled Alice. And the Queen seemed to guess her thoughts, for she cried, "Faster! Don't try to talk!"

Alice looked round her in great surprise. "Why, I do believe we've been under this tree the whole time! Everything's just as it was!"

"Of course it is," said the Queen, "what would you have it?"

"Well, in our country," said Alice, still panting a little, "you'd generally get to somewhere else—if you ran very fast for a long time, as we've been doing."

"A slow sort of country!" said the Queen. "Now, here, you see, it takes all the running you can do, to keep in the same place.

If you want to get somewhere else, you must run at least twice as fast as that!"[9]

Species usually stay constant, "staying in the same place" by using sexual reproduction to their advantage, because that introduces new genetic combinations into every individual, and it allows for mutagenic changes to offer selective advantage. Each new organism is a dice throw, with half of the genes in an individual coming from each parent.

First described in 1866 by a monk named Gregor Mendel, the conventional rules of inheritance, also known as Mendelian inheritance, dictate that offspring have on average a 50 percent chance of inheriting a gene from one of their parents. With Mendelian inheritance, not all offspring will inherit any one particular gene, and so the frequency of that gene in future generations will be similar to the frequency of that gene in the parents' generation—a dice throw each time, unless a gene confers a notable survival advantage. In that case, over very long periods of time, a population can accumulate advantageous mutations. Evolution is also affected by other forces: the migration of populations, sexual selection advantage, and drift.

But Burt had noticed something else—what he called "a fifth force" in evolution, in addition to mutation, migration, selection, and drift. In looking at a range of species, Burt noticed that evolution was marked by genes that seemed to be in conflict: "The genes in an organism sometimes 'disagree' over what should happen. That is, they appear to have opposing effects. In animals, for example, some genes may want (or act as if they want) a male to produce lots of healthy sperm, but other genes in the same male want half the sperm to be defective. . . . In plants, too, there can be internal conflicts . . . indeed, in the extreme case, some genes want to inactivate half the genome, while the targeted half prefers to remain active."[10] By 2003, Burt proposed thinking about manipulating the genome to engineer natural populations genetically.[11] Three years later, writing with Robert Trivers, an evolutionary biologist, he noted that some of these "selfish" elements were only in a few species, but others were in virtually all. Some were, at that moment, theorized but not yet confirmed, like mate or progeny preferences. These genes are called "selfish" because they are designed to spread—even if they confer no survival or adaptive benefit, even if they would be harmful to the organism. They act for their own interests. "The evolution of selfish genetic elements inevitably leads to within-individual or intra-genomic conflict. This occurs over evolutionary time, at genes at different locations within the genome are selected to have contradictory effects. It also happens in developmental time as organisms experience these conflicting effects. In this sense we speak of 'genes in conflict' that is genes within a single body that are in conflict over the appropriate development or action to be taken."[12]

Inheritance and function usually work in an orderly fashion, in a manner that Burt and Trivers call "fair." Diploid individuals, meaning creatures that reproduce sexually, and have two sets of chromosomes, one from each parent, transmit the two copies of their genes with equal likelihood, and the frequency of any one genetic element—the gene for of red hair, for example—has the same frequency from year to year, unless red-haired couples suddenly begin to have far more red-haired children than black-haired couples do. This is important, for most species have evolved to function well—to "run in place," or to increase the chances of survival or capacity to reproduce in a steady fashion. Mutations are rare, and if they are harmful, they do not persist. "But some genes have discovered ways to spread and persist without contributing to organismal fitness. At times, this means encoding actions that are diametrically opposed to those of the majority of the genes. As a consequence, Burt and Trivers explained in their book, most organisms are not completely harmonious wholes and the individual is, in fact divisible . . . selfish genetic elements are a universal feature of life, with pervasive effects on the genetic system and the larger phenotype. . . . a truly subterranean world of sociogenetic interactions, usually hidden from sight."[13]

Not only is their ubiquitous nature and their survivability impressive, but selfish genes are also transmitted to a disproportionate or "unfair and not transparent" fraction of the organism's offspring. Selfish elements are transmitted, they argue, or "driven" to a biased ratio—51 percent, 60 percent,

99 percent—even when harmful. Three major types of drives have evolved. The first of these is interference drives, where the gene biases by disrupting the transmission of a particular allele—or by killing the 50 percent of the offspring that lack that allele, increasing the survival of "their" allele. The elements can target genes, chromosomes, or entire haploid, meaning the cells of the egg or sperm, which have only a single set of chromosomes. A second type of drive happens when genes get themselves replicated more often—adding extra cell cycles, or making extra copies of themselves, or "jumping" across the genome to a new place and getting copied again there, or by increasing the replication rate of the entire cell.[14] The final type of drive uses the process of meiosis during reproduction. Instead of replicating into a gamete and a somatic cell, the chromosome replicates twice into a gamete in a process called genotaxis n which the genetic element has now doubled its chance of being transmitted to the next generation.

There are, as Burt and Trivers explain, a "whole zoo" of possibilities. There are selfish elements that occur across families, ones that suppress the frequency of males or females. There are a variety of transposable genetic elements, called names like gamete killers, maternal effect genes, and homing endonuclease genes (HEGs), to list but a few, all of which are segments that can enhance their own transmission at the expense of other genes in the genome. Of course, these selfish elements will eventually induce other suppressing genes to emerge, mitigating the harm, but also of course potentially making other changes in the organism.

Burt and Trivers point out that the "zoo" is far more than merely an interesting curiosity with obscure names. They argue that: "There is also a practical reason to be interested in the effects of various selfish genetic elements on population productivity. Despite much effort, many species harmful to humans are beyond current methods of control. Selfish genetic elements seem, in many ways, ideal tools for population control and our ever more detailed molecular understating of how they work to make such control increasingly likely." To scientists who studies these effects, like Burt and Trivers, these new capacities suggested an almost immediate utility: finding a sophisticated genetic mechanism drawn directly from observed natural processes that could alter a species phenotype, or perhaps edge it toward rapid elimination.

In characteristic fashion, Burt and Trivers give credit to the iterative nature of this scientific insight by listing the fifty-eight researchers who, since 1887, reported the curious features of these odd genetic elements.[15] Even leaving out

many of the details of each discovery and giving only a brief history here of
the development of gene drives and many of the researchers in this abbreviated account, one can trace the many examples of how this insight was slowly
built, the careful work that led to the possibility of the practical utility of their
suggestion. From 1887 to 1960, the selfish elements were simply observed in
the lab and the field and reported in the scientific literature. The first selfish
elements were ones that could be easily noticed—a plant that did not make
pollen or the t-haplotype in mice. In 1928 Gershenson noted their presence
and again in 1936, Sturtevant and Dobzhansky documented their existence.
There were papers that discussed genes that increased in frequency purely
because of biased transmission, involving what turned out to be the "driving
Y" chromosome. In 1938, Alexander Sergevich Serebrovsky, a Russian geneticist, published an elaborate theory of human breeding based on selecting the
sperm of the most robust men to improve the socialist state (a theory whose
eugenicist implications was too extreme even within the Soviet state and that
got him removed from his several prominent posts and the leadership of his
lab in the Moscow Zootechnical Institute.).[16] He turned to researching insects
and, in 1940, published a plan for releasing genetically altered sterile males
into insect pest populations in order to suppress and control them. It took
some time between the discovery and the realization that scientists might
actually manipulate populations using genetic manipulations. For much of
the 20th century, as scientists slowly became to understand molecular genetics,
conceptual advances in the field were only loosely correlated with empirical
discoveries. As scientists gained more control over genetic alternation, they
began to consider how the altered insects might be useful. "In 1960, George B.
Craig, a mosquito biologists, and two of his colleagues, W. A. Hickey and R. C.
Vanderbilt, suggested using a breeding program in which a 'male-producing
factor' that is naturally present in some male *Aedes aegypti* mosquitos would
be harnessed to control mosquito populations. When male mosquitos with
this male producing factor breed, most of their offspring develop as males."[17]
Here was a genuinely new way to control the population of insects. But how
to actually do this proved more difficult.

In 1966, Hickey and Craig published a paper to show this newly discovered
phenomena—the "driving Y" chromosome might be utilized by releasing
males altered in this way, which would reduce the number of females below
that needed for disease transmission. A year later, W. D. Hamilton speculated

about the Y chromosome being "freed from the inhibitory control of the rest of the genome," which could control sex selection, and a year after this, Chris F. Curtis,[18] a medical entomologist long interested in how mosquitoes developed resistance to malaria control measures, published a first mathematical model demonstrating how a naturally occurring "desirable" gene, such as a gene to make mosquitoes non-infectible by pathogens, could spread to fixation in a population, "preventing the parasite from ever re-infecting the mosquitos."[19]

A flurry of others followed. Then, in 1972, another paper by Hamilton was published with a description of how genes are selected to act as if they are maximizing their inclusive fitness, extending the understanding of population genetics. Fifteen new papers, each describing new genetic elements, and new ways that genes are selected to act as self-promoting strategists appeared over the next several years.[20] The use of PCR testing, which amplifies a tiny stretch of DNA based on sequence specific primers, allowing scientists to study mutations fare more accurately, and DNA sequencing which reveals the order of the sequence of DNA, uncovered other new genetic sequences in the "zoo" of genetic elements of interest. The 2006 book by Burt and Trivers, included a taxonomy of these elements at the molecular, genetic, physiological, behavioral, populational, and evolutionary levels. Much of the biology of each element was not as yet fully understood, or not understood in all its complexity, Burt and Trivers noted, but they asked a set of questions about each element: "How does it gain its advantage? How did it arise? How long ago? What are its effects on the larger organism? How fast is it expected to spread? What is its frequency within a species? What determines this? Why is it found in some species and not others? What counter-adaptions has it stimulated in the rest of the genome. What other effects has it had on the host lineage?"[21]

Burt and Trivers explored several of these elements. For the purposes of this chapter, I am going to discuss only some of them: so-called killer gametes or "driving Y" chromosomes, homing endonucleases, and female sterility genes, since these were the ones first explored in the Crisanti and Burt labs at Imperial College years later and they are elements that it is anticipated will be used in *Anopheles* mosquitoes, and explored (initially) as a way to change or suppress populations with a gene drive. Killer Y or X-shredder elements placed on chromosomes in the gametes of *Diptera* (including flies and mosquitos) are intended to be used to eliminate or "shred" targeted sections of DNA on the X chromosome during spermatogenesis, disabling it.[22] Burt is particularly interested in killer Y chromosomes, as we shall see, because the reduction of females is key for interrupting malaria transmission. This idea is noted only in a small paragraph in Burt and Trivers's book:

> Y-linked loci that disrupt the formation of X-bearing sperm have been reported in 2 mosquito species, *Aedes* and *culex* . . . For several reasons, Y drive is expected to more easily cause populations extinction than X-drive. Y drive is 3 times stronger than X because it recurs every generation, while an X-drive only every third (Hamilton, 1967.) X-drive also leads to population expansion, while the Y-drive leads to population contraction. In addition, in a population without suppressors, a Y that spreads through a population would bias the sex ratio toward males and each male would have fewer chances to mate with a female.[23]

Far more detailed is a section in the book on gene conversion and "homing."[24] Which is based on the understanding that genes have the capacity for repair, in some cases, after they are damaged. DNA is a double strand of coded sequences, base pairs of nucleotides (cytosine, guanine, adenine, and thymine) represented by letters CGAT, that are complementary to letters on the other side, which store and transmit biological information. In most cases, a matching sequence is on each of the double strands of the chromosome. So, if part of a chromosome is damaged only on one strand, the "letters" of the DNA rendered unusable, the undamaged strand can be used to make a copy of itself and replace the damaged section on the other strand. If the damage affects both strands, then a matching chromosome is copied, and that copied section moves into the repair site. In a gene drive, some alleles or "letters" of the DNA can be favored and transmitted to the repair more than others. This is called "biased gene conversion" and happens only occasionally and weakly. But there are other sorts of repair mechanisms: write Burt and Trivers: "At the other extreme are homing endonuclease genes (HEGs) a class of selfish genes that are anything but passive. These are optional genes, with no known host function, that spread through the populations by exploiting their host's DNA repair system. They encode an enzyme that specifically recognizes and cuts chromosomes that do not contain a copy of the gene; the cell then repair the damage and in so doing copies the HEG onto the cut chromosome. HEG cause minimal damage to their hosts even when homozygous, and can sweep through a population with minimal hitchhiking effects on flanking DNA."[25] It would be this capacity for "cutting" in a relatively sophisticated manner, at a specific 15- to 20-bp site, that would interest Burt. HEGs—among the smallest of the "selfish genetic elements"—are widely spread across different species. They target a very specific part of a genome, and they have the capacity to cut the DNA at a target site, while maintaining their own stability. Then the chromosome will repair the break as it does any other, inserting the element along with the repair in a process called homologous repair, because then, the two different alles would be identical, in which the HEG and the sequence are both copied. This capacity would allow the HEG, in theory, to be used as a tool in gene editing. "The homing mechanism converts an organism that is heterozygous in of the drive into a homozygote in the germline, and thus transmits it to offspring at a rate above 50%."[26] Homing occurs only in heterozygous organisms, when individuals carry two copies of alleles for a particular trait. Homing drives are efficient and move steadily through a population. Burt and Trivers then speculate that "A strong drive combined with minimal harm to the host should lead to an HEG spreading through a population and going to fixation. But then what? Once fixed in the population, there are no more empty targets to cut and so no selection against mutations that destroy the enzyme's ability to recognize and cleave the target site . . . How then can functional HEGs persist over long evolutionary time? . . . The answer appears to be that HEGs occasionally move from one species to another."[27] It had become clear, thought Burt and Trivers, that transposable elements and HEGs could move between species, even without fixation. In fact, they were capable of moving between much more distantly related host groups than would be possible by hybridization. These elements can far outlast their hosts simply by transferring to another host before they degrade.[28] Burt theorized that the HEG would target highly conserved parts of the genome, making it possible to transfer to another highly conserved space in a new genome.

By 2003, Burt was using all of these features to work on a question: Could HEGs be used to drive modified genes through a mosquito population? He noted: "One of the many pleasures of working on selfish genetic elements is the possibility that they may one day be used to ameliorate human suffering. There are a small number of species that cause substantial harm to the human condition—species that cause disease, transmit disease, or reduce agricultural output—and there has long been the hope that selfish genetic elements could be used to reduce population numbers or otherwise render these species less noxious."[29] Burt and Trivers, again, first cite the work of other researchers: Belfort, Bibikova, Chevalier, Silgman, and Guo. Then, they describe Burt's idea for a project: engineering a HEG that would kill four-fifths of zygotes in a mosquito population. Even if only 1 percent of the population was initially affected, in twelve generations, 90 percent of the population would carry this construct. In 2006, Burt and Trivers were convinced that this intervention would be both evolutionarily stable and reversible—an position that they would interrogate by 2015. They also raised and considered the possibility of horizontal transfer to other species, which, in 2006, they believed could be dealt with by genetic engineering or directed targeting.[30] Almost as an afterthought, Burt and Trivers note another possibility: the use of a Y chromosome to show drive and spread to fixation, making the sex ratio male biased. They theorized they could "insert onto a Y chromosome 1 or more endonuclease genes that recognize and cut sequences specific to the X chromosome . . . Then, during spermatogenesis the X chromosome would be cut and as there would not be an appropriate template for repair, the Y chromosome would show drive."[31] Burt and Trivers consider, in later chapters, transposable elements, female drives, B chromosomes, genomic exclusion, and selfish cell lineages. All of this categorizing and cataloguing would be useful for exploring new directions. But over and over is repeated the phrase: "Much is still unknown, or much else remains unknown. Even with the new tools of molecular biology, PCR, large genetic data sets, complete genome sequencing, it was still unknown how to find the physical traces of many selfish elements, like gamete killers, maternal effect killer, or other elements."[32]

"Nothing surprises us more," they say, "than the steady discovery of a vast, hidden, world of genetic elements, inhabiting every species studied."[33] What we think we knew about evolution is challenged by this "parallel" universe, claim Burt and Trivers. And it was to that universe that Burt would now turn. The trick would be not only to find a way to insert a new genetic sequence into an insect gamete or egg, but also to insert one of these driving elements with it, so that in each generation, the driving element would be inherited, ensuring that the trait would be passed on in more than 50 percent of the offspring, spreading persistently In the population.

2.2   Imagining Designed Mosquitoes: The Technological Imaginary

By 2003, Burt, along with a handful of others—Margaret Kidwell, an evolutionary geneticist; Jose Ribeiro, a vector biologist who proposed using transposable elements to drive in the 1990s; James (2005); Rasgon and Gould (2005); Adelman (2007); and Windbichler (2011)—began to conceptualize building gene drives using these newly available "tools," and as new technologies began to be developed in the field of genetic engineering and synthetic biology, they too were rapidly developed for this project. All of these tools, with growing efficiency, were able to allow researchers to "make" or manipulate the genetic sequence, using the enzymes to cut and then to link two genetic pieces together, and all allowed them to affect the genome of targeted species—they had names such as chimeric antigen receptors (CARs), zinc finger nucleases (ZFNs), and transcription activator-like effector nuclease (TALENS), CARs, ZFNs, and TALENS were slowly moving into human clinical trials and were beginning to be used on the mosquitos in the Burt laboratory. Burt was now joined by Andrea Crisanti, an Italian researcher, at Imperial College London. Together, they began the painstaking work to genetically engineer and then raise mosquitoes to test the theory that Burt had first proposed in 2003. In that paper, Burt posited three reasons for conducting research on gene drives: "to motivate more rapid development of the technology; to warn of containment issues that ought to be addressed during development; and to stimulate discussions of the desirability of eradicating genetically modifying particular species."[34]

Their work was slow and deliberate—the genetic construct had to be "made" in the laboratory and then carefully placed inside the extremely tiny fertilized egg laid by a female mosquito, which is the size of the period at the end of this sentence. Eggs have a top and a bottom, and there is only one place to insert the genetic construct so that is properly aligned. It was a difficult and uncertain process.

While it had long been known that organisms can be genetically modified using viral vectors and then the new tools of genetic engineering, and existing DNA can be removed or new DNA inserted, "knocking in" or "knocking out" a specific genetic set of instructions the process was complex, even for the most skilled researchers.[35] But in 2012, a new gene editing technique was developed and rationalized by two scientists, Jennifer Doudna and Emmanuelle Charpentier. When studying the defense system of bacteria, they noted something that other researchers had described: the ability of bacterial DNA to recover and defend against viruses by using a cut-and-copy mechanism to repair damage caused within cells, Because DNA is double stranded, when an area of DNA is damaged, that mechanism scissors the damage out and replaces it with a copy of the same stretch from the other strand which is similar to the same mechanism used by the HEG I just described. They described a mechanism called CRISPR (which is short for Clustered Regularly Inter-spaced Short Palindromic Repeats) which is a bacterial genetic segment, and Cas9 (just one example—there are other Cas proteins) is a CRISPR-associated protein that makes the cut and guides the proper new segment to the DNA strand in question. Doudna and Charpentier were interested in how to hijack the system of the repeating genetic elements that bacteria used in the process. They were able to use their construct to make the cuts, which they could target to specific places within the genome, and the cell then replicated the bacteria's process of replace and repair after the cuts. Their experiment was intended to see if this worked in cells in other organisms. Unlike bacteria, all animals, plants, and fungi, are called eukaryotes, because their cells have a nucleus. Could this bacterial mechanism work in eukaryote cells? Indeed, it could. Thus they had made a remarkable genetic tool. This tool could then be used to make far more precise alterations within cells, cutting the DNA sequences in more deliberate ways than could be done in earlier recombinant techniques such as viral vectors and then inserting other sequences, called transgenes, to replace them, making genetic engineering far easier. They called it the CRISPR-Cas9 system, and for this advance, they won the Nobel Prize in Chemistry in 2020. Later work showed the robustness of this system. It was adapted by George Church to work in yeast, by Feng Zhang to work in mammals, and by many others to work in fish, flies, plants, nematodes, monkeys, and human cells. What was once laborious and time consuming was now "facile and rapidly achievable," noted Doudna.[36] It is known now, a decade later, that CRISPR-Cas9 is not quite as facile as the newspaper images of little scissors or the linguistic metaphors ("like spell-check; cut and paste") would have one believe because not all cells take up the CRISPR intervention, creating what is called a mosaic organism. At times, like in all earlier gene editing methods, the new genetic construct placed in the nucleus inserts in the wrong place in the chromosome Yet, it clearly created a new set of pos-sibilities for genetic engineering.

Burt and Crisanti's groups at Imperial began to use the new technique as one of their methods to build a gene drive in *Anopheles*. In 2016, they published proof of a gene drive in mosquitoes. Other researchers—Anthony James, Valentino Gantz, and Ethan Bier, at the University of California, Irvine—published in 2015, with Gantz and Bier working on the fruit fly, and James, like the Imperial group, working on mosquitoes, primarily *A. stephensi* and showed how CRISPR-Cas9 could work in a mosquito.[37] In less than four years, that new genetic engineering tool, CRISPR-Cas9, paired with advancing knowledge about selfish genetic elements, enabled a breakthrough in what scientists had been studying for more than fifty years and which Austin Burt and his colleagues had been thinking about for decades: gene drives to alter the population of *Anopheles* mosquitoes, with the specific aim of eliminating malaria.

2.3   Imagining the Translation of Basic Research

> Will applications of gene drives be safe? Will they be effective? Will they have unintended consequences for the environment or public health? Do we know enough to release gene-drive modified organisms into the wild? Is using a gene drive to suppress or eliminate a pest species a good idea? What can scientists do to reduce risks to humans, other organisms, and the environment? How do we decide where gene drive modified organisms might get released? What should governments do? Who gets to decide?
>
> —National Academies of Sciences, Engineering, and Medicine, "Gene Drives on the Horizon"

In 2016, the NAS convened a group of experts to testify for their report on gene drives. While the concept was still largely theoretical in that no gene drives had been released, much less perfected, even in the laboratory, several projects had begun. Kevin Esvelt, the MIT scientist whom I had met the year before, had held a series of small meetings to discuss his murine immunity enhancement drive on the basis of his mathematical models with the Martha's Vineyard community, while the Burt laboratory was steadily moving through the stages of community engagement and laboratory testing that Burt had described the previous year.

Now, Burt was here explaining to the committee how he had come to understand the power of the "fifth force"—the hidden world he had first described more than a decade earlier. "There occurs in nature, many examples of selfish genetic elements that can 'drive,'" he noted, "for example gamete killers, t-haplotypes in mice, driving sex chromosomes in mosquitoes, homing endonuclease genes (HEG) and others." It was his whole "zoo" of genetic elements. He explains that these drives can be used in two different ways. They can be used for either population suppression—in which fewer organisms are conceived or born—or population modification—in which the same number of organisms are born but have new characteristics or lack key characteristics that make them able to transmit disease. Both strategies might be used to eliminate organisms that are disease vectors or pests, or invasive species that are destroying habitats by, among other options, altering their capacity to reproduce or survive, or to change their fertility rates or the sex ratios of their offspring, or to alter immunity to parasites or capacity to carry them. Genes that control traits or capacities can be "knocked out" or "knocked in" (which had been done for several decades) and vectors could be given an alternative phenotype. The age profile of vectors can be altered, since, in the case of mosquitoes, only older females need to seek a blood meal before they can lay eggs, or they could by modified simply to die on becoming infected. One could change host feeding preferences for animals, as opposed to humans, or simply change the vector competence. Because malaria transmission is such a chancy business, it is perhaps the case that a slight alteration might upend the chain of transmission long enough for the parasite to be eliminated from the human population.

There were many unknowns, even then, before scientists were as aware as they are now about the problems of genetic error, off-target insertions, and mosaicism in the use of CRISPR. That day, in subsequent talks, Burt stressed the fact that we do not yet know which tool will be the best to use to create the genetic changes, that CRISPR-Cas systems are new, and perhaps there will be other new methods developed to alter genes. Moreover, he emphasized that we do not yet know which strategy—modification, reduction, changing feeding preferences, reducing competence, or some other yet-to-be-discovered target—will be the best one. The point is, he noted that molecular biology gives a far wider range of possible responses to the problem of vector control, than had been available to earlier generations of malaria researchers and public health administrators, and at this stage, all ideas should be tested and welcomed. "It is premature to say which is best, and combinations of several are possible," Burt stressed. Yet, he made a case for the value of suppression—the main thrust of the work of the Imperial laboratories.

Burt took a moment to compare suppressive and modification strategies using a gene drive to alter mosquito populations, comparing suppressive strategies and modification provides an interesting look into both the hope and the risks of gene drives, and each raises different sorts of issues. In strategies of suppression, in which the goal is to dramatically reduce the population of mosquitoes in a given area, Burt argued, there are uncertainties on several fronts. For example, what was the propensity for the drive to "burn out" or self-extinguish? How possible would it be for the drive to eliminate or "crash" the entire population after several generations? Or would the population of mosquitoes continue to exist, with the driving elements, and the transgene, but without the parasite, because the altered biting rate cannot sustain the transmission of the gametes, but it was uncertain if the male mosquitoes who were heterozygous for the drive, would remain fertile and viable in the wild, thus able to mate successfully and spread it.[38]

In this lecture at the National Academy, Burt thought that suppression drives would tend to be relatively evolutionarily stable, for he believed that mutations that would destroy drive function would be expected to disappear as they move through populations, for the equilibrium of the construct would be low. In that case, Burt thought, to "undo" a suppression drive, a second drive would not be needed and might in fact create new problems. He argued then that natural selection could be used instead. Suppression drives were to be directed at the vector, hoping that reducing the mosquito population would reduce the biting rate and thus reduce the possibility that the parasite would be transferred to another person, which is necessary for the parasite to exist and reproduce, continuing its life cycle. Suppression is not aimed at changing the characteristics of the mosquito, with the exception of the addition of the transgene, but at preventing the birth of viable females, resistance would eventually develop in the mosquito itself. In this sense, suppression drives are "the genetic equivalent of insecticides."[39]

Modification drives, "in which an altered allele that will lead to a specific trait is spread by "hitchhiking" with the drive to a wild-type chromosomes using a CRISPR-Cas9 system with and a guide RNA to target the desired location, have as their target the parasite (which would be where resistance would be found) argued Burt."[40] Modification drives, are "intended to change the insect vector to prevent it from transmitting the pathogen which leaves the insect in place, and the population at the same density in the environment, but blocks disease transmission.[41] Modification drives, he argued, are intended give a high abundance of the new trait in the population, and the drive is unlikely to self-extinguish or burn itself out. A modification drive had uncertainties as well. First, mutations have to alter the mosquito, but not in ways that would deter mating, or make it less likely to compete with a wild-type mosquito, which has been exquisitely difficult in the past, according to Burt. And because of this, successful modification drives must have small fitness effects. Thus, to "undo" a modification drive, one would need to release a second drive, also with small fitness effects. While the species would not "crash" or be depleted as in the suppression drives, the "new" genetically altered mosquito species would replace, ideally, permanently, the original wild type species (which, as an aside for moral philosophers reading this, recalls classic debates in ontology about identity and change).

Each idea will need to be thought about on a case-by-case basis, Burt noted, and he told the committee that scientists and the regulators who will oversee the project eventually, need to be wary of over optimism or a "cavalier" attitude about the safety of the project, of either suppression or modification and replacement drive, if they were thinking that because of the possibility of a recall, reversal, or remediation drive, any serious safety issues could be undone. This idea—that a second drive could undo the effects of a first gene drive gone wrong—might tempt researchers or regulators away from the serious need for strict controls on safety at every single stage of the process which he argued is critically important. Then, Burt described the two main strategies that his laboratory, and others at Imperial were working on at the time: homing drives and "driving Y" sex chromosomes.

Homing drives, as I explained above—also called "mutagenic chain reaction"—use the same strategy of naturally occurring HEGs and replicated it by using a CRISPR-Cas9 and a guiding RNA to direct the DNA cleavage to the correct site, which is then repaired and the homologous chromosome then carries the new sequence adding the cutting mechanism to the genome in the germline cells. A gene of interest can also be bound to the cleavage construct. It will be pasted back into the genome, along with the copied construct. Thus, the strategy can be used either to knock in or to knock out a gene in addition to the driving element. CRISPR-Cas9 with gRNA made this possible and ease of engineering is important, but Burt suggested that day that different tools that met other criteria may also be needed based on the factors he listed: specificity, type of DNA repair that is stimulated, stability of activity and specificity, and robustness against resistant alleles.

Another strategy they were exploring was to create a gene drive using a "driving Y" chromosome, or he explained to the committee. "Here, the goal is to achieve genomic cleavage without homing, by placing a gene for enzyme on the Y chromosome that is specifically active when the male is making its sperm. That would find the X sequence that is only found on the X chromosome. Ideally, a repeated sequence, and would shred it. Thus, the functional sperms that are produced are those carrying the Y chromosome, and those will also carry the transgene for the drive, and this which will spread through the population."[42] This drive, modeled as a proof of principle in the Burt laboratory, which mimics a naturally occurring drive found in Aedes mosquitoes, which while it is not completely understood, he noted, creates meiotic X breaks. In their modeling, this leads to 95 percent of the offspring being males with normal fertility in the population in twenty generations. The different dynamics of the enzyme—its expression, its activity, its half-life, and the differences in the target gene (whether it is in the germline or not, if it is recessive or dominate, where the construct is located)—all might give tremendous complexity to the possibilities of genetic engineering. By the winter of 2016, the Crisanti laboratory was clearly exploring many of these possibilities and researching new applications of CRISPR-Cas systems that might interfere with female fertility, which would eventually, two years later, yield the most promising results.

The laboratory was also considering the process, safety concerns, and regulatory issues, as they imagined the gene drive project succeeding. He described two ways in which the approach of the project would proceed in a stepwise manner. First, by the release of sterile males, then, fertile males with a self-limiting genetic alteration, prior to releasing the actual self-sustaining gene drive, and second, by doing the research first in London, then in large cages in Italy, then in the labs in the country where the drive would be used, and finally doing field trials. In the next chapter, you will see how these Burt and Crisanti plans and protocols became part of the final NASEM report as best practice concepts.

One of the most thoughtful parts of Burt's presentation was an analysis of one of the critiques of gene drives: its complete novelty as a concept—that nothing had been done like this—meaning releasing a scientific project out of the laboratory and into the wild. Burt then noted while genetically created gene drives had not been used before, other genetically engineered organisms had been. In particular, two aspects of research that were closely related to gene drive research had in fact been used with extraordinary success and could be used as useful lessons. The first was the history of the capacity for containment. Burt pointed out that scientists around the world work on a daily basis with dangerous pathogens and have developed a sophisticated system of biosafety based on physical containment, caution, protective barriers, and laboratory safety.

Biosafety has long been a concern for genetic research, and molecular geneticists use the same international systems to study infectious diseases. A biosafety level is a set of biocontainment precautions required to isolate dangerous biological agents in an enclosed laboratory facility so that they can be handled without escape or contamination. The levels of containment range from the lowest biosafety level (BSL-1) to the highest (BSL-4). In the USA, the Centers for Disease Control and Prevention (CDC) have specified these levels.[43] In the European Union (EU), the same biosafety levels are defined in a directive.[44] In Canada, the four levels are known as containment levels.[45] There are broad levels of agreement on safety levels, and organisms are grouped by scientific consensus regarding their infectivity, which is largely shared between scientists globally.[46]

Research proceeds without incident daily because there is international agreement and training that protects the public. At higher biosafety levels, these include precautions such as airflow systems, multiple containment rooms, sealed containers, positive pressure personnel suits, established protocols for all procedures, extensive personnel training, and high levels of security to control access to the facility. In fact, many of the pathogens that ordinary members of the public consider dangerous are contained at lower levels of protection—severe acute respiratory syndrome, tuberculosis, yellow fever, and West Nile virus among them—because scientists feel secure in their capacity to work at that level. BSL-4 viruses include smallpox, monkeypox, Marburg virus, Ebola virus, Middle East respiratory syndrome, and viral hemorrhagic fevers, among several others.[47]

One can see the careful containment protocols at the Imperial laboratories in London. The insectary at the Imperial laboratory is in the basement of a secure floor, with locked doors and restricted access, with two other doors separating the mosquito room, which houses the insects on a special closed metal shelf with glass doors, on which sit small white mesh cages—they look like the lace doily covers for cakes at a county fair—for the mosquitoes. Visitors need to be escorted, and gowned. Burt argued that entomologists, both in London and in large-cage experiments in the laboratories in Terni, know how to contain insects effectively and have done so for decades, using multiple systems of control.

Second, he pointed out that it is not novel to release genetically altered or displaced and relocated organisms into the wild for use as vector control, and Burt turned to describe this in his talk. There have been a series of releases into the wild of insects that, it is hoped, will reproduce and spread—not at the rate of a drive, but nevertheless at a rate intended to affect wild-type populations. Burt in his testimony mentioned the conventional biological control release of the wasp that fed on the destructive cassava mealybug. Later in this book, I will expand on this example, and others which use genetically altered sterile male insects (SIT) for population control of screwworms Let me mention it here for a just a moment so that you, reader, can understand why Burt mentioned this in his presentation. It was his contention that while the mechanism he was proposing was novel in some ways, in others, it is not: gene drives occur in nature, and humans have manipulated insects to control diseases in the field before.

2.4 Imagining Collaboration: Target Malaria

Burt mentioned that his laboratory worked with others in a collaborative academic, nonprofit consortium called Target Malaria. Target Malaria is a not-for-profit research consortium whose goal is to develop and share not-for-profit technology for malaria control. Target Malaria started as small, university-based research program, but by the time of Burt's talk, it had grown to include scientists in African, European, and North American laboratories, stakeholder engagement teams with specialists in community communications, modellers, mathematicians, field entomologists, ecologists, quality assurance teams, risk assessment specialists, stakeholder engagement teams, and regulatory experts from Africa, North America, and Europe. From the beginning, the teams were optimistic about the possibility of gene drives. The plan was to use the new genetic engineering tools to create a gene drive to reduce the numbers of female mosquitoes, and the teams were open to a variety of ideas about how to do this. The partner institutions included the CDC Foundation, USA; the Fred Hutchinson Cancer Center Research Group, USA; Imperial College London, UK; Institut de Recherche en Sciences de la Santé (IRSS), Burkina Faso; Keele University, UK; Malaria Research and Training Center, Université des Sciences, des Techniques et des Technologies de Bamako, Mali; Polp d'Innovazione de Genomica e Biologia (Polo GGB, the Terni labs), Italy; Uganda Virus Research Institute (UVRI), Uganda; University of Cambridge, UK; University of Ghana, Legon, University of Notre Dame, USA; University of Oxford, UK; University of Pergula, Italy; and the University of Washington, USA. The deeply international reach of the team is indicative of the commitment to being rooted in the Africa countries—Mali, Burkina Faso, and Uganda—where the releases of the mosquitoes are intended to take place. Here is how the project describes itself on its website:

> Target Malaria is a not-for-profit research consortium with a mission to develop an innovative approach to malaria control. It was established in 2005 as an academic research programme and now includes scientists, stakeholder engagement teams, risk management specialists and regulatory experts from Africa, North America, and Europe. The project aims to reduce mosquitos' population, vectors of malaria in sub-Saharan Africa in order to reduce transmission of the disease. There are more than 3,500 species of mosquitoes in the world, of which about 840 occur in Africa. Within this diversity, only a small group of species are responsible for most malaria transmission cases—three species of the kind *Anopheles gambiae* (*Anopheles gambiae*, *Anopheles coluzzii* and *Anopheles arabiensis*) and the species *Anopheles funestus* s.l. The technology suggested by Target Malaria specifically targets mosquito vectors of malaria of the *Anopheles gambiae* kind. The aim of the project is to develop a technology based on genetic modification of mosquitoes that should be complementary to other anti-vectorial control methods and offer a long-term, cost-effective, and sustainable solution.[48]

The project is not only a collection of basic scientists—there are teams of academic experts in a variety of areas. Here is how they described themselves on their website in 2017:

> The scientific teams bring together experts in protein engineering, molecular biology, population genetics, entomology, and modelling. The protein engineering and molecular biology teams are focused on developing the different stages of the technology, looking at how the modifications can best be built and most efficiently inserted in the malaria mosquito's genes. The entomologists and population geneticists are studying local mosquito populations, to understand their composition and behavior and also working with the teams responsible for maintaining and evaluating the modified mosquitoes in the insectaries to see how their behaviors compare. We also have teams of expert modellers, who are helping us think through population dynamics and how, if our research is successful, the technology may one day be deployed.[49]

One notable aspect of Target Malaria is their public commitment to transparency and to open access to the research itself, as well as to any product that they might develop if the research project proves successful. Each member has publicly pledged that any technology resulting from their work be made available for free or for a very low cost. Because they are based in universities, they were funded in part by grants from foundations and national agencies, and they list these sources on their website: "Target Malaria receives core

funding from the Bill & Melinda Gates Foundation and from the Open Philanthropy Project, an advised fund of Silicon Valley Community Foundation.
Individual labs also received additional funding from a variety of sources to
support each lab's work, including DEFRA, the European Commission, MRC,
NIH, Ugandan Ministry of Health, Wellcome Trust, UNCST."[50]

The project was at that time also exploring new ways of doing what they
called "codevelopment." I will turn to examine this claim in some detail in a
subsequent chapter, but that day, Burt explained that Target Malaria had not
only delivered classic public education, held structured community engagement in which they listened to the local stakeholders in places where they
anticipated the building of insectaries and releases of mosquitoes. These,
concerns and insights about the research, were a part of the widespread and
specific community consent in the villages in which the mosquitoes will be
studied, but they had also initiated a program to train villagers—men and
women—to catch, identify, and categorize mosquitoes. The villagers, who
knew the mosquitoes' behavior most intimately, were trained to study and
report behaviors to the scientists. How do the mosquitoes swarm? When and
where? When do mosquitoes bite? Inside or outside? This was a key part of
the research, as is noted in all of their literature:

> Stakeholder and local community support for our work is essential. Our teams are
> working to develop an innovative technology to reduce the number of malaria
> mosquitoes and therefore reduce the transmission of the disease but this can only
> work if those affected are supportive of our approach. Stakeholder engagement is a
> priority. We have teams working at various levels: with international and national
> stakeholders, working with the local communities in which the baseline fieldwork
> is taking place, with the communities around the insectary, and with local and
> national authorities. Our teams are committed to explain the project and its phases,
> answer questions and address any concerns that may arise.[51]

Not only was there local participation, he noted, but every local, state, and
federal regulatory body was also consulted at every stage of the work, for regulations about genetically modified (GM) organisms and, indeed, fieldwork
in Africa needs to meet specific standards for approval. This includes obtaining both regulatory licenses to transport eggs and larvae (which is how the
insects travel between sites) giving permission to enter the country and area
and social licensing from the various NGOs and civic organizations. As this,
too, is described on the website: "At each step of the way, we are committed
to abide by international guidelines and comply with national legislation in

all the countries involved and to observe best practices. We have a regulatory affairs advisory team that helps us understand what the requirements in each country are and what information we need to provide."[52] In addition to the scientific, engagement, regulatory, and operational teams, Target Malaria had an external, independent Ethics Advisory Committee. This is the board to which I was served from 2016 to 2023, which gave advice (not always, but most often, followed) about ethical dilemmas that arose in the course of the research.

Target Malaria was moving ahead with the work in an iterative fashion and, by 2017, had gained approval to move the first genetically altered mosquitoes "made" in London to the large cage laboratories in Terni, Italy. That day, at the hearing, Burt explained how the complexity and multiplicity of the targets and behaviors, and the complexity of the new tools, allowed for a careful, step-by-step exploration of various pathways toward, in Target Malaria's case, a suppression strategy.

Next, Burt outlined his plans for the ultimate release of the mosquitoes into the wild. It was to be a multiyear project, now staged elaborately in computer models. First, the laboratory, under strict safety and containment guidelines, would work on the basic science and technology of creating a genetic lineage either of the homing drive elements, or with the driving Y, or, in a third team, by targeting a gene that would alter the reproductive integrity of females, all doing the work in the insectary in the basement of Imperial College London. In addition to the strict containment practices, it was theorized that the African *A. gambiae* mosquitoes that might somehow escape would have to confront the London climate, which is fairly unforgiving to mosquitoes, even to British anopheline species. Next, the laboratory in Italy, under strict containment, using sophisticated large cages, which would more closely replicate conditions in the wild than could happen in the London laboratories, would see how the genetically modified mosquitoes did in that habitat. These cages, as I later saw, are large enough that they can mimic the *A. gambiae* mosquito habitat, warm and humid, with space and a "horizon point" to allow males to swarm, and realistically simulated dawn, day, dusk, and night. Here, in the unlikely event of mosquito escape (past the doubled doors, the special outfits, the air blowing backward, the routine outdoor spraying) *A. gambiae* might well survive in the southern Italian air, so extraordinary care was taken to prevent this from happening.

Finally, the African entomologists in the project, collaborating with their universities, were building insectaries in the African countries that had agreed to participate, under strict containment and under the jurisdiction and leadership of the local scientific, ethical, and legal community.

The mosquito release itself would be similarly "staged." First would be a release of sterile males, without the gene drive elements, primarily to practice the technical aspects of releasing genetically altered mosquitoes to train the teams, build operational capacity, continue the discussion about the work locally and internationally and to prepare for any problems that might arise.[53]

Then, after the sterile male release was studied, there would be a release of males that were genetically altered to have a male bias but not a drive. "These are genetically modified males that can successfully mate and produce offspring, but in which the genetic modification would only persist for a limited period of times before disappearing."[54] This modification produces mostly male mosquitos, which is why they are called "male bias" and the modification is similar to one made to the sterile males, using a nuclease gene that fragments the X chromosome of the sperm, resulting in a mosquito that has only Y bearing sperm and produces predominately male offspring in each generation.[55] Because the nuclease gene is inserted into a mosquito autosome, not a sex chromosome, the alteration is not "driven" but is only inherited by 50 percent of the offspring.

Finally, if all had gone well, there would be the final gene drive, where males would be released with a self-sustaining drive, engineering using one of the ideas still being explored, intended to begin population suppression. This drive would, once released into the field, continue to spread out of direct human control, and its success would rest on the capacity for the genetically altered mosquitoes to not only survive, but mate successfully and spread the drive, reducing the first, the number of breeding females and then, the number of mosquitoes in the population. It was intended of course, to have, in addition to this entomological endpoint, ideally, a clinical endpoint as well, which would be apparent only if malaria rates went down measurably. At every stage, in what Burt imagined as more than a decade-long process, there would be an ongoing assessment of the basic molecular biology, the entomology, the technical and regulatory issues, the risk assessment, and the environmental impact. The project was also committed to sustained community engagement at every stage, in the villages most affected by these releases.

Finally, in addition, the project has contracted with independent, outside experts in social sciences, economics, and ecological research to undertake independent assessments at each stage of the escalation of the research plan—before the release of sterile males, before the release of male-biased, non-drive males, and before the gene drive release. These groups review the stakeholder work, and the environmental, economic, social, and policy status before, during, and after each stage of the research. The project was alert to any critique that it operated alone and without oversight, for there was extensive oversight, with external and internal groups that used the Environmental, Social, and Health Assessment (ESHIA) environmental, socio-economic, and health impact assessment practices, developed by the mining industry in Africa, and now used more extensively by policy makers "to look at the broader impacts of human or environmental activities such as socio-economic dimensions, both negative and positive.[56]

The committee that listened to Austin Burt would go on to approve continued gene drive research tentatively and within careful guidelines, using many of the concepts used by Target Malaria, as we will see in the next chapter. Approbation of the research by the House of Lords and the African Union in support of the project was even more robust as I will describe in the next chapter.

Meanwhile, research on gene drives continued, and not only in London. In Southern California, at the University of California at San Diego, Ethan Bier and his postdoctoral students and his laboratory, funded by a 70 million partnership with the Indian company, Tata Trust,[57] were working first with fruit flies and then with *Aedes*, the mosquito species that is the vector for a host of human diseases, including yellow fever, Zika, and dengue fever. In 2015, working with Anthony James, a Distinguished Professor of microbiology and molecular genetics at the University of California, at Irvine, who had been long working on this possibility, he too turned to the problem of malaria, targeting *Anopheles stephensi*, a species that is responsible for Asian malaria. Using a CRISPR-Cas9 method, this group, as mentioned before, created transgenic mosquitoes that carried, in the laboratory, anti-pathogen effector genes that could target human malaria parasites, and carried a driving element that they theorized could be the basis for a strong modification drive, aimed at changing or replacing the mosquito species with a genetic variant that cannot transmit the plasmodium.[58] Thus, the research target is a different *Anopheles* strain, and Bier has spun off companies to develop the technology: Synbal, Inc., and Agragene, two a companies that intend to develop agricultural uses for drives, should that be possible. Bier holds equity and sits on both boards and the scientific advisory board of the companies. Bier argues for first use only on islands, as a safety measure, and has argued for the possibility of drives to undo drives. He is a firm believer in the replacement strategy. So, I was interested to speak to him about these differences.

I spoke at length with Bier,[59] a Distinguished Professor of cell and developmental biology, about the choice to modify rather than suppress populations. His office and his laboratory were crowded with projects, gifts, mounted specimens, plants, photos, and new ideas for projects, and he was eager to explain his work to me and was quite generous with his time. He took pains to show me why he thinks that he, too, might be able to end malaria. And that would be just the beginning, he tells me. "We would have control over so many terrible diseases, and not just disease, but food production."

Altering the phenotype (the observable genetic characteristics) of the mosquito, as was done in the 2015 experiment, seemed to him to be the better strategy for a few reasons. The first reason was because suppression drives would be imperfect, he thought because mosquitoes would hide or evade the drive by mating and breeding in remote places and would then return to repopulate an area with wild types. The second reason was because suppression drives would be more highly resisted by the mosquitoes, he argued in our conversation because they were reproductive drives. Thus, the selective pressure was greater, and the resistance to the drive would develop faster. Replacement drives, in his opinion, since they would still allow for mosquito reproduction, would not have this feature, and thus their subtle effects (a change in a body part, or enzyme) might persist in the population in a more stable fashion (although the selective pressure on the Plasmodium would still play a considerable role). Bier raised the problem of suppression drives leaving a ecologic niche empty, which might create a risk of another, troublesome species inhabiting it. He also argued that replacing mosquitoes with new ones that simply could not successfully harbor the P. falciparum parasite but were otherwise unchanged and which left the species intact in the wild, but still in the niche in the same numbers, for example, was "more natural" (although the removal of the pathogen could change vector populations dynamics and ecological relationships too). In the years since, although I have focused on the laboratories within the Target Malaria consortium, I have also followed the progress of the Southern California groups because, as Burt himself has repeatedly pointed out, it is not clear which strategy will work best in the field, and it is possible that many ideas could be used at the same time. In 2022, for example, Bier published a new paper about a different way to use CRISPR, by switching out the Cas9 protein scissor for another protein, nickase, which only selectively cuts one of the two DNA strands, leaving the other chromosome intact. Nickase showed promise in fruit flies, with high efficiency and far fewer off-target mistakes than Cas9, but Bier's laboratory had not yet used it in mosquitoes.[60]

While other laboratories began to work on gene drives, the consortium of university centers in the Target Malaria project continued to proceed along the plan laid out by Burt, that afternoon in Washington, DC, step by step. And importantly, they continued the work in the villages where they planned the releases, training villagers to work in new insectaries built to house the mosquitoes once the countries had been selected for the eventual release, which were now Mali, Burkina Faso, and Uganda. Eventually, they would add projects in Ghana, where they would do very specific research on insect and animal food networks and habitat ecosystems, and for a time in Cape Verde.

By the early summer of 2018, the approval for the first small-scale release of sterile male *Anopheles coluzzii* mosquitoes was granted to the project and the Institut de Recherche en Sciences de la Santé/Centre Muraz IRSS by the National Biosafety Committee of Burkina Faso. This release, while not intended to reduce the incidence of malaria, was to be the first release of GM mosquitoes of any type in Africa, and the first intended to be eventually used to research the vectors against malaria anywhere. Even though the sterile mosquitoes were not expected to produce any viable offspring, and since mosquitoes usually die after two weeks in the field, and would disappear shortly after release, the release site was monitored for seven months. The release was designed to yield data on the longevity of the modified mosquitoes and critical lessons about operations and to allow the newly trained local workers experience in releases that would be valuable when gene drive mosquitoes were released in the coming years. Most importantly, the villagers and regulators could think about and critically assess this stage before the project moved to the next stage in the plan: releasing the male bias, non-drive strain.

The summer of 2018 also marked the publication of a major new scientific publication by the Imperial laboratories, where an ingenious solution to interrupting female fertility had been discovered, when researchers were able to target a mosquito gene that resulted in female sterility. The first author was a young graduate student Kyros Kyrou and the second, Andrew Hammond, a postdoctoral fellow at the Crisanti laboratory, who had done the molecular biology that supported the work in 2016, using CRISPR-Cas9. They created a successful gene drive made from a CRISPR-Cas9 complex targeting the gene that researchers call *doublesex*.

How did this work? Let me turn to their paper in some detail. First, the alert reader will see that this strategy used neither the "driving Y" nor the homing originally proposed which, as the authors of the study note had proven to be elusive to create.[61] It turned out that while these ideas work in theory and in modeling studies, in practice, the authors wrote that the use of the "driving Y" in mosquito breeding "has proven difficult because of the complete transcriptional shut down of the sex chromosome during meiosis, which prevents the expression of an Y-led sex distorter during gamete formation."[62] And the use of CRISPR-Cas9 homing drives other than *doublesex* has been more complicated in vivo as well, for rapid and significant resistance mutations arose as quickly as in the second generation and blocked the spread of the drive—the problem of resistance once again. Both strategies had hit technical roadblocks, which is what led Hammond and his colleagues toward another idea.

Aware of the problem of resistance, the team turned toward strategies for disruption of new genetic targets, ones with functional or structural constraints, a place on the genome in which mutations would be rare—for the sequences would need to be essential for the organism to allow the drive to spread long enough and widely enough to affect population. Thus, they turned to the highly conserved *doublesex* region.

In insects, sex differences arise, as much as is understood in mosquitoes, when a primary genetic signal is turned on that sends instructions for "alternate splicing" of the *doublesex* gene, hence the name. One pathway will become male, but the other, female: *dsx*.

During meiosis, Kyrou and Hammond used a CRISPR-Cas9 complex to cut, or "knock out" the female specific isoform of the wild-type *dsx* variant of the *doublesex* gene, and during the repair, they offered the drive cassette of the CRISPR-Cas9 plus the altered female *doublesex* gene, *dsxF*, to make homologous—matching—DNA pairs in the embryo. Females with this altered repair are completely infertile. Females with one normal gene and one altered gene were fertile and could pass the drive construct to the next generation, and this worked whether the break was made in the gene that was inherited from the mother or the father, with no effect on the males. Moreover, in the first eleven generations, no mutations emerged that could not be cut and repaired in the same way. Interestingly enough, when the female mosquitoes with the altered gene emerged, they had a "male-like" phenotype and could not bite effectively. Thus, not only did this render them unable to get enough human blood to mature their eggs, it also inhibited the homozygous females efficacy as a vector for the transmission of the *Plasmodium* back to humans. It offered a path to complete mosquito population suppression. The new transgene reached 100 percent prevalence in seven to eleven generations, or just under five months in Kyrou and Hammond's caged laboratory mosquitoes, where the populations of insects were substantially and then completely diminished in the laboratory cages. The drive was targeted at *A. gambiae*, the most lethal of all the mosquito species in Africa and the most effective carrier of *P. falciparum*.

The development of success in a cage population is not, of course, the same as a gene drive in the wild, and thus this experiment, while centrally important as a proof of principle, was clearly only the beginning. But the paper represented a significant advance. Finding an elegant technical and practical solution to reduce both the efficacy and fertility of female mosquitoes and ensuring the continuation of the drive in the population, and using that as a suppressive strategy, was very promising. In the careful language of the report: "The gene drive *dsxF crisprh* targeting exon 5 of *dsx* has several features that make it suitable for future field testing. Specifically, this drive has high inheritance bias, heterozygous individuals are fully fertile, homozygous females are sterile and unable to bite, and we have found no evidence for nuclease-resistant functional variants at the drive target site."[63] Unlike other experiments, this one seemed, at least at first, not to evoke resistance genes. However, on paper, the authors argued for further testing, and as of the writing of this book, this testing has continued. The gene drive would need to be repeated in the large cages in Italy the authors noted, to see if there would be a reduction in fitness that did not appear in the small-cage studies, when confronted by competition for food, climate alterations, and other stressors. But the authors were cautiously optimistic, for even with up to a 40 percent fitness reduction, the suppression still worked in the caged mosquitoes.

It was at this point that COVID-19 paused the world for a long while, and international meetings went online, but in Mali and Burkina Faso, the research continued, despite extraordinary challenges. By July 2021, the experiment had been refined and repeated extensively in small cages and then with colonies of mosquitoes raised in the laboratories at Terni, so close to the lovely human-engineered falls that I visited in 2019 to see the "large-cage" experiments.

The laboratories at Terni are a modest affair by American standards. Along one corridor, behind sealed doors, a reverse airflow lock, and a special transitional antechamber lie four large "rooms" the size of huge walk-in closets. They are intended to look—to a mosquito—as close to an African habitat as possible, with timed light and dark phases that match the hours of sunlight, with open spaces for male mosquitoes to swarm, and with horizon foci for them to locate. It is hot and moist. The researchers are extremely careful. I cannot go in to see the cages, even wearing the full body gear that all the researchers wear, because I have recently been in Africa to see the Ghana project and may inadvertently be carrying malaria in my bloodstream. These cages are the last step in the iterative process before the eggs these mosquitoes lay are transported after an application for import and contained use was approved by the regulatory authorities in each African country, and raised in the African purpose-built insectaries. Here in Terni, unlike in cold London, if the genetically engineered mosquitoes somehow escaped, and evaded the monitoring and spraying, they would survive. So, just as Burt had promised the National Academies years before, they are exceedingly careful.

In the paper, "Gene-drive suppression of mosquito populations in large cages as a bridge between lab and field,"[64] Andrew Hammond, who at the time was a post-doctoral student, I met in Crisanti's laboratory, reported suppressive activity here too, in population that had a variety of ages, complex feeding, and reproductive behaviors that were permitted in the large-cage areas, and that could not be seen in the small cages. The paper noted:

> Indeed, previously developed genetically modified mosquito strains have shown strong fitness costs when tested in large-cage or semi-field experiments that were not observed in initial small cage testing, including severe mating disadvantages that precluded further testing of the strain. We refer herein to the initiation of these indoor large-cage experiments with the gene drive strain as releases, given that this is what they are designed to emulate, albeit they are performed in fully contained chambers that comply with appropriate arthropod containment guidelines. Many of these fitness challenges and complex behaviours can be reproduced in large cages by allowing overlapping generations so as to reveal potential differences in life-span and fecundity over time that cannot be captured in discrete-generation studies. As such, large-cage release experiments are now considered an essential bridge between laboratory and field testing within the tiered testing approach.[65]

For this to work, the males that carry the gene drive must be fit and must be attractive to the females.[66] They proved to be.

> Ag(QFS)1 males are introduced at ~12.5 or 25% initial drive frequency and key measurements of drive invasion and population fitness are monitored over time. We observe increases in frequency of the transgenic mosquitoes within the populations in all four cages initiated with the drive that lead to complete population suppression by 245–311 days after introduction. We compare these results to the output of a stochastic model using the method of Approximate Bayesian Computation, in order to infer key life-history parameters that are difficult to measure in dedicated assays. Our findings represent the first successful demonstration of efficacy for a gene drive in the second phase of testing which focuses on acquiring information under challenging ecological conditions, provide a platform for generating key evidence to inform initial go/no-go operational decisions, and pave the way for the first field trials of gene drive technology.[67]

Within one year after the introduction of a gene drive, the population had dramatically reduced, without selection for resistance to the drive.

> As with other forms of vector control, gene drives designed for population suppression will exert a strong selection for resistance. The force of selection for resistant mutations is proportional to the fitness cost imposed by the gene drive itself, but it can apply even to population modification gene drives that are intended to drive an anti-parasitic effector gene into a vector population, with the intention of changing its competency to transmit pathogens. The most likely form of resistance is a change in the target sequence that can prevent cleavage by the nuclease. Various strategies exist for reducing the probability of resistance arising against both population suppression and population modification gene drives. In the case of Ag (QFS)1 the gene drive is deliberately designed to target a region of its *doublesex* target gene that is under high functional constraint and cannot readily generate or accommodate sequence variants that confer functional resistance.[68]

This was a remarkable finding and, for the researchers, a very hopeful indication that the drive might achieve the goal theorized for it. But of course, the optimism needed to be tempered. Nevertheless, these experiments marked a significant move in the stepwise plan outlined in nearly every ethics document, moving genes drive closer to reality in Africa.

2.5   The Question of Resistance

But almost as soon as the paper was published, the researchers knew they had to be alert for signs emerging in the Terni laboratory that mosquitoes may have developed resistance even to the *doublesex* gene drive. This was expected—and the idea of a drive being clinically effective is contingent to some extent on not only on how quickly the drive is taken up, but how durable it is, allowing time for the intervention to work. It if can work well enough, fast enough, before resistance can occur, as, for example, DDT did in North America, then enough people would clear the parasite from their blood and could not reinfect mosquitoes. So, even when mosquitoes later developed resistance to the construct, it would not impact the disease dynamics or transmission, because the human link in the chain of the Plasmodium life would be broken. But it is this very durability that is in question. One issue is based on the way that CRISPR-Cas9 works, which is by cutting and then inducing repairs using an inserted snip of code. But it is an imperfect biological process. On occasion, the gene repairs incorrectly, or in the wrong spot, or deletes another snippet, or randomly mutates within the process—and any of these may create an unstable change in the genome of the mosquito embryo, and any of these might, in fact, allow the driving element to be overcome. A mutation may simply make it impossible for the CRISPR-Cas9 element to "recognize" the spot of insertion, and these varieties may overtake the population.[69] As in every population suppression strategy, from Paris Green to DDT to Quinine, and even draining the swamps and using bed nets, there will be resistance. A few mosquitoes will survive the intervention, whatever it is, and with that selective advantage, their offspring will, of course, spread the trait that led to that advantage. In the wild, this could lead to the development of isolated pockets of gene-drive-resistant mosquito populations that diverged and did not mate with the mosquitoes that were the target of the gene drive, and that could allow the parasite to escape the drive, and this is only one way the gene drive could mutate out of stability.

The investigators have been thinking of strategies to overcome this, and this research is still ongoing as I write this book. Because anopheline species of different sorts already exist, targeting several genes that are common to all, such as *doublesex*, but that exist on two different loci on that gene might slow resistance just long enough for eradication of the parasite. This is done using a technique called "multiplex genome editing," in which simultaneous expression of multiple guide RNA molecules (gRNA) are generated.

Currently, the Target Malaria teams are working on inserting two or perhaps three CRISPR-driven genetic changes into the mosquito genome instead of one. The idea is that making several single-allele changes, and linking them to the drive, will make resistance extremely difficult without creating a lethal or otherwise fecundity-destroying mutation. To create successful resistance would mean successfully mutating around several alterations, which would be evolutionarily more difficult.

But targeting *doublesex* raises another interesting challenge. Kyrou and Hammond, in the original paper, were also aware of this issue when they used *doublesex* as a target since their first caged experiments, that is, the ubiquity of the target gene beyond mosquitoes. They tell the readers this in the first paper: "Our results may have implications beyond malaria vector control. The role of *doublesex* in sex determination in all insect species so far analyzed, and the high degree of *doublesex* sequence conservation among members of the same species (in gene regions involved in sex-specific splicing), suggests that these sequences might be an Achilles heel present in many insect pests that could be targeted with gene editing approaches."[70] All insect species.[71]

Indeed, there certainly are implications. Success in this strategy would open the door to the concept in general as a way to control every single variety of insect. Although (as we shall see) the researchers were very excited about the possibility of using this target widely and optimistically to hobble the Achilles heel in the natural order, I as a watching ethicist did have some concerns about the very ubiquity and possibility of success. I was not the only one. Mark Benedict, who works with Target Malaria, raised the issue, and in a paper critical of gene drives, Virginie Courtier-Orgogozo and others worried that the possibility of horizontal transfer between species was "not insignificant." As they wrote:[72]

> One obvious risk associated with gene drive is that the sequence may escape from the target species and spread into other species. Such spillover could have devastating effects, such as the extinction of a species, or the modification of a large number of individuals, with potentially important ecological consequences. Compared to natural bacterial CRISPR systems, gene drive cassettes are more compact and contain eukaryotic cis-regulatory elements, so that they are one step closer to potential contamination of non-target eukaryote species. The risk of gene drives contaminating another species has been mentioned by several authors.[73]

The authors of this paper admit to "needing six consecutive steps"[74] for a drive to transfer horizontally. They confess to the unlikelihood of this.[75] Importantly, this would require hybridization of two different species—something that they note has not happened over millennia of evolutionary history and centuries of cohabitation of the same ecosystem. (Flies and mosquitoes do not mate, for example, even though they are related species.)

Moreover, it would be highly unlikely for the hybridized entity to be a disease vector. Given that the mosquito/*Plasmodium* construct has been in place for millennia and has not spread in the wild in the past, it remains extremely unlikely it would suddenly be adapted now. But clearly, these possibilities, even if remote, needed to be carefully understood and well monitored, especially in a ubiquitous genetic pathway. Yet, even these authors realized that they do not know exactly what to look for in their further research. I will return to this issue of uncertainty in my final chapter.

As I write, of course, because I am writing about a moving target, what I tell you here may well be out of date by the time you read this book. The science proceeds new tools and new insights, added to the project steadily, but it does not always proceed in a forward direction. Women and men bent over the trays with the white mesh tops, rather tenderly caring for mosquito generations, pouring over the tiny eggs to insert the gene sequence in just the right spot, or working on careful mathematical models or counting the number of living insects, in a particular habitat, is slow and tedious work, both within the Target Malaria group and in several other laboratories that are also working with gene drives, including the University of California groups at the Irvine and the San Diego campuses. Watching them, one remembers Ross and his obsessive, deliberate dissections, repeated a thousand times over the investigators who are the subject of this chapter are not the only ones working in quiet laboratories. Other projects are now under way at the Liverpool School of Tropical Medicine, Ifakara Health Institute in Tanzania, and the Akbari laboratory at USC in Los Angeles, all on a variety of mosquito targets. Although Target Malaria is the first laboratory to advance this far, and the only laboratory that has coupled its basic science research with the large projects in stakeholder engagement that I will address in a later chapter, it is not the only project, and laboratories are exploring other insects, birds, and mammals as potential populations that could be controlled using a gene drive. Other applications for gene drives are being suggested for ecological remediation, for example by the GBIRd group, which is exploring how nonnative species introduced to Pacific islands by nineteenth-century sailors, such as house mice, could be controlled without poisons on fragile island ecosystems so that the mice do not eat the endangered native bird populations. Esvelt remained interested in the mice in New England, which are a key part of the Lyme disease chain of infection. And of course, Target Malaria is not the only effort to eliminate malaria, as the project always reminds people who listen to its presentations or read its papers. There are dozens of new research projects at various stages of development to combat malaria, which I know about because my colleagues and my family, knowing that I am writing about malaria, send me clipping after clipping of other promised breakthroughs. Who knows, one of them could in fact be so monumentally important that it would render gene drives unnecessary.

Here is one example, announced in the summer of 2022 and published in the prestigious *New England Journal of Medicine*, which describes a challenge trial in which a small group of people showed promising results for a mono-clonal antibody injection given once every six months:

"A next-generation monoclonal antibody against malaria performed well for safety, efficacy, half-life duration, and ease of delivery in a phase I study. **Could this be the holy grail for the eradication of the mosquito-borne disease?** (emphasis in original) Just one dose of the antimalarial antibody L9LS conferred protection to 15 out of 17 recipients challenged with con-trolled human malaria infection. In contrast, the six controls not receiving the treatment all showed parasitemia on PCR testing within 21 days of expo-sure to infected mosquitoes."[76] It is, perhaps, not the holy grail, for even a drug needed only every six months is both logistically challenging and expen-sive. One can still see the appeal of a gene drive that is self-sustaining and, once initiated, continues to suppress the parasite without any further human intervention, but as the researchers in the Target Malaria project always argue, every single strategy is useful and important, and needs to be pursued.

I am writing because, as a member of the Target Malaria Ethics Advisory Committee, I had a front-row seat to watch the development of this science, and because the way that the gene drives are being investigated was itself interesting and important, and because I have long been interested in the larger issues that surround this particular project: befallenness, and response; justice and health-care research; and the way we understand and live within the natural world: I know that like Celli a century before them, the research-ers in the labs knew that the social, economic, and political terrain of each community was an important part of malaria eradication, which means understanding—and changing—structural issues at a broad scale; and I know that because of what was hinted at in the Hammond paper—the very power-ful capacity of human intervention in the order of the world, in all the com-plexity of that statement, is inevitably at stake as well. Every creature in the swarming, flying, buzzing, and biting world of insects—every single one of them—carried that *doublesex* gene coiled in its body. Insects in their fecundity, brittle brilliance, chanciness, danger, and necessity, all at once, and it was that gene that was targeted.

But I was not the only one who raised questions about how to assess and regulate the science that Burt had described and that Kyrou, Hammond, Bier, and James were beginning to work out, and who wondered what it would mean for the future of nature and the order of the species they were engineering in their laboratories.

It was precisely these sorts of questions that led to a swift reaction to the first announcements of gene drives' potential. Right after the science, and long in advance of its application, came the regulators. It is to this aspect of our story to which we will now turn.

3   The World as We Order It: A Review of Regulation

3.1   The Language of Genetic Regulation

When the idea of using a genetically engineered gene drive to replicate those found in nature was first proposed, it was still a computer-driven, mathematical concept after several years of thinking, only enacted in tiny pilot studies in laboratory insectaries. Insectaries have had a careful code of safety for years. So, the regulatory issues in the research[1] were quite narrowly defined. Austin Burt's and Andrea Crisanti's laboratories and other labs worked in relatively obscurity, with an article or two in the press about the ideas they were studying. However, almost as soon as the research became linked to the words "genetic" and "CRISPR," it began to draw the attention of national and international bodies, the House of Lords, the African Union, and the WHO, as well as the world's press. To be sure, it was not the first time that a pilot project had attracted immediate attention. Consider the cloning of Dolly the sheep and the immediate panic that humans would "soon" be cloned, which attracted congressional hearings, national commissions, and the full attention of scholarly academies from including Royal Academy of Sciences, the US National Academy of Sciences, the Chinese National Academies of Medicine, the President's Bioethics Commission, the Wellcome Trust, fifteen international religious bodies, and dozens of quickly assembled conferences, complete with grant funding—all for a process that was actually unlikely to be possible in humans.

In part, this careful attention to genetic research is the result of modern regulatory processes that began in 1972, when graduate students and assistant professors raised questions about a new technique being studied in their laboratories, which had its roots in earlier discussions about science and genetics in the 1940s. In particular, the graduate students were concerned about the new work by Paul Berg, Stanley Cohen, and Herbert Boyer. In a two-year period, between 1972 and 1974, Berg and Cohen at Stanford and Boyer at nearby University of California, San Francisco, began to extend Berg's work on recombinant DNA, experimenting with techniques to manipulate it and reorder it in simple bacterial organisms. Boyer had expertise in working with restriction endonucleases, and Cohen was an expert on plasmids.

Since 1959, scientists knew that bacteria contain extra loops of DNA called "plasmids" in addition to their chromosomes. In nature, bacteria can swap these plasmids with one another, quickly transferring beneficial genes such as those that code for antibiotic resistance. By the early 1970s, investigators had isolated several plasmids as well as special enzymes known as "restriction endonucleases" that work like scissors to cut open the loops of the plasmids.

After meeting at a conference in 1972, the two decided to combine their research efforts. After preliminary experiments in 1973, the Cohen–Boyer team was able to cut open a plasmid loop from one species of bacteria, insert a gene from different bacterial species, and close the plasmid. This created a recombinant DNA molecule—a plasmid containing recombined DNA from two different sources. Next, they inserted the plasmid into bacteria and demonstrated that the recombinant DNA could be used by bacteria. The team had created the first genetically modified or GM organisms.[2]

But the younger researchers were somewhat alarmed by the possibilities of this odd new capacity. Raising the question of how these GM *Escherichia coli* bacteria and, by extension, other organisms might affect human society, they called for a meeting of all the laboratories able to recombine DNA and transfer it into other organisms. Here is the letter from Maxine Singer and Dieter Soll to the head of the NAS, Philip Handler, whom they wanted to sponsor the meeting. Soll and Singer represented this concern after a meeting on the topic at a Gordon Research Conference:

Dear Doctor Handler,

Several of the scientific reports presented at this year's Gordon Research Conference on Nucleic Acids (June 11–15, 1973) indicated that we presently have the technical ability to join together, covalently, DNA molecules from diverse sources. Scientific developments over the past two years make it both reasonable and convenient to generate overlapping sequence homologies between DNAs of, for example, bacteria and animal viruses. Such sequence homologies can then be used in order to combine the diverse molecules by Watson-Crick hydrogen bonding. Application of existing methods then permits covalent linkage of such molecules. In this way new kinds of viruses with biological activity of unpredictable nature may eventually be created.

Certain of these hybrid molecules are potentially hazardous to both laboratory workers and the public. This possibility was recognized and agreed upon by a majority of those attending the Conference, who voted to communicate their concern to you and to the President of the National Academy of Medicine (to whom this letter is also being sent). We suggest that the Academies establish a study committee of appropriate individuals to consider this problem and to recommend specific actions or guidelines should that seem necessary. Related problems such as the risks involved in circuit large-scale preparation of animal viruses might also be considered.[3]

The meeting was small—the technique still quite new. All the researchers who could accomplish it could fit into one room at a retreat center called Asilomar, a windswept California State Park just down the coast from the University of California, San Francisco, built on sand dunes, which had rustic buildings designed by Julia Morgan, a group dining hall, and windows that faced the cool gray Pacific. The organizers decided to invite a reporter (for public inquiry), some nonscientists, and some lawyers to join the discussion, and valuing transparency, they made their recommendations available, hoping to begin a "larger social dialogue" about the new powers of genetic scientists.

This was an innovation, these meetings about science and its new direction, and the philosophers, lawyers, and theologians who just began to call themselves "bioethicists" were included in a series of such meetings. It was not the first appearance of a field that would be called "bioethics." For example, just north up the coast in the city of Seattle, the new lifesaving machines for kidney dialysis were introduced at the University of Washington Hospital. But there were not enough apparatus or skilled teams for everyone in end-stage renal disease. So, they had to be rationed, and committees of "leading citizens" were included in the deliberations. At the same time, in newly built neonatal ICUs, pediatricians sought advice about which babies to allow to die and which would receive aggressive care, and they invited theologians and philosophers in to help decide. Of course, debates about abortion, heart transplants, and end-of-life care were all just coming to the fore, with a flurry of new literature about ethics, medicine, and science. All of this activity was in part a reaction to the new technological prowess of science and medicine, and in part because of a series of revelations about the failure of that science and medicine to protect subjects of research. The Nuremberg Doctors' Trial had conclusively demonstrated why the enormous power of science ought not to be wielded, especially by the state, without careful and rigorous oversight, and it also showed that experts with power and the backing of their government needed outsiders to oversee their activities. The revelations about the Tuskegee syphilis experiment, where penicillin was withheld from subjects with syphilis for decades in a misguided and unethical effort to maintain an observational trial, and the Willowbrook hepatitis studies, where disabled children living in a state school were given hepatitis so that a vaccine could be tested on them, raised similar questions and called for similar oversight. By the time Singer and Soll raised the issue, there was a new field called bioethics, and it was clear that recombinant DNA research would have to proceed with some sort of bioethical oversight to be considered ethical.

But the actual results of the meeting were, in retrospect, quite modest and entirely focused, by design, to avoid contentious philosophical concepts. Here are the final points of advice:

- Don't insert pathogens.
- Don't insert cancer sequences.
- Don't insert genes for drug resistance.

There was no real advice about the problem of justice or access to a powerful new technology, nor who should own it or control it. There were no guidelines about avoiding enhancement or concerns about the mastery of nature or ontological shifts—just advice about safety. To make the point that safety concerns would be the focus, the group recommended that all subsequent recombinant DNA research was to be done in BSL-4 biocontainment facilities, and certain applications were held in moratorium for ten years. Nevertheless, the research was banned as unsafe in Cambridge, Massachusetts, after a contentious city council meeting—a precursor of what would be constant public opposition to genetic research.

Why was the research finally allowed to proceed? In large part, it was because of science self-regulation. The handful of scientists at the meeting were able to agree on norms for research and to assure one another of their commitment to enact them. The (perhaps apocryphal) narrative about this aspect of the story includes a scene in Senator Edward Kennedy's office, just as he was about to go to the Senate chamber to argue for a bill to regulate the research federally, when scientists burst in to tell him that the first successful use of recombinant DNA technology—Humulin, Eli Lily's recombinant insulin made from Genentech's specially modified bacteria—had been developed and was going to be submitted for trials. Suddenly, supporting new research and leaving regulation to normative processes run by scientists themselves was more plausible than federal restrictions. Artificial growth hormone followed next, then erythropoietin and other blood clotting products for hemophilia, all of which reassured the public of the safety and dramatic benefits of recombination.

It was decided that a national Recombinant DNA advisory committee, the RAC, would be established, and would review any and all proposed experiments in genetic manipulation in humans, in special sessions at the NIH, open to the public. The criteria for judging the ethical permissibility of the research were written largely by bioethicist Leroy Walters, who was on the first committee. This led to what was called "Appendix M" of the Human Subjects Guidelines, or "Points to Consider in the Design and Submission of Protocols for the Transfer of Recombinant DNA Molecules into One or More Human Research Participants." The establishment of the RAC also led to local biosafety committees and guidelines for accidents in the laboratory at every institution that received federal funds to do this research. Soon, these became standards that were widely accepted, even in the growing private sector of biotechnology where, increasingly, as the decades went on, most of such research was carried out. The first meeting of the RAC was held two years after Asilomar in 1975.

By 1978, under President Jimmy Carter, a new National Commission on the Protection of Human Subjects met to consider the issues and produced what would be called the Belmont Report.[4] The report stressed the need for informed consent for participants, justice in the selection of subjects, and a broad series of principles—beneficence, non-maleficence, justice, and autonomy—to guide research processes. It called for national oversight and local regulation of all research projects. By 1980, a new commission with a broader mandate, the President's Commission for the Study of Ethical Problems in Medical and Behavioral Research, took on a variety of bioethical issues. In

1982, it issued a comprehensive report on recombinant DNA, called Splicing Life,[5] which emphasized, as had the Asilomar meeting, the need for safety and the need for oversight.

This was widely considered a foundational text. It drew on far wider ethical, theological, and social sources and considered implications for the research. Although it had taken Asilomar for its framework and, like that meeting, its ultimate normative focus was on safety, it established an IRB process designed to regulate the technical aspects of experiments but allowed the RAC to review for "broader issues." Both the Belmont Report and the Splicing Life report relied on the consent and withdrawal rules for human subjects as the best method to protect subjects, underlining the strong autonomy bent of bioethics in that period. They both delineated extra care when treating vulnerable populations (a loosely defined term), and they suggested a carefully structured decorum in regard to publication practices, designed to protect the work of graduate students and post-docs. The Splicing Life report set in place concerns and guidelines for tissue use, largely supporting the need for privacy of the subject in genetic research. It set in place a process that suggested that ethical responses to emerging technology should not happen a priori, based on abstract principles, but rather by waiting until actual research cases could be proposed with specific features that could be analyzed and then compared to cases where the field had more assurance, experience, and familiarity. Judgment in this way would use a process called casuistry in ethical reasoning.

In 1984, the RAC created a new group with the sole purpose of looking closely at human gene therapy, called the Human Gene Therapy Working Group. The first task of the group was to create a mechanism for how scientists looking for approval from the RAC should structure their proposals, taking into account ethical as well as scientific issues (those "Points to Consider"). The RAC first worked to approve all the basic research projects involving recombinant DNA in all US laboratories, then all gene marking research, and, finally, all gene therapy protocols.[6] The RAC approved the protocols only in conjunction with the US Food and Drug Administration (FDA), which was primarily concerned about safety, as it is with standard drug protocols. By 1991, the FDA, too, had published its own Points to Consider, and the RAC committee was then guided by Appendix M ("Points to Consider in the Design and Submission of Protocols for the Transfer of Recombinant DNA Molecules into One or More Human Research Participants"). The RAC review of all individual gene therapy protocols became standard. The RAC was then moved into the NIH process to review new technologies and recommend new regulatory changes should these be understood as necessary for clinical gene transfer research.[7]

The RAC then began a robust period as a part of complex regulatory system, which included the Office of Biotechnological Activities Office, the FDA, biosafety (IBC) committees (producing guidelines for accidents in the laboratory) at federally funded institutions, IRBs, and voluntary compliance oversight by non-federally funded companies. Leroy Walters, chair of the first RAC Clinical Gene Transfer Research (CGTR) committee, noted: "Gene therapy research was clearly a hybrid field. On the one hand, it was highly technical and required the expertise of molecular biologists and human geneticists. On the other hand, gene therapy research was human subject research which was governed by its own set of rules and which was quite comprehensible to laypeople."[8] In addition to human research, a significant change was occurring in plant biotechnology and this drove another comprehensive regulatory regime. The first GM plants were developed in the early 1980s from the work of Mary Del Chilton, and the FDA approved both Calgene and Zeneca's tomato products for human consumptions in the early 1990s.[9] The federal rules were complex and reached across many agencies. The Environmental Protection Agency (EPA) created computer modeling for the accidental release of synthetic microbes and studying Toxic Substances Control Act implications. The Department of Agriculture undertook the inspection and certification of recombinant DNA for diseases that affected animals or plants, for example foot-and-mouth disease, nematodes, and plant germ plasm. The Federal Trade Commission regulated deceptive practices. The CDC had a twenty-four-hour hotline for reports of leakages in shipping of agents if interstate travel is involved. The National Institute for Occupational Safety and Health and the Occupational Safety and Health Administration did research on worker safety, with no specific regulatory plans. The Department of Transportation regulated recombinant DNA as hazardous material. The Department of Commerce and National Board of Standards is also allowed to regulate by-products in feedstocks, patents, and trade secrets standards. The state department worked with the UN when it considered recombinant DNA. The Department of Energy (DOE) had a research protocol on Chinese hamsters. Several National Science Foundation committees suggested regulations (the Law and Social Sciences Committee and the Ethics and Values in Science and Technology). The NAS set up grants and committees. It also regulated and oversaw certain recombinant DNA projects, and the Office of Technology Assessment (OTA) also conducted its own studies. Currently, all clinical GTR protocols connected with institutions that receive federal funding were submitted to the Office of Biotechnological Activities for RAC review (simultaneously with local IRBs, so that the RAC review went first). They were then passed via email review or went to full public hearings, and also hade IRB and IBS committees at each university. New rules involved efforts at "harmonization" of oversight, including attention to data monitoring, research ethics education, and conflict of interest issues. RAC protocols that were not selected for full review are published, as is all the email correspondence about each protocol. Adverse incidents are reported to both the FDA and the OTA using the same form when they occur.

Also of critical interest to the genetic engineering community was the creation of two entities. The first is the Gene Transfer Safety Advisory Board, a "nontraditional super-data safety monitoring board,"[10] composed of some RAC and some FDA members, ad hoc consultants, and others as needed to review all data comprehensively that emerges from all CGTR, in order to see larger trends, error patterns, or paradigms and to present these at public RAC meetings.[11] In addition, the government set up what is now a massive database called the Genetic Modification Clinical Research Information System, which contains information on protocols, available online, with some protected and some public access.[12]

Since the 1980s, gene transfer research was established as being among the most heavily regulated of any scientific intervention. All clinical gene transfer research protocols connected with institutions that receive federal funding use the casuistic model at local and national levels, and they have to submit written justification to the national RAC, including responses to these questions:

• What are potential harms and benefits to research subjects?
• How will potential harms and benefits be communicated so they can consent?
• How will selection among research subjects be made?
• How will privacy and confidential be preserved?[13]

In short, recombinant DNA protocols are without a doubt the most heavily regulated arenas of modern medical technology, as Alta Charo notes, and far more regulated than many other arenas, such as fertility clinics or surgical trials.[14]

Many of the current regulations reflect efforts to correct the mistakes that emerged in 1999, when a patient in a Phase I Gene Transfer trial died at the University of Pennsylvania, after a number of errors in such regulation and oversight.[15] The year 1999 marked a tragic turn in gene therapy, for the death of eighteen-year-old Jesse Gelsinger shook both the scientists and the bioethicists who had been overseeing the project, with both groups being sued for negligence by the Gelsinger family. Jesse Gelsinger had a rare metabolic disorder called ornithine transcarbamylase deficiency syndrome (OTCD), in which ammonia builds up to lethal levels in the blood. Babies born with OTCD usually fall into comas soon after birth and suffer brain damage. Half of them die within a month, whereas for other children, the disease is relatively mild, albeit hard to manage. Jesse Gelsinger's milder version of the deficiency was diagnosed when he was two years old, and he managed the condition with a low-protein diet and a regimen of nearly fifty pills a day. Still, he had occasional health crises. When he was seventeen years old, he stopped taking the drugs regularly. One day, his father came home to find him curled up on the couch, vomiting uncontrollably. He had to be intubated and kept in an induced coma until his ammonia levels were brought under control. So, when a doctor told eighteen-year-old Gelsinger, a year later, that a clinical trial for a potential OTCD treatment was in the works, he was very interested, and was flown to Philadelphia—and as an 18 year old, he could consent to the trial himself. It was his first plane trip. Researchers at the University of Pennsylvania in Philadelphia were developing a fix for the *OTC* gene, which produces an enzyme that prevents ammonia buildup. Patients would be injected with working copies of the gene that had been attached to an adenovirus, a type of cold virus. The virus, genetically altered to be harmless, would infect the patients' liver cells and integrate the added gene into their chromosomal DNA.[16]

But Gelsinger had a dramatic reaction. He suddenly became extremely ill, eventually becoming comatose, and needed ICU care and mechanical ventilation. In total organ failure, he was taken off life support, stunning his doctors with the rapidity of his fatal collapse. They at first claimed not to know what had happened. But journalists and federal health officials discovered several troubling lapses in the conduct of the study. For example, the researchers had earlier told the FDA they would tighten up the trial's eligibility criteria, but they never followed through. When two patients suffered serious side effects, the scientists did not immediately inform the agency or put the study on hold as required. It turned out Jesse's pretrial test results showed he had poor liver function, indicating he arguably shouldn't have received the *OTC* gene injection.[17]

But perhaps the most damning were failures in the informed consent process. Researchers hadn't told Gelsinger about the earlier patients' side effects or about two laboratory monkeys killed by high doses of adenoviruses. Wilson was also accused of a conflict of interest: he had a stake in the company that owned the gene transfer technology and stood to benefit if the trial succeeded.[18]

Wilson denied that financial considerations affected the study and said it was impossible to predict that Gelsinger would suffer such a bad reaction. Nevertheless, the Gelsinger family sued, and the university quickly settled for an undisclosed sum while declining to take responsibility for Jesse's death. In January 2000, the FDA suspended human research at Penn's Institute for Human Gene Therapy, and the university eventually shut the program down.[19]

Further research revealed systemic problems in reporting adverse incidents, all of which raised the index of suspicion for the public not only for gene therapy but also for clinical research in general. The FDA and NIH revealed that 691 volunteers had either died or had serious adverse reactions in the seven years just before Gelsinger's death, but only thirty-nine had been reported. This led to increased monitoring, more site inspections, and a new reporting system for serious adverse events. The role of the bioethicists, who were also sued by the parents, came under scrutiny, and new norms prohibited "curbside consults" on cases and the separation of funding for bioethics review and bioscience enterprises. The field also began to focus on the problem of conflict of interest, for both ethicists and researchers, especially since it was more and more common as NIH funding was cut and private foundations became to be the main funding sources for such research. The Gelsinger case deeply troubled the field. Yet, over the next several decades, research continued, with careful reviews—scientific, clinical, and ethical—for each protocol. As many as three different bioethicists were members of the RAC at any given time. From 2013 to 2018, I was one of these members. Definitive scholarly books were written about gene therapy, and to read LeRoy Walters and Julie Gage Palmer's 1997 work, *The Ethics of Gene Therapy*, is to see every subsequent concern of the next thirty years raised and considered carefully. Very little has changed, as you will see, reader, in the ethical analysis since the last 1970s, where much of the philosophical, theological, and ethical apparatus was worked out for medical uses of genetic engineering. Meanwhile, after the passing of more than twenty since Walter and Palmers wrote, the debates continued and were renewed with every new change in technology or method. In particular, even though no real "gene therapy" had been successful in humans, even at the somatic level, and even though bioethicists had taken to writing those words in scare quotes, the idea of unjust or untoward heritable genetic changes continued to be raised as problematic. If, the arguments went, it is ethically permissible, under situations of constraint allowed by the RAC and the Points to Consider, to alter the genes of an individual, then why not alter the genes of embryos or gametes, so that the alteration could be passed on—so-called germline gene therapy. Bioethicists still agreed on two "bright lines" in genetic alteration in humans: first, that it was permissible for therapy but not enhancement; and second, that it was permissible for somatic use in an individual but not for germline use in embryos or gametes. But both of the "bright lines" were getting somewhat murkier. Was correcting for short stature an enhancement or a therapy, for example? What was the point of allowing the selection of embryos with and without specific alleles, such as in Tay–Sachs disease, but not allowing their correction?

In late 1999, the American Association for the Advancement of Science (AAAS) convened a group of theologians, philosophers, bioethicists, legal scholars, and scientists to consider this question of heritability. I was a part of those meetings, which took place over a two-year period, and there was much disagreement about exactly those issue. (Remember, this was prior to CRISPR-Cas9, and yet the bioethicists were told that the viral vectors used for genetic engineering at the time would work efficiently to alter the human genome—a claim that, in retrospect, was not the true.). The two "bright lines" did in fact hold, and a moratorium was called on any heritable gene therapy in humans that has held to the present, despite the remarkable changes in the technology itself, with CRISPR. Of course, the alert reader will know that there was one notable violation by a Dr. He of China in 2018. Dr. He used CRISPR-Cas9 to alter three embryos, a set of twins and a singleton, to knock in genes thought resistant to human immunodeficiency virus infection.

For this, he was universally condemned and served three years in prison in China, which reinforced the seriousness with which the scientific community took the moratorium.

In 1999, while we did not agree on many concepts, the group did agree that four questions needed to be asked about any genetic technology, which I have mentioned in the introduction to this book. These are:

(1) Are there reasons in *principle* why using this technology should be impermissible?

(2) What contextual factors should be taken into account, and do any of these prevent development and use of the technology?

(3) What purposes, techniques or applications would be permissible and under what circumstances?

(4) What procedures, structures, involving what policies, should be used to decide on appropriate techniques and uses?[20]

I tell this long story about the history of regulation because understanding the regulations clearly comprises the third set of facts, along with the history of malaria and the science of gene drives, that are critical to have in place before we consider the question of whether gene drives are indeed ethical. Let me now turn to think about how the foundation of regulatory policy in genetic intervention sets the stage for the current regulatory landscape.

3.2 The Languages of Risk, Benefit, and Precaution

After Mr. Jesse Gelsinger's tragic death in 1999, the arguments against genetic engineering tended to coalesce again around two issues: safety and individual consent. For example, in the National Academies (NASEM) a review about a brand new use of genetic engineering—whether to allow mitochondrial DNA transfer from the eggs cells of one woman to the egg cells of another for the therapeutic purpose of allowing prospective mothers who carried damaged mitochondria to use their own eggs for reproduction—the former "bright line" regulation about not allowing heritable DNA applications was crossed, and this was done because of arguments about parental desire and autonomous requests for the procedure. If it was safe, it was decided, it was a personal decision, a very American solution, based on the principle of autonomy that had become, by then, fundamental to American bioethics.

It had taken another decade for gene therapy to slowly deliver its promise, with the discovery of CARs, TALENs, new and more precise tools for genetic manipulation, and, of course, CRISPR-Cas9 and gRNA. With these new tools, the debates began again, returning to the original arguments of the 1970s. In 2017, the first clinical protocol for the use of CRISPR-Cas9 in humans was sent to the RAC and approved. It was a protocol to treat leukemia, from the University of Pennsylvania, bringing the narrative full circle. Shortly thereafter, despite protests from the field of bioethics, in 2019, the NIH disbanded the RAC, arguing that now that gene therapy was normalized, it should be regulated just like any other clinical trial, with the FDA and a system of IRBs and DSMBs and without special national expertise or oversight. The NIH then set up a new committee that would look at emerging technologies that sought to enter the clinical trial system. Somatic gene transfer protocols, no longer novel or in need of special national review, had become, in the view of the NIH, commonplace. In fact, by 2022, when this book was written, not only had severe combined immunodeficiency due to a defective OTC gene (SCID), Gelsinger's disease, been successfully treated, twenty years after his case had rocked the field, but so had several cases of sickle cell disease, making a strong proof of concept for somatic gene therapy for disease to be actual at last. The techniques are still evolving. The sickle cell treatment required significant funding, a full team of experts, and a sophisticated hospital, little of which is possible to access even for most Black Americans who have the disease, much less the millions in Africa.

Gene research in the USA had focused on human interventions and had carried the optimism and entrepreneurial spirit of its California roots into the clinic. Despite year after year after year of initial failure, the American public largely supported the concept, still trusting in the powerful promises of medical researchers. Agriculture uses of genetic engineering too, initially had the support of the majority of American consumers, most of whom happily munched on genetically altered tomatoes, rice, and breakfast cereal, and whose cows ate GM grain, for decades, despite a steadily growing concern with Monsanto's work that I will address in the next chapter. In the USA, genetically engineered plants are subject to regulation by three federal agencies: the USDA Animal and Plant Health Inspection Service, the Department of Health and Human Services' FDA, and the US EPA, under a plan called "the Co-ordinated Framework" as determined by OSTP in 1986 and amended in 2017. If a major federal action results, there might also be a requirement for public review and consultation under the National Environmental Policy Act.[21]

And, as Charo and others noted, genetic research had, from the time of its birth to the development of CRISPR, been scrutinized by the regulatory gaze on a number of levels. Charo gave an account of the taxonomy of regulation at a meeting called by the NAS in 2018: "Governance of Dual Use Research in the Life Science: Advancing Global Consensus on Research Oversight."[22]

Governance is a layered system, she noted. It is not only understood by considering the actors involved, such as governments, universities, private sector bodies, and the public as consumers or critics, it can also be understood by looking at the different regulatory issues, such as intellectual property rights, public information, food health and safety, and consumer choices. Different legal, economic, or educational challenges offer different paths to regulation. Citing the work of Robert Paarlberg, who created a taxonomy of regulations along a spectrum from promoted through permitted to prohibited, which itself is drawn from older theological and philosophical norms for moral action, she noted that such regulations allow a range of complex responses to any given intervention.[23] This creates, noted Charo, an "ecosystem" for research, in which formal legal instruments regulate some actions, marketplace constraints others, and academic norms still others. Science self-governance, as we have seen, journal policies, and funding priorities also shape the terrain. Finally, Charo pointed out that research has patterns that define its progress, and that regulations and norms exist at every stage, from initial conceptual planning, through funding, operational conduct, and the dissemination of results, to the final phases of translation into technology licensing.[24]

Charo's argument describes how complexly genetic research is regulated, including its initial and continuing impulse to self-regulation. We will see how this impulse is a part of gene drive research, as scientists undertook a number of pledges promising to abide by norms as the research proceeded, just as they had done since Asilomar.

To understand this ecosystem it is useful to turn to the seminal work of Helen Longino, a philosopher of science known for her 1990 work on values and objectivity in research.[25] Genetic research would of course be deeply affected by conceptual framing and value-laden decisions, she notes, but it could and would also be subject to some external standards for regulation, which would be the measure of any self-regulatory capacity. Longino articulated four criteria for criticism that a scientific community must ensure to be valid. First, there had to be shared avenues for criticism, including scientific journals, conferences, and the peer review process. Second, there had to be shared standards for criticism. These are the values of what counts as good science, she argues—such as fruitfulness, truth, and consistency. Third, researchers had to demonstrate responsiveness to criticisms. Grants are awarded; textbooks are adapted according to criticism. So, this requires the community also to be aware of what is happening in the critical conversation. Finally, there had to be a system of shared respect for qualified authorities. All authorities and voices that are qualified must be able to participate in science. To allow only some voices, argued Longino, anticipating the fundamental need for expanding the conversation far beyond a small room at a California conference center, will lead to a lack of crucial insight.[26]

In the next section of this chapter, I will turn to the question of how this history of regulation led to current policies about gene drives. But first, I will consider another feature of the debate and another aspect of the history of regulation: its globalization. For the discussions about genetics in Europe took a somewhat different turn, and thus the regulations reflected a certain wariness about agricultural and animal uses of genetic technology. Let me turn to one particular aspect of that debate: the precautionary principle.

The Discussion as Global

European discussion about the regulation of genetic research followed close on the heels of the American model, with one exception. A principle was entered into the bioethics debate about genetic alteration in addition to autonomy, justice, beneficence, and non-maleficence. It was the principle of precaution, long a part of the European tradition in ethics—a principle developed in the environmentalist's debates about the safety of extraction processes that might threaten fragile ecosystems.[27]

The discussion of the principle of precaution is so fundamental to the next part of our story that I will turn to it in some detail at this juncture. It is a central part not only of scientific norms in many areas of research, also of the EU Treaty: "The precautionary principle is detailed in Article 191 of the Treaty on the Functioning of the European Union (TFEU). It relates to an approach to risk management whereby if there is the possibility that a given policy or action might cause harm to the public or the environment and if there is still no scientific consensus on the issue, the policy or action in question should not be pursued. Once more scientific information becomes available, the situation should be reviewed."[28] The first use of the precautionary principle was made in 1992 at the UN Summit on Environment and Development (the "Rio Declaration").

Principle 15 of the Rio Declaration on Environment and Development, adopted by the UN Conference on Environment and Development in Rio de Janeiro, Brazil, 1992, states that: "In order to protect the environment, the precautionary approach shall be widely applied by States according to their capabilities. Where there are threats of serious or irreversible damage, lack of full scientific certainty shall not be used as a reason for postponing cost-effective measures to prevent environmental degradation."[29] In other words, in this understanding of the precautionary principle, it was intended to protect the public when, for example, extraction companies wanted to create a large project—mining, say, or oil drilling—and environmentalist and community members were concerned that that might despoil the environment. The environmentalists could not exactly prove scientifically all the details of how harm might result, but the precautionary principle said that they did not have to—because full scientific proof was not needed if the threat was serious, even in the face of uncertainty. Thus, some action had to be taken: either the project had to be stopped until they could prove their extraction completely safe, or companies had to protect in advance against any damage they might (or might not) cause.

By 2000, the EU Commission solidified the principle, in the words of the Commission, as "better safe than sorry." Necessary in situations where is "incomplete information, inconclusive evidence, or public controversy over the appropriate response to hazardous substances or activities . . . regulatory intervention may still be legitimate even if the supporting evidence is incomplete or speculative and the economic costs of regulation are high."[30] This double concept meant that a new principle could both block processes or technologies that carried any risk of harm and enact protective provisions, even if these had not been fully tested, establishing two separate standards of evidence. Further, the EU Commission added: "Recourse to the precautionary principle presupposes that potentially dangerous effects deriving from a phenomena, product, or process have been identified, and that scientific evaluation does not allow the risk to be determined with sufficient certainty."[31]

The precautionary principle (or precautionary approach) generally defines actions on issues considered to be uncertain, for instance those applied in assessing risk management.[32] The principle is used by policy makers to justify discretionary decisions in situations where there is the possibility of harm from making a certain decision (e.g., taking a particular course of action) when extensive scientific knowledge on the matter is lacking. The principle implies that there is a social responsibility to protect the public from exposure to harm when scientific investigation has found a plausible risk at any level. These protections can be relaxed only if further scientific findings emerge that provide sound evidence that no harm will result, or in some cases, where a lower level of protection is found to be sufficient, or when social views about risk and uncertainty change significantly.[33]

In some legal systems, as in laws of the EU, the application of the precautionary principle has been made a statutory requirement in some areas of law; in others, it is simply part of the assumed equipment of regulation. The principle that the WHO, too, sums up as "look before you leap" stresses that as science becomes increasingly complex and outcomes increasingly uncertain, it is better to avoid a change, especially one that could be permanent. Intended initially rather narrowly as a way to allow protective innovation before a complete data set was in place to justify it, it is now a feature in both genetic and nongenetic interventions across a wide array of topics and new technologies. It is a central feature of the Cartagena Protocol, which is concerned with species diversity, as this summary of the law notes: "The Cartagena protocol to the 1993 Convention on Biological Diversity (see summary) is based on the precautionary principle. It aims to prevent any harm to biological diversity when living modified organisms are transferred, handled or used, especially across borders (Regulation (EC) No 1946/2003—see summary). It takes into account risks to human health. The Council decision gives the EU's legal approval to the protocol."[34] The term appears in the EU Community Treaty where "Article 174 of the EU Community Treaty provides that all Community Policy on the environment shall be based on the precautionary principle."[35] In December 2000, the Nice European Council meeting that approved the Declaration on the Future of the EU extended it to all health and safety policy. Many American philosophers (included this author) saw serious problems with the principle, however.

Frank Cross, writing about the problems with the principle in a legal sense,[36] pointed out that the premise of asymmetry of consequences implied by the principle—the classic formulation that a false negative could cost lives, whereas a false positive would have only economic consequences—was asserted without proof and was likely wrong. "The truly fatal flaw of the precautionary principle," he argued, "is the unsupported presumption that an action aimed at public health protection cannot possibly have negative effects on public health . . . Because the precautionary principle counsels for action even against those uncertain hazards that might be nonexistent, the presence of real health effects consequent to the action will often cause more harm than good."[37]

H. Tristram Engelhardt, Jr., and Fabrice Jotterand also objected, pointing out that economic reasons sometimes have profound public health effects, so that positing health against economies is a false dichotomy. Those who have defended the precautionary principle in the past have focused upon the dangers of a narrow range of technological development, for example, arguing that industrial plants which released sulfur dioxide and nitrogen oxides into the atmosphere, combined with oxygen and water, to fall as sulfuric nitric, which led to what was called acid rain, which left unchecked, turned out to threaten the health of forests. According to Engelhardt and Jotterand, people have, however, ignored considerable information showing that many other new technologies have prevented significant catastrophes around the world, for example by helping people who would otherwise starve or die of diseases. They conclude that it is plausible to use the precautionary principle to forge ahead with technological development, business interests, and biotechnology.[38]

Bioethicist Loretta Kopelman worried that "the precautionary principle was introduced by people favoring proof of safety to human health and environment before adopting new technologies." She pointed out that new technologies might cause irreparable harm and defended the commonsense approach of "look before you leap." Typically, the private sector makes the profits, she argued, leaving it up to the public to face the damaging consequences of too hastily introduced new technologies and to pick up the costs of restoration or repair. Environmentalists claim that if nations had waited for clear proof that acid rain was destroying forests, the forests would have been lost. One area of dispute concerns whether or when the shift in the burden of proof is politically motivated. The precautionary principle calls for more studies to resolve questions regarding new technologies, policies, or other issues. Critics claim that advocates of the precautionary principle may be trying to use it as a ploy to attack capitalization, globalization, and technological advancements, as well as to set up trade barriers or otherwise advance people's own self-interests on politically divisive issues.[39]

The House of Lords, writing from the UK in their report on GM insects, offered this critique of the regulatory regent, including the principle:

> The EU regulatory regime does not take into account the benefits of a technology: regulation is entirely on the basis of risk. Any rational approach to deciding whether or not to pursue a given technology should include an assessment of its net benefits. At the moment, moreover, no consideration is given to the risks of alternatives to the GM application. A potential new GM insect technology to reduce an agricultural pest population, for example, would not be compared alongside the insecticide currently used to tackle the pest. As such GMOs are effectively considered against an idealized, risk-free alternative. For many GM insect technologies, the alternative may present a number of risks and problems and in many cases, such risks and problems may be the imperative behind the development of GM insect technology in the first place. Considerations of the benefits of a technology and acknowledgements of the control methods currently in use, should be incorporated into the regulatory regime in order to address this illogical situation.[40]

Finally, some question the "look before you leap" and "better safe than sorry" folk wisdom that seems to define the principle. What is the standard of judgment of complete knowledge, and how is that different from scientific risk assessment?

However, it is perhaps too facile to reject the precautionary principle as muddled philosophy or to make a dramatic distinction between European and American ideas of precaution. Arguing these points in a series of influential articles about the complexity of the principle, Jonathan Weiner noted that while the principle has a three-decades-long history and is so widely adopted that it "is ripening into an enforceable norm of customary international law, a kind of legal doctrine of which no nation can dissent,"[41] it is more complex. Weiner believes that the concept that the USA is hostile to precaution, waiting instead for evidence of actual risk, proven scientifically, and Europe welcoming, seeking to prevent harms by informal decision making unfettered by science, is incorrect both descriptively and normatively:

> In a world of multiple risks, the reality is more complicated. First, although precaution can be warranted, it is not universally desirable. Sometimes it is for the best, but sometimes precautionary regulation is too costly, and sometimes—given multiple risks—precaution can even yield a perverse net increase in overall risk. Context is crucial. And different versions of the PP imply different outcomes, some

superior to others. Second, when multiple risks are examined, it becomes clear that Europe is not more precautionary than the US across the board; sometimes Europe does take a more precautionary stance than the US, but sometimes the roles are reversed and the US is the more precautionary regulator. Again, context is crucial. Ultimately, the PP offers important insights but remains too simplistic for a complex multi-risk world.[42]

Weiner describes at least three different versions of the principle. The first, "uncertainty does not justify inaction," is the most straightforward. It makes it clear that imperfect knowledge should not stop our action to block risk, and that it is better to act preventively, before deaths occur. So, science needs to become involved to establish the nature of the risk. A second version is more "aggressive." Here, preventative action is impelled by uncertainty. Some regulatory action is needed, even if a "clear cause and effect relationship cannot be established, because such relationships are never "fully" or "conclusively" established." The final version of the principle of precaution is "even more adamant," for it shifts the burden of proof to the proponent of the activity and forbids the potentially risky activity until it can be conclusively proven to be safe.[43] Then, there is the problem of setting standards for harm, the complexities of what state action to take, and, above all, balancing the risk of false negatives (allowing some risk and causing harm) and false positives (prohibiting some things and overregulating.) Finally, in the real world, regulators have to consider multiple risks all at the same time, some of which are connected, some of which are tangential, and all of which may create latent harms across the timescale it takes to sort all of this out. His final point is of particular interest as one considers all the factors that surround interventions for malaria, for example.

One serious problem with precaution as a principle is its basic underlying moral claim, which is that the status quo is to be protected and that the wrong act would be one that changes the status quo. This of course is problematic on two counts. First, it bootlegs in an account of natural law that assumes the moral goodness, and perhaps the purity, of an abstracted "nature." Let me expand on this. Natural law, an important feature of Catholic moral theology, as in the work of Thomas Aquinas, is largely based on the theory of Aristotle's ethics. Aquinas argues for the essential goodness of God's creation, with creatures acting in accordance with their natures. The natural world is Edenic, pure, only brought to ruin by sinfulness, and since, citing Aristotle, he says "nature does nothing in vain,"[44] the order of the world also teaches us the values of the world. All rational humans, in this view, inherit an internal moral law, a set a moral rules, that, indeed, for Immanuel Kant, are one of the proofs of God's existence, as ordered and obvious as the order of the stars and planets. But we know that many critical values are in fact not at all universal, or obvious, just as we have come to see and understand the non-Edenic nature of the natural world in an era of COVID-19.

Second, and of particular importance, it ignores the ethical horror of our present situation. No ethicist would permit a technology whose outcome leads to the death of a child every two minutes. Yet, this is our present situation, living under the burden of malaria, and it would seem that needing to wait until every outcome can be made "safe" raises the question: Safe for whom? How safe is our present situation for vulnerable populations that may desperately need the intervention and would be willing to forego some other good to have it? This question turns our attention not only to justice considerations but also to one of the central problems of regulation: What is the warrant for judgment and enforcement? Who makes and who enforces this judgment?

Finally, it is true of course that some unknown terrible consequence could happen as a result of any human gesture at all. But humans are fated always to live in the grip of time. Thus, there is no place in which our actions are morally neutral. If the precautionary principle is to have any validity, it would need to be applied to our present situation as well as to imagined futures. Every single action in which we choose and partake is an action against an unknown horizon. There is no perfect knowledge. It the case of malaria, "we" are surely not "better safe" unless the "we" in question excludes African and Asian people who live with the daily threat of a malarial death.

We live, it is true, in a condition of uncertainty, precarity, and contingency, and yet we must act. By prohibiting technology, regulators also risk harm, and they set in place a nearly impossible epistemic quandary: How can we know the future consequence or either action, leaping or standing there, looking. I will return to this important issue in my final chapter where I will give you a more extended philosophical account. But let me bookmark it here, without such a principle, most American regulatory bodies turn to the idea of risk and benefit. But because the risks are unknown, this approach presents challenges as well. I will explore this problem of uncertainty in my final chapter as well.

However, until 2014, as I have noted above, genetic engineering was really focused on first-in-human medical interventions on individual patients, often patients with single-allele rare mutations that offered a ready target for gene therapy, such as SCID, or muscular dystrophies, or it was targeted toward making alterations and adaptations of crops for agriculture, such as making tomatoes that resisted frost by adding an arctic fish (flounder) (ATP) gene to resist ice crystallization or altering crops to protect them from harmful pests, or to alter herbicide tolerance.[45] In both of these situations, the way to ensure safety was to tighten all possible restraints where the work was done, and all possible rules were put in place to ensure that genetic alteration was contained. Remember, the first agreements at Asilomar required BSL-4 laboratories. In personal medicine, care was taken to isolate genetic changes away from gametes. But gene drives are intended to do the opposite—they are intended, eventually, to spread as widely as possible.

3.3   Gene Drives under the Regulatory Microscope

Now that I have reviewed a very brief history of the regulation of genetic intervention, and you, reader, have had an opportunity to see how carefully it has been considered over the last forty years, I will explore, in the next section, the interesting phenomena of the robust regulation process that surrounds gene drive technology, including the Target Malaria project, all of which has begun with eagerness and earnestness and become widespread, long, long in advance of the project's instantiation, and perhaps even before researchers could know whether it would work. As one body after another met—sometimes governmental, sometimes based in ad hoc, self-organized, private groups, sometimes foundation funded, sometimes just academic scientists self-organizing as they did at Asilomar—all of the groups had similarities in their epistemic and normative project, despite their constitution or funding. They considered the new ideas about gene drives, they worried about the concept of nature, and they erected structures of moral norms long in advance of any actual science. It was argued, in each forum, that it was critical to do so at the very earliest point in the process, which is an important and defensible point to be sure, but once again, you will see that most of the elaborate structures focused on the same issue: safety.

Target Malaria was concerned about that issue as well. What would the implications of a genetically altered mosquito be on a place and its people? In the first years of the project, Target Malaria sought experts who could suggest ways of thinking about risk. Risk assessment was already an integral part of internal regulatory structures based on the Cartagena Protocol on

Biosafety, and was required. Thus, the project turned first to the Australian National Academies of Science and the Commonwealth Scientific and Industrial Research Organization (CSIRO) for guidance. CSIRO is an independent Australian federal government agency responsible for scientific research with expertise in environmental impact studies. This was a proactive step, and indeed, it would become part of the regulations later suggested by every organization that sought to regulate gene drive research. To be certain, the risk assessment was limited to the first phase of the sterile male mosquito release, but since this method forms a great deal of the language of regulatory standards that were created later, I will turn to an evaluation of this report as an example of how risk assessment is done.

Next, Target Malaria went to their African stakeholders to listen and collect the local and state communities' concerns about the staged field release, starting with the sterile male release, to identify risk assessment endpoints.

The community subsequently identified four human health concerns and five environmental concerns that were deemed to have plausible adverse outcome pathways:

(1) The probability that the dominant sterile male (DSM) construct will increase the vectorial capacity of female mosquitoes for three pathogens (*P. falciparum*, o'nyong'nyong virus, and filariasis, relative to wild type mosquitoes).

(2) The probability that incidentally released female genetically altered mosquitoes will be a vector for some novel pathogen.

(3) A longer-term survival of genetically altered mosquitoes both for incidentally released females and for genetically altered males.

(4) The probability that DSM mosquitoes will spread and persist in wild type anophelines.

(5) The probability that DSM mosquitoes will make female genetically altered mosquitoes more resistant to the insecticide used in Bana village in the Kou Valley.[46]

The CSIRO noted that the insectary in Burkina Faso had been set up close to the village of Bana, one of the study sites, and it was to that insectary that the genetically altered mosquito eggs had been sent under an Burkina Faso import permit for transporting the GM eggs and a second national permit from Burkina Faso for their contained use and rearing. The insectary had successfully backcrossed the transgenic mosquitoes with local wild-type strains—the mosquitoes were *Anopheles coluzzii,* and the final strain to be released had this wild-type genetic background. In Bana, female *A. gambiae* s.l. account for 77.8 percent of all samples, and male *gambiae* account for 21.4 percent, with numbers peaking in September and October at the end of the wet season that lasts from May to October and with numbers of mosquitoes ranging seasonally from 500,000 to 10,000 in the target area. And while the number of DSM would be far less, there were several technical steps that had to be defined, regulated, and stipulated in the report. First, the project had to be sure that it was releasing males and not females. Mosquitoes, prior to release, have to be sorted by sex, and it impossible to avoid accidental mistake. (Think for a moment of the difficulty of even that one task.) But the Project was committed to a limit of a 5 out of 1,000 error rate, and so far, they had been able to maintain that standard, which was confirmed in subsequent analysis. Given that, and comparing the population to wild-type populations, the CSIRO risk assessment determined that there would be a 70 percent chance that the genetic mosquitoes would be *less likely* to transmit *P. falciparum* and o'nyong'nyong virus, and a 90 percent chance that they would be *less likely* transmit filariasis. The second goal was about the likelihood of accidental, catastrophic release. Here the CSIRO advised that the likelihood of accidental release is between 0.03 and 0.05, and likelihood of them transmitting a new pathogen is 1.3×10^{-8} (less than one in a million). Finally, they anticipated that mosquitoes would persist at the most for sixty-five days (including accidentally released females) and ten days (for males only), and that the probability that the construct would persist was 8.87×10^{-4} to 1.96×10^{-3}. And finally, testing of the colonies revealed empirically that mosquitoes with this construct have the same or higher susceptibility to insecticides, just in case of any unforeseen error.

Would the model hold when it was tested in the field? The project had written the plan long in advance, years prior to implementation. They could not be known until the release, which had been planned for the summer of 2019, three years after the report was completed. Of course, COVID-19 slowed but ultimately did not stop the process. And the sterile male release indeed turned out as planned.

Computational models surely do not promise that risks can be entirely avoided. They cannot. However, the use of complex regulations to try to anticipate all risks has its own intricate ethical challenges as well. The risk assessment statement and the project plan were just the beginning. There would be a complex set of new regulations that would unfold as the project became more widely understood.

3.4 The Regulatory Imaginary

As we have seen, an elegant regulatory and bioethical structure has long been in place for human clinical trials of genetic alterations. However, there was far less structure, and far fewer norms, for the agricultural use of genetic alterations in plants and animals, and the rules that existed were largely on containment and efficacy. In the case of animal research, the focus is largely on avoiding animal suffering and, in a few cases, a concern about the status of chimeric animals. But no norms or structures had been anticipated for the use of a genetic alteration whose entire intent was to spread in the wild as widely and durably as possible and of course perhaps, affecting unknown numbers of plants and animals in unknown and, to some extent, unknowable ways. Even the widespread spray campaigns, which of course, also affected entire ecosystems, started out as interventions that were always held directly in the hands of public health authorities or troops, placed wall by wall, stream by stream, field by field.

Thus, the assessment of gene drives to eliminate malaria was immediately of interest, not only to the academic scientific community but also to government commissions, who, by 2015, had a history of commenting on science, especially where there would be the sort of far-reaching economic impact that a gene drive for malaria control promises. Internationally, as news of gene drives began to emerge, several important regulatory commissions were immediately formed and began to convene, some quite consciously modeling themselves after Asilomar but with televised testimony and multiple meetings. Reading the reports ex post facto, one can see the broad similarities between the meeting in 1973 and those in 2015. Unlike Asilomar, nearly all of the commissions and ad hoc groups include a wider array of experts in the discussion. Sensitive to issues of ethics, they hear testimony on that topic.

However, many of the initial gatherings had some epistemic lacuna. The meetings were similar in design, in that they constructed an imaginary, in which the research does not begin with nor seriously confront any of the realities of the African context in which the drive is intended or the background of malaria, its history, and its record of spectacular failures. Many of the attendees wrote articles carefully and seriously suggested measures that were already in place in the work of Target Malaria, including its iterative approach, its community engagement, and its risk assessment apparatus, all of which the authors were unaware. Some ignored fundamental realities of work with insects, an odd echo of Ross's confusion. Like many such efforts, the reports were speculative, based on concerns that they must imagine, and anxieties about what might occur and then imagining how to avoid imagined outcomes with regulatory protections set up in advance—a difficult and speculative project.

To critique is surely not to say that the efforts were in vain. On the contrary, they were extremely important because they sincerely expressed a desire to work to make science safe, and they had several substantial ideas about how to do so. There is something hopeful and poignant about such regulatory imaginaries. They recall the detailed plans laid in advance of World War I, in which each alternative was carefully spelled out only to face completely different conditions in the real world. And for a generation of bioethicists and regulators, who had been saying and writing that it was important to be consulted *prior* to the use of controversial technologies, it was exactly what we in our discipline had been asking for. The process was important because ethicists complained that we were usually not brought in for comment until after the technology was in place, too late with our objections, which were unable to be addressed after the fact. Thus, we saw that it was a very good opportunity to try to ensure that best practices could, in advance, make the research on gene drives ethical from the beginning. This has largely taken the form of gatherings of experts, sometimes governmental and public; sometimes of foundations, self-appointed, in private; sometimes of groups of scientists alone; sometimes with a wide group of disciplines; sometimes with activists; sometimes without.

There have been meetings, gatherings, and reports about gene drives from 1991(WHO); 2009 (WHO) and a flurry in 2025, until [47] to today, and as I write in 2023, while researchers are still at the very beginning of this project and far from any deployment, I anticipate that by the time this book is published, such meetings and such reports will continue.[48] For the purposes of my discussion, however, I am going to discuss only three reports, after making a note about the report that emerged from an early group of scientists at a meeting convened by Kevin Esvelt and others. These three reports, I would argue, are the three most important regulatory projects. One is from a scientific working group made up of members from Burkina Faso, Durbin, Mali, Canada, the USA, Kenya, Tanzania, Scotland, England, and South Africa. One is the NASEM report, "Gene Drives on the Horizon." The third is the report on gene drives from the African Union, arguably the most important perspective on the topic, since it is the people from that continent who are most affected by malaria and who are most likely to bear both the burdens and benefits on the use of gene drives.

The Report from the Scientist Working Group

Before I discuss those three reports, let me begin by describing a very early report, most like Asilomar, convened by Keven Esvelt. Esvelt's call for caution and his commitment to convening was one of the many efforts to understand and regulate gene drives between 2016 and 2018. This report, which was one of the very first, is also the one that represents scientific self-governance in a traditional form: a small group of insider scientists, themselves concerned about the implications of their work, figuring out the methods and criteria for a new research enterprise. A later article by James et al., who participated, highlighted the considerations that ought to be involved in the planning of any deployment of a gene drive:

(1) Establish a team with appropriate expertise and experience

(2) Develop/refine the target product profile and criteria for advancement

(3) Conduct modeling to inform experimental study design and understand potential benefits

(4) Develop processes for information and data sharing to promote transparency

(5) Establish partnerships as necessary

(6) Characterize the field testing site (ecology, vector and clinical)

(7) Undertake environmental risk and biosafety assessments

(8) Address ethical issues

(9) Plan for and conduct stakeholder engagement at multiple levels

(10) Plan for and meet regulatory requirements

(11) Design remediation/mitigation plans.[49,50]

What is interesting is that these eleven steps are drawn directly from any standard health and safety environmental checklist. These emerge from another regulatory system, not from genetic regulation. What is distinctive is

the emphasis on community engagement (step 9) and community partnerships (step 5). The report goes on to define what is meant by community—
the people directly affected by the gene drive as opposed to communities of
interest who live far from both the problem of malaria and the effects of the
intervention.

For this project, they argued, transparency is key: "The working group
members noted that development of gene drive technology carries an obligation for transparency and accountability. This is important for earning public
confidence, ensuring that the product meets stakeholder needs, encouraging
inter-project coordination necessary for responsible field testing, and mini-
mizing any risks to human health or the environment. Gene drive researchers should commit to being appropriately[51] transparent about their work."[52]
Like all of the groups interested in advising regulations, the Scientist Working Group called for a standard pathway to deployment—as is being done,
as we saw in the last chapter, by Target Malaria, beginning with laboratory
studies and modeling and moving on to large cages and then to small-scale
and large-scale releases with surveillance. For the section on ethics, the group
largely discusses the need for safety and consent: after a process of community
engagement, "practices undertaken to inform such persons about the project
and to understand, respond to, and learn from their perceptions and reaction
in a way that makes it clear their opinions have influence."[53] They also suggest
the formation of an independent ethics advisory committee, in addition to
the ethical oversight provided by countries, and IRBs, a committee made up
of both ethics experts external to the project and in-country experts to advise
on their projects throughout the research and field testing trajectory.

The report ends with the key points for implementation of a gene drive as
a comprehensive public health tool and a scientist's pledge to follow all the
recommendations, in every country in which they work. Because a drive will
be, if successful, steadily broadened to include entire regions, it will need to
be evaluated in different climatic, geographical, and social areas and be part
of a national and cross-border effect that uses all the tools—bed nets, spraying, vaccines, larvicide, swamp reduction, better housing, and ACT. The plan
also raises the issue of how the mosquitoes would be "created" and distributed if gene drives are massively implemented, and it ends with a comprehensive and highly technical call for a surveillance plan.

But soon, the scientists would be joined by others, and as we will see, the
science became a matter for the state to consider and regulate. What follows
is a review of some representative policies and their rationales.

The House of Lords

The House of Lords, under whose general British jurisdiction the Austin Burt laboratory worked also invited Burt and others to give testimony there in November of 2015 about what they saw as "British science", noting that since Ross, the UK had been a leader in research on tropical diseases. They wrote a document in advance of what they perceived as the problematic views of the EU and their precautionary principle, which I quoted above. After noting that GM technologies are not a panacea and that there are one of a number of experimental techniques and already existing ways to combat malaria, they state: "Despite inevitable uncertainties, we conclude that GM insect technologies should be afforded an opportunity to play a complementary role in helping to meet the global challenges of disease control and food security."[54] First, they mention that the UK is the leader in the field, not only due to Burt and Crisanti and others, but also a for-profit company, Oxitec, which distributes sterile Aedes male mosquitoes for control of other diseases. But they worried, in their report, that their new research could be blocked by over-regulation: "Unfortunately, we are very concerned that the benefits offered by GM insects may not be realized. The EU regulatory regime for genetically modified organisms [GMOs] is not functioning effectively. Although no EU-level GM insect applications have been received to date, the regime has seen many applications for GM crops. In these cases, the regime is failing lamentably."[55] Like all of the other commissions that would look at the issue, the House of Lords invited public comment. But despite the strong anti-GMO NGOs in London, none came to protest or participate. It was a pattern that would be repeated. "We note our surprise and regret that individuals and groups who are sceptical of the merits of GM technologies did not engage with our inquiry. No written submissions were received from groups known for their concerns about GM, and there was seemingly little appetite from them to give oral evidence to us. There was, of course, no obligation on this community to engage with our inquiry, Nevertheless, it was puzzling that they did not wish for their voices to be heard.[56] Nevertheless, the House of Lords report set their own restrictions on gene drive technologies. The report set out three principles (taken from a Pirbright Institute report[57]) that would limit the target of the drive to:

(1) One species of insect that is exclusively or almost exclusively responsible for transmission, because the technique only directly affects the target species.

(2) The insect can be readily reared and mass-reared in captivity.

(3) Only one sex is responsible for the impact of the insect species.[58]

The third caveat is intended to make sure that insects that cause disease by blood exchange—*Aedes*, anopheline mosquitoes, sandflies, and ticks—can be eliminated but that those insects that primarily infect or eat agricultural crops would not be a target in the hope of limiting the use of gene drives to insects that cause fatal illness. The first requirement may be difficult to uphold if the target is a highly conserved gene such as *doublesex*, for it would be available in many insect species and could potentially be affected by a drive in a neighboring species. As early as 2003, Burt and Trivers raised the problem of horizontal transfer. This unanswered question is of course key to serious ecological concerns and needs careful research. It may or may not be a rate-limiting step. The second requirement is logical: for all studies are done in the laboratory settings.[59]

Again and again, the Lords express concern that lack of leadership at the international level and EU regulation of GMOs will keep the technologies from the people and countries who need it most and whose suffering under a "catastrophic disease burden"[60] is most acute. In the void left by the lack of leadership, they suggest the UK government, "in light of its strong commitment to international development," take the leadership role.

They note a central problem—all current regulatory schemes rest on one assumption—that the goal for regulation is containment, using biological, temporal, or geographic methods. Yet, gene drives are the very opposite of containment—they fail unless they spread and persist. Thus, new sorts of conversation would need to take place. In the opinion of the Lords, this will be difficult if not impossible with the precautionary principle in place. One idea, they noted, was to place risks in a different category from benefits. Benefits should not be weighed against risks but rather against non-benefits (the term I would suggest here is "benefits and harms," which, the Lords are correct, is different from risks.)

The Lords noted eight anxieties that were brought to their attention:

• Horizontal gene transfer within the environment [as discussed above];

• Potential impact on ecosystems;

• Effects on predator/prey relationships and the food chain;

• Evolution of more virulent strains of particular pathogens following GM control;

- A general feeling that GMOs are unsafe and create risks for individuals and the environment;
- The potential for unknown and unintended consequences;
- Questions about intellectual property, patenting and excessive corporate involvement; and
- Lack of confidence in scientists, companies, and governments to understand and appropriately regulate the myriad possible implications of GMOs.[61]

The report ended by thinking about applications, not only for malaria but also for dengue, "the world's fastest growing disease . . . half the world's population is now at risk."[62] In general, this report is the one with the strongest approbation of gene drive technologies, welcoming them into the general struggle against vector control, foregrounding the problem of malaria and other diseases, and, not tangentially, noting the potential for an enormous new market for the technology, a market led by British scientists.

The NASEM's "Gene Drives on the Horizon"

The Americans had followed the debates closely as well and did not miss the significance of that final point—convening an expert panel to consider gene drive research and technology. While in theory, National Academy Reports are guidance documents intended to influence regulations, they are generally understood as having normative authority, setting standards across a broad range of research projects. To a large extent, the NASEM report is the largest and most comprehensive of any of the regulatory projects thus far, even though it was one of the first, and it covers the wide range of science, existing regulations, concerns, and proposals in the field. Their meetings are where Austin Burt, Kevin Esvelt, and others made formal presentations in Washington, DC, which I described in the last chapter of this book, all of which were videotaped and placed on a website for continuous viewing.[63] One can also download the PowerPoint slides to see firsthand the pictures of a gene drive modeled in little mosquitoes or little mice. Additionally, after the meetings, NASEM wrote a 271-page report, which is also publicly available and can be downloaded or ordered by mail for free.[64] It is the report to which others refer, and it has already, by 2023, achieved nearly canonical status. First noting the historical course of research that discovered gene drives in nature, the committee describes why the matter of gene drives now had some urgency: "Preliminary evidence suggests that gene drives developed in the laboratory with CRISPR-Cas9 could spread a targeted gene though nearly 100% of a given population of yeast, fruit flies, or mosquitos."[65] The report notes that research on the molecular biology of gene drives has outpaced research on population genetics and ecosystem dynamics, and it calls for more research to learn if the fitness of GMOs is stronger or weaker than wild-type ones, how steady the conversion rates are, how to describe gene flow between different populations of the target species, and the persistent question of horizontal gene transfer. The authors raise the same questions as their predecessors did at Asilomar: Will it be safe? Will it be effective? Will it have unintended consequences? Do we know enough to release into the wild? Who decides? Many of the questions were about ecology: What species fill the gap created by eliminating a species from its ecological niche? How would resistance work?

The authors attempt to defend their choice of the term "public values" in a section called Charting Human Values, but the content of the argument returns to the same questions: What are the benefits and harms to people? What are the harms to the environment? And who will decide? At stake in the report is that many drives have been conceived, they note, to solve difficult problems—for example non-native rodents on an island that are destroying native species, or malarial mosquitoes in villages out of the range of campaigns—and thus many of the alternative solutions (pesticides, etc.) are actually more harmful than a gene drive appeared to be. The report is honest about the limits of knowledge, calling again and again for more research, in particular for research on ecologies. Yet, the authors are deeply aware of the enormity of the public health benefits of the concept of gene drives. For malaria alone, not to mention the problem of dengue fever, for which there is no curative agent, it has the potential to save close to half a million lives a year. In addition, the report also advocates for the value of basic research, even without its translation implications:

> The capacity of research on gene drives to foster advances in science and technology might be considered valuable for a more immediate and less tangible reason. It may be rooted, to some degree, in an intrinsic value sometimes given to knowledge, understanding and innovation. To possess knowledge is to have a belief that is not only true but justified by evidence and reason. To gain understanding is to develop an overall picture of the thing one understands, putting different pieces of knowledge together and critically reflecting on their relationship to each other. Innovation is valuable in good part, of course because it often leads to economic benefits, but it may also be valued in itself . . . Finding intrinsic value in knowledge is also very much a part of the tradition of science.[66]

The report discusses harms and also the problem of dual use, although it suggests that all research can involve gain of function. Much more time is given to the problem of the harm to what they call an "intrinsic value of nature." Thus, in the report, the authors note the long history of arguments about the term nature and consider how human participation as beings with agency who both live within nature and can alter it have been considered. However the report, while noting that there are competing values at stake, explicitly does not "side with any particular way of understanding these issues."

The report, unlike many regulatory projects, raises explicit concerns about justice, and although it does not suggest an answer to how to make the research just, or the implementation of the eventual technology just, it surely raises the question of justice in a way that is striking in a scientific report:

> Questions of justice differ from questions about potential benefits and harms in that they are more about who than what. They are about who would be affected by the benefits and harms, who will be able to conduct research into gene drive technologies and study the release of gene drive modified organism, and who will make the decision about whether to pursue the benefits and risk the potential harms. They are questions about the distribution of potential benefits and harms, about liberty, about the nature of legitimate decisions making for matters affecting the public. They are about how communities and nations are affected by gene drive technologies, the ability of scientists and funders to undertake the research and the relationship of citizens to nations and of nations to each other.[67]

The report makes the obvious observation that the funding for gene drive research and much of the expertise comes from the wealthier West (Gates, Tata) but that the burdens for the research—and potentially the benefits—will all occur in poorer nations, and that these nations will live with the consequences forever. There is no discussion about what theory of justice it would be best to use under these conditions. The implied theory is of course utilitarianism. The report explicitly rules out the possibility of a "strategy" to resolve injustice, but instead suggests that full community engagement will lead to the best results, offering if not a just distribution plan then a plan for procedural justice.

Like their plan to empower communities to create a procedure for the just distribution of the goods and the harms of the research, the authors of the report similarly turn to "empowered communities" for the best way to deal both with uncertainty and with the unease felt about "human power over nature" which is mentioned in the report. It is this point that the report offers some hint of who, until now not identified, is raising these concerns. It is the "existing scholarly commentary."[68] And here, the alert reader ought to pause, for it is clear that the "existing scholarly commentary" to which this refers is the entirely Western (even American) bioethics scholarship. This commentary is "in agreement" that gene drives might have broader environmental harms that need assessment, but the range of concern apparently does not extend to the humans in the actual environment, but rather to a theorized "human" who is concerned about "human impact on the natural world" and is fearful it may become too "Disneyfied."[69] And here again, the report calls for a "broader public discussion." The report is very careful to remind its readers of the perils, however, of public discourse, when a public may not understand risk or fear some types of things (genes, sharks) more than is actually warranted, if they are associated with a "marked sense of dread and unfamiliarity."[70]

The report stresses the need, given this problem, to assess the risk of gene drive organisms accurately, and has a long section about the nature of risk. It settles on this definition: "Risk is the probability of an effect on a specific endpoint of set of endpoints due to a specific stressor or set of stressors."[71] It also considers the problem of uncertainty in ecological risk assessments—a field that began in the late 1980s. Uncertainty has both linguistic and epistemic aspects. Epistemic uncertainty is based on the problem of measurement and its instability, and the lack of determinate facts. There may be variability in sampling in a field environment, or the inability to construct an accurate model. Linguistic uncertainty occurs when there are differences in definitions of terms, such as "health."[72] This concept of ecological risk is of course critical and, as described in a subsequent chapter about Africa, will be a central task for the research about gene drives in the Target Malaria consortium.

The report moves forward by using several case studies: gene drives for Palmer amaranth, a plant with both a useful species and a harmful invasive one; *A. gambiae* mosquitoes; *A. egypti* mosquitoes, which spread Zika, yellow fever, chikungunya, and dengue fever; and invasive mice from islands where they eat native birds. This led the authors to focus clearly on the specifics of the scenarios, recommending the use of models, small field trials, and the study of cause-and-effect pathways.[73]

One of the most interesting aspects of the report is the delineation of "public" and "community" for engagement into three groups. The first group is called "communities" and is defined as groups of people who live in or near candidate release sites for gene drive organisms. The next group, "stakeholders," defines the people who have "direct professional or personal interest in gene drives." The third group, called the "publics," refers to the large groups of people who contribute to democratic decision making but may lack direct connection to gene drives.[74]

The report is focused on the centrality of engagement and proposes it for every level of these groups, asking which groups have a sufficient "stake" to be "stakeholders". And it is honest about the problems with engagement across cultural educational barriers and authority. It proposes a framework to build an "evidence-based framework" and includes the need to set goals by the organizers, to have enough funds for the process, and to have a method for gauging the success of the process. As you would now expect, reader, the report does not "attempt to proscribe an engagement plan," and calls instead, again, for more discussion first, and for transparency, open acknowledgement of diversity and the basis of exclusion, if any: "Researchers . . . should design engagement activities to respect different points of view. Such deliberations may enable participants to reflect on their own beliefs and understandings in new ways. Dissent should be captured and considered carefully but engagement does not require the dissenters to be convincing or convinced."[75]

The report then turns to issues of governance and considers how the process of exercising oversight through regulations, standards, or customs through which individuals and communities are held accountable could be enacted. This, as the reader will recall, had also been one of the four points that the AAAS had raised in 1999. This includes: the process by which authorities are selected, monitored, and replaced; the capacity of governing authorities to formulate and implement sound policies; and the respect of the governed community. Here, the report references the Nuremberg Code, which was created after the Nazi Doctors' Trial mentioned in chapter 1. The code, which regulated how research subjects are to be treated, has but the most general applicability for research in which the "subject" is entire regions or entire populations. Yet, the example seems to have been given to illustrate the differing levels of the governance of science at play. "The governance of science is both a set of policy tools for self-governance developed by the scientific community and mandatory policy tools developed by entities outside the scientific community. There are also cultural norms at stake, things such as "don't take credit for another's work."[76] In reading the reports detailed in this book for example, there is a range of concepts, from the promotional support in the House of Lords and African Union document to the neutral support or non-interference of the NASEM documents, which feature dozens of comments declining to take a position, oppositional, precautionary or preventative plans put forward by NGOs such as Greenpeace.

It is not until page 150 that a small caveat of interest is quietly mentioned and not developed as a "general principle for governance of gene drives . . . ." The release of gene drive modified organisms requires predicting the consequences of genetic modification in complex environments. This is and will likely remain an imperfect task; sources of uncertainty and ignorance will need to be clear to decision makers."[77] This is a critically important point, uncertainty, and it is one to which I will return in the final chapter.

The report then turns briefly to the question of mistakes and dual use: There are several types of concerns related to safe, ethical, and secure research: "unintended and unforeseen consequences of release; unintended releases due to negligence or natural disasters; release of information that could be used for intentional misuse and intentional release or misuse of a gene drive technology."[78]

In 2016, as this report was being written, the Worldwide Threat Assessment of the US Intelligence Community, under the auspices of the US Director of National Intelligence, classified genome editing as a weapon of mass destruction and proliferation. The assessment states that "given the broad distribution, low cost, and accelerated pace of development of this dual use (genome editing) technology, its deliberate or unintentional misuse might lead to far-reaching economic and national security implications."[79]

This rather astonishing assertion has its first-and-only mention at the end of the report. The reader is referred to an NRC report on biosecurity— Understanding Biosecurity: Protecting Against the Misuse of Science in Today's World—and is assured that measures are in place because the research is being carried out largely in academic centers.[80]

Leaving this quickly, the report next considers the issue of biodiversity. Biodiversity, a critical topic globally, whose intricate politics and economic I can only briefly mention here, not only refers to a field of descriptive research with policy implications, charting how species of plants, animals, and insects thrive or collapse, especially in our era of climate change, but is also a community of activists, conservationist, wildlife biologists, and others who are a part of the movement that seeks to protect the diversity of species on our planet, arguing that species diversity is essential to a healthy ecosystem. It is a difficult task, and every year, more and more species are threatened or blinkered out entirely.[81] For many countries—but not the USA, which is not a signatory—the norms about best practices in this regard are regulated by the UN Convention on Biological Diversity (CBD). This is a global agreement to cover all aspects of biological diversity for the UN Environment Programme. Their work also includes attention to the issues of poverty, food, water, indigeneity, and climate change. There are 193 nations that have agreed to abide by three principles: the conservation of biological diversity, the sustainable use of the components of biological diversity, and the fair and equitable sharing of the benefits arising out of the utilization of genetic resources. While there is no mechanism for enforcement, signatories are supposed to create "means to regulate manage or control the risks associated with the use and release of living modified organisms resulting from biotechnologies that could have adversely environmental impacts that could affect the conservation and sustainable use of biological diversity by taking into account the risks to human health."[82] The target imagined was GM crops, but the meetings have become a rather contentious forum on synthetic biology, genetic editing, and, in 2017, gene drives. The Convention on Biological Diversity (CBD) Conference of the Parties annual meetings, called the COP, were interrupted by the COVID-19 pandemic, but had served as a very large, international public space for vigorous debate on the topic since 1994 (meetings are now held every other year). In 2018, a working group on the topic of gene drives began its study, and by 2022, it had presented this report to the meeting. Meanwhile, the WHO, an institution that is especially important in countries with no or weak governance structures for public health, also considered this topic in relationship to its health-care goals, and in their case, the WHO does often serve as the de facto authority for action, especially for interventions that have proven successful and improved public health and need to be recommended by national ministries of health. The WHO has written its own guidelines on vector control, the use of GM mosquitoes, and relevant guidance structures for gene drives. But after this brief mention, the NASEM report goes on.

The NASEM report concludes with a long series of recommendations, and with a very American nod to the personal responsibly of the individual: "The governance of research begins with the personal responsibility of the investigator, is formalized in professional guidelines, and often extends to legally binding policies and enforceable regulations."[83] The report then stresses the inadequacy of the existing US regulations for genetic research, either because the regulations cannot fully capture the characteristics of the novel gene drives, or because regulators lack a way to engage the public, or because the regulations as written are too vague. Turning to the role of the Institutional Biosafety Committee (IBC) at the National Institute of Environmental Health Sciences, and to the NIH as critical in regulating research, the report then edges again toward safety. The general thrust of the many recommendations, all of which are earnest moves toward aspirational goals, is that only laboratory proof-of-concept research ought to be conducted, which should then proceed through small, iterative steps, until all the recommendation can be put in place and the ecological consequences more fully understood. In general, the report stands as a written record of the current debates around "nature," risk, and engagement, and is a critical step in defining much of the scientific road[84] to be followed as the science proceeds.

In response to the report, a group of funders, (including the private foundations such as the Bill and Melinda Gates foundation) supporters, and practitioners in the field met and then wrote a pledge in *Science* to indicate their commitment to the principles and practices that had been recommended:

> The signatories to these principles have come together to provide a coordinated response to the NASEM recommendations in the form of commitment to a set of guiding principles intended to (i) mobilize and facilitate progress in gene drive research by supporting efforts of the highest scientific and ethical quality; (ii) inspire a transparent atmosphere of conscientiousness, respectfulness, and integrity wherein the research can flourish; and (iii) support existing biosafety requirements and best practices as minimum standards for research. Endorsement of the principles represents a pledge to advance the foundational elements of efficient and responsible research conduct: evidence, ethics, and engagement, which are also important themes represented throughout the NASEM report.[85]

The principles were rather general, things such as: "advance quality science to promote the public good"; "promote stewardship, safety, and good governance"; "demonstrate transparency and accountability"; "engage thoughtfully with affected communities, stakeholders and publics"; and "foster opportunities to strengthen capacity and education." In general, they allowed the work to proceed, but they were not really defined. For example, who decides what is a public good and what is not? Or what does good governance mean in states where there is no democracy? Or who exactly are "the publics" and what is their relative weight in decision making? Thirteen organizations and foundations as well as many individual researchers have signed up to these principles.

In November 2016, several authors who were members and staff of the NASEM committee published a separate commentary on their work, which both defended and then extended their arguments some of which were not agreed upon by the larger official group. This was published in *Science*, as "Precaution and Governance of Emerging Technologies."[86] Here, the authors defended the NASEM report as a strong example of how the precautionary principle might work staking a space between "risk panic" and "innovation thrill."

Sincere progress in the debate over precaution is possible if we can reject the common assumption that precaution can be explained by a simple high-level principle and accept instead that what it requires must be worked out in particular contexts, argued the authors. The 2016 report, they added, from the US NASEM on gene drive research illustrates this position. The report shows both that precaution cannot be rejected out of hand as scaremongering and that meaningful precaution can be consistent with support for science.[87]

The authors then suggested four additional "broad constraints" if gene drive research is to go forward. These were, first, to "understand that research is related to values" and that questions about economic, social, environmental, and health effects are just as central to the research as the scientific and technological aspect; next, that community engagement about the questions of value, done with "relevant publics" needs to precede any releases; third, that a phased testing approach with post release monitoring should be used; and finally, that an ecological risk assessment should be used to define the long-term environmental and health outcomes further (Alert readers will immediately notice that these features had already been built into the Target Malaria plan.). It would be these "off-ramps, checkpoints, and flashing red lights" instead of a moratorium that would act as a safeguard as the work unfolded, argued the authors.

Within the year, other experts would weigh in to consider the NASEM report. Typically, the science and technology studies (STS) scholarly critique of technology is quite earnestly hesitant about new technology, and this case was no exception, for the STS scholarly association devoted their entire journal, the *Journal of Responsible Innovation*, to their critique of gene drives. At an STS Association meeting held to discuss this issue, Austin Burt and Kevin Esvelt, from the George Church lab presented, and both of them wrote articles about their work for the journal, discussing the need for regulation in the issue dedicated to discussing the meeting's results.

Esvelt, who has been initially both extremely and publicly eager to promote gene drives (his drive was intended for the mouse in the deer, mouse,
tick, human chain of Lyme disease, as you read in the Introduction, and
presented at the NAS/Royal Academy meeting where I first was introduced
to the topic) and then extremely and publicly worried about their use, was
concerned about the difficulty of containment. Thus, he suggested developing self-limiting or regional drives, and began pursuing research on reversal·
drives or "immunizing drives" (a strategy that has subsequently proven far
more difficult than first supposed using mathematical models). He argued:
"Any efforts to develop interventions that fail to take such precautions may
be viewed as less responsible. Future advances capable of perfectly restoring
the population to its original genetic state could be transformative for both
safety and public acceptance."[88] Esvelt and his collaborators were also the
first to write about the serious problem of misuse of gene drive technology.
"The extent to which CRISPR gene drive could be used as a weapon was
carefully considered prior to public disclosure of the technology" (by which
they mean in their laboratory). Esvelt then called for "a new kind of science,"
an idea mentioned in this paper, which he has developed more completely
since, calling for the end of patenting or licensing and complete transparency: "Successfully balancing these conflicting demands (preform experiments with caution, yet accelerate development in order to reduce human
suffering) will require a new approach to science and technology development that emphasizes openness, responsiveness and community guidance
of interventions designed to impact on the shared environment. Awareness
of the issues, the availability and need for safeguards and the strengths and
weaknesses of different gene drive systems can help scientists walk this delicate tightrope. We are, at long last, learning to speak the language of nature.
With sufficient cooperation and humility we might even use it wisely."[89] Setting aside the claim that there is a language of "nature" to which access has
hitherto been inaudible, the claim also raises the familiar problem of subject
and object (Who is the "we?" Is it just scientists? Or does it include the community of others?). However, Esvelt has consistently argued for caution in
this work, for the inclusion of ethics, and for a reduction in the role played
by the marketplace.

Austin Burt and his colleagues, in the same journal, begin, as he did in
the House of Lords, with an emphasis on malaria and its intractability, even
when using all possible available tools, and scaling up existing interventions.

"Expert opinion suggests that without additional tools, malaria elimination with be out of reach in some locations, no matter how much effort we deploy. According to the WHO Global Technical Strategy for Malaria, under the most optimistic scenario of increased investment in existing interventions (with the resources available increasing to about $8.7 billion a year—about three-and-a-half times more than is currently available), death rates and case incidence could be reduced by 90 percent and malaria eliminated from thirty-five countries, but it will still exist in fifty-eight countries, requiring ongoing expenditure."[90]

Instead, Burt suggested that all strategies should be urgently pursued, and that the research on a gene drive should proceed, but he proposed first raising a series of questions prior to its deployment, after successful proof of principle in the laboratory setting:

(1) Is the phenotype (e.g. male bias, female sterility) maintained in diverse genetic backgrounds; in realistic, viable environments; in other members of the *A. gambiae* complex?

(2) Is there a genetic basis for escapees?

(3) What is the potential timescale over which the target mosquito population(s) might evolve resistance and what would be done if it did evolve?

(4) What are the effects and dynamics of the construct in cage studies?

(5) What are the effects and dynamics in a self-limiting (non-driving) open field release?

(6) What release strategy might be needed to ensure spread and prevent re-invasion; what are the logistical and cost implications?

(7) What are the likely community or ecosystem effects (e.g. competitors, predators)?

(8) More generally, what are the human health and environmental risks and can they be managed or mitigated to an acceptable level?[91]

Unlike some of the authors more critical about gene drives, who focused solely on adverse effects or risks in their articles for the journal, Burt and his colleagues stressed the unique value of gene drives as an additional tool in vector control. Not only do they offer the best hope at contributing to disease control, he argued:

Drives are widely applicable, able to act in diverse, settings, whether hypo or holo-endemic areas, in rural and urban settings, against mosquitos that feed indoors or outdoors, during daytime or nighttime, and can control mosquito populations that are otherwise difficult to access. They provide area-wide control, and therefore protection without obvious biases relating to a person's age, wealth, or education. They should be compatible with and complementary to other disease control measures both current (e.g. chemical based vector control) and under development (e.g. vaccines) and they can be relatively easy to deliver and deploy with little or no change required in how people behave and as a result have the potential to be highly cost effective.[92]

Americans in the STS field were not as sanguine. Mitchell, Brown, and McRoberts, writing in the same journal, raise the economic issues to consider for gene drives. They imagine an unregulated, for-profit world in which gene drives create a commercial industry, adding, "we expect a wide range of public and private individuals" to be involved in this market.[93] This is a far different imaginary than Esvelt, with his scientists "speaking a new language," or Burt, with his careful questions. Rather, they worry that "the monopoly or market power large corporations can exert would also likely reduce the supply of gene drive deployments to be less than socially optimal."[94] Why do they worry that there would not be "enough" gene drives? Because of the failure of GMOs to be approved: "As a result, many valuable crop and agricultural biotechnology applications remain underutilized or unavailable."[95]

Rehearsing a nineteenth-century argument—one that weaves in and out throughout the long history of malaria, one that also played a sub-rosa role in 1956–1960, as I have noted—the authors warn that "social gains arising from eradicating diseases would be offset to some extent by negative changes on other measures, such as equity and environmental degradation from increased resource use." By this, they explain, they mean that more people would survive, especially in Africa, where they doubt that Africans would have the same demographic shift as that which has occurred in every country as infant mortality went down, inspiring the birth per woman rate to also decline as people began to trust that their children would grow to maturity. They are similarly worried that these new people would fall subject to what is called the "Easterlin Paradox"[96] or the crisis that ensues when people, newly freed from conditions of abject poverty, begin to wish for more. They are then trapped by a "hedonic treadmill," never seeming happy, despite a rise in income.[97]

Rejecting these scenarios to focus on the existing regulatory structures, a different set of authors, Kuzma, Oye, and others, attend to the rules that already govern the USDA and the FDA as models. Yet, the authors note the problems of definition: Are GM mosquitoes classed as animals? Or are they more like an insecticide? What goals should be defined? What values do these goals most clearly articulate?[98] These authors believe in the concepts of community consent and advocate this strongly.

Following this argument in a closely argued essay by Paul Thompson[99], then set forth six key "domains" of ethics for all new technology:

(1) Standard research ethics (by which he means honesty, careful record keeping, cautions against plagiarism, and disclosure of potential conflicts of interest, the protection of human subjects, the use of an IRB, and the protection of informed consent).

(2) The identification and interpretation of risk (the values in the selection of risks, the social amplification of risk, meaning the impact of perceptions by the public, the role of race, age, and gender).

(3) Fiduciary responsibility (meaning the presence of a scientist's duty to serve the overall public good, and the commitment of a promise to stakeholders).

(4) Democratizing technology (here, he argues that even public discourse can be understood as important but not fully be able to control technology, but that "engagement in these political issues is an inevitable aspect of the social ethics for developing gene drive technology").[100]

(5) Epistemology and power (he mentions here the problem of standpoint epistemology and of how minority viewpoint, or that of the women's perspective, can be ignored to create a science that is defined by the maintenance of dominant power structures).

To this last point, he could have added that many of the contributors to the effort were in fact Africans. He also makes the claim that the Tuskegee research, widely seen as unethical, is "an error that would not have been made if black scientists had been adequately represented,"[101] missing the fact that there were many Black scientists and doctors and that the main study nurse was a Black woman. They all participated in the observational experiment and in the withholding of the penicillin that could have cured the disease under study, which paradoxically shows how errors in ethical judgment are disturbingly possible, even within such structures.

Other essays focus on potential risks of CRISPR-Cas9 cleaving to another similar gene and creating a new lethal phenotype,[102] the problems if gene drives are used in agriculture, and how to handle anomalies.

Sam Weiss Evans and Megan Palmer, for example, long familiar with the synthetic biology community, in their essay asked both whether gene drives are actually novel and whether current governance strategies can adequately cope with them if they are. Gene drives are "anomalies" that can slip out of regulatory norms. Figuring this out is a political act, they argue, and an ontological one: "Up for contention are decisions about the ontology of gene drives (i.e. what is the nature of gene drives) who should work with them, and for what purposes. By outlining strategies to construct and handle gene drives as anomalies, within discussions concerning regulatory systems, we invite more nuanced consideration of the multifarious goals these strategies served. In the absence of such considerations, changes to regulatory systems are likely to be enacted reactively and within a narrow framing."[103] Evans and Palmer comment on the Kaeback et al., article in *Science*, with the concern that it could be considered a version of a moratorium by another name because it seemed to advocate pausing until some essential problems of irreversibility can be worked out:

> In it, the authors call for counteracting a long-standing desire in science to "get an innovation thrill." This term originally referred to J. Robert Oppenheimer's comments before Congress on why he and his team developed the atomic bomb: 'When you see something that is technically sweet, you go ahead and do it and you argue about what to do about it only after you have had your technical success.'[104]

Of course, this quotation does a great deal of work: it raises the comparative specter of the atomic bomb in the same paragraph as gene drives, and it attributes Oppenheimer's view—that you need first to have proof of principle before you reflect on how to manage a technology, a reasonable idea, to be sure—to a sort of boyish "thrill." But Evans and Palmer do not take a position on the use of gene drives or the problem of malaria. They are interested in framing analysis and the way that systems "order both the technical and social world[105]" (such as determining who has the power to decide what attributes of gene drives are considered in governing their development or use).

And in 2021, lawyer George Annas, along with Andrea Crisanti and a group of other commentators, published an online set "code of ethics for gene drive research," with a similar intent: "At the dawn of an era in which gene drives are advancing toward applications in the field, it is increasingly important that scientists developing these technologies adopt and agree to follow a code of conduct to reassure the public (and themselves) that ethical values will be at the core of their actions."[106] A series of other statements and codes continue to be written, largely by Americans and Europeans. There is an important exception to this trend, and it is the report of the African Union.

The African Union

Since the gene drive of interest in this book is the gene drive to alter malarial mosquitoes, *A. gambiae*, which only exist in Africa, the report of the African Union is of primary importance, for it was in Africa that malaria first evolved and that colonialism was most fiercely extended. It is there that the dreadful burden of malaria has historically been most acute and fatal, and of course, it is there that the first impacts of gene drives are likely to be felt.

The African Union is a continental union consisting of all fifty-five countries on the continent. It is a relatively new political formation, begun in July 2002 in South Africa after an initial conference in Addis Ababa, Ethiopia, replaced the Organization of African Unity (OAU). All decisions are made collectively by the Assembly, which then represents Africa in its documents.

> The AU was established following the Sirte Declaration of the Heads of State and Governments of the OAU. The AU is based on a common vision of a united and strong Africa and on the need to build a partnership between governments and all segments of civil society, in particular women, the youth, and the private sector, I to strengthen cohesion and solidarity amongst the peoples of Africa . . . it focuses on the promotion of peace, security and stability. . . . Guided by the AU agenda 2063 which is a 50 year plan to harness Africa's comparative advantage to deliver on the vision of "The Africa We Want."[107]

The African Union set up a separate development arm, the New Partnership for Africa's Development, which was a codeveloper of their position on gene drives. Not only is this report strongly supportive of gene drive technology, it also urges African participation—despite the NASEM, Africans are the proper stewards of the technology: "Given the potential for rapid development in this technology space and the potential for misuse and improper trials, researchers and developers should establish a network of Africa-based scientists and developers to register their studies, self-regulate, share information regarding their technology, and peer-review all ongoing development and field testing of the technology on the continent. They should also adopt a 'co-development' approach that emphasizes collaboration between the partners and the teams, from research design to the creation of standard operating procedures."[108] While, like all reports, they call for a risk/benefit analysis, the African Union is more intensely aware of the devastation of African lives by malaria. Despite the successes, they too are aware that the problem is far from solved, and that progress seems to have leveled off. But they assert that they maintain their goal, stated in the 2063 agenda, to have eliminated malaria by 2030. Malaria is heavily concentrated in fourteen countries, with 111 million people at high risk for malaria. The war and the poverty, which are always both a cause and a consequence of malaria, remain high. Economic losses from malaria varies from 0.41 percent to 8.95 percent of GDP, and countries severely affected by malaria have up to a five times lower GDP than those without.[109] All of this drives interest in high-impact technologies.

The African Union is ready to look to WHO guidelines, since many governments are not able to do all the functions needed to develop, evaluate, implement, regulate, and survey gene drives. In some cases, countries collaborate to oversee science, for example the "Eliminate 8" countries (Angola, Botswana, Mozambique, Namibia, South Africa, Swaziland, Zambia, and Zimbabwe) work across borders for malaria control. Obviously, regional alliances will be better able to cope with mosquitoes as they cross national borders. Other organizations are Pan-African, such as the Pan-African Mosquito Control Association, a professional body for researchers. Additionally, there is an African Biosafety Network of Expertise, which is working to build functional regulatory systems, and the African Medicines Regulatory Harmonization program, which is working to increase access. And even less visible in the public domain, there is also the West African Integrated Vector Management Group that is developing guidance documents for the use of gene drive mosquitos in vector control, with ambition to be a pan-African group.

Finally, most countries have strong institutional national ethics committees with the capacity to assess research related to the development and field testing of novel vector control programs. One is reminded, reading the African Union report, that none of this was mentioned in the NASEM report or in the *Journal of Responsible Innovation*.

The report regards two factors not fully considered in the NASEM report as important. The first is the sociocultural aspects of community engagements, where risks may be considered differently in different settings and where the process of engagement—a (hopefully) empowering conversation about the future of one's village—can itself build practices of citizenship and ownership of the technology, if it begins early in the process. The second is the attention to gender. Gene drives have the potential both to treat all genders equally and to avoid the painful choices women often make when bed nets cannot cover every child. In villages where women lack power, gene drives would treat all without bias, allowing for agency to be directed toward other decisions.

The African Union begins by writing: "Expert views currently indicate that no major risks are foreseen that cannot be mitigated in the application of gene drive technology for malaria elimination, and that the potential benefits will almost certainly outweigh any minor risks served. However, developers, regulators, and any risk assessors must remain vigilant a should update available information on the state of development, risks, and benefits of this technology."[110] Thus, this statement is the strongest of any regulatory body. It is my contention that it is also the most central to the debate.

The report also comments on the issue of biodiversity with immediate practical observations:

A. *A. Gamblae* is not a keystone species in the environment and is not known to provide any non-redundant ecosystem service.

B. Changes in population size or even elimination of *A. gambiae* from a particular environment are unlikely to harm biodiversity of ecosystem services. This is based on existing knowledge and experience with vector control programs.

C. *A. gambiae* interacts with other species by feeding on them, being consumed or competing with them.

D. These interactions may require consideration for species of relevance to the assessment such as threatened, endangered or valued species, Incidental contact between organism and *A. gambiae* carrying gene drives is not likely to lead to harm those organisms compared to interactions with other *A. gambiae*.

E. *A. gambiae* is not known to be the sole or primary food source for any organism, with the possible exception of a few species of spider known to prefer *Anopheles*.

F. Removing *A. gambiae* from the environment is unlikely to harm species that feed on it due to the availability of other prey including *Anophelines*

G. Consideration should be given to any proteins introduced into *A. gambiae* including gene drive components or markers for toxicity to other species.

H. Gene flow to other species within the *A. gambiae* s.l. complex though hybridization is likely and does not create additional pathways to harm.

I. Horizontal gene transfer is not likely to occur to other organisms on any relevant timescale and is not a pertinent pathway to harm.

The African Union writes with confidence about issues concerning mosquitoes based on long experience with elimination strategies. To that end, the document reminds readers that, like any elimination or control strategy, failure to sustain a successful control plan will cause a rebound effect and must be avoided. It stresses the importance of continuing to use all possible tools against malaria, considering this a complementary effort, and adds that stakeholder engagement is important not only at the village level but also for senior policy makers, who have to be educated and involved in the early stages of research design. This report also calls on the need for anthropologists to explore how gene drives will be understood. Unlike the NASEM report, however, the African Union report did not produce a reaction. In fact, outside of the scientific community, it went largely unnoticed.

In the years since I began to write this book, in 2018, more than two dozen other committees of various kinds, with varying levels of information, some privately funded, some connected to scholarly organizations, some to governments, some who invited the researchers to give testimony, some who did not, have published regulations, guidance, or advice. With minor exceptions, they all match the norms suggested by the reports of the House of Lords, the NASEM, and the African Union, which are logical and reasonable, and which are followed quite closely not only by Target Malaria, but also by other laboratories that are also working on similar technologies.

In 2020, a new group of forty-two authors—, "a multidisciplinary group of gene drive organism developers, ecologists, conservation biologists, and experts in social science, ethics, and policy"—signed up to a second gene drive pledge, this time proposing standards for field releases. It was published in *Science* as "Core commitments for field trials of gene drive organisms," and it, they promised to "ensure that trials are scientifically, politically, and socially robust, publicly accountable, and widely transparent."[111]

In 2021, the WHO also weighed in on the issue with a report about gene drives and other genetic technologies, which also reinforced these same norms, stressing ethical concerns, stakeholder engagement, and the phasing of research.

Of course, this book is not a handbook or a book of regulations but rather a meditation and reflection on the use of gene drives for malaria in Africa—a set of linguistic qualifiers whose specificity matters. I will return to this in my penultimate chapter.

However, even now, in the very early days of the science, the problem of malaria and its vectors is not the only one for which gene drives are being researched.

Another set of norms, guidance and regulations has been published about the second major gene drive project currently under discussion in the scientific and environmental communities, called GBIRd. GBIRd is a conservation drive, whose purpose is to restore native habitats on Pacific Islands, where native birds have been decimated by house mice inadvertently brought to the islands in the eighteenth and nineteenth centuries by European seamen and settlers. These mice now have taken over and happily and successfully dominate the islands, eating the eggs of the birds and fledglings and competing for food. The drive aims to eliminate the mice and thus save the native bird species. Because much of the opposition to gene drives has come from conservation NGOs, conservationists who want to use them to save endangered bird species have to confront a deep divide among people who worry about diversity and habitat preservation, some arguing for the development of a gene drive, some against. For readers wishing for more information on this aspect of gene drives and their regulation, I recommend the excellent book by colleague Kent Redford and William Adams, *Strange Natures: Conservation in an Era of Synthetic Biology*.[112]

But what a philosopher finds interesting and worthy of consideration is the activity that creates the regulatory imaginary itself. This was surely not the first time that Western intellectuals gathered in earnest groups to define and debate and then structure the norms for technology said to be "soon" emerging. As an American bioethicist, I have been involved in a series of such imaginaries. As stem-cell research was first proposed, the field spent a great deal of time setting the norms in place for its regulation. We wrote rules for chimeric animals, and for the structure of clinical trials and for just distribution of the benefits of the technology itself. This happened again when nanotechnology became the next technology to excite our interest. Then, developments in neuroscience alarmed the field of bioethics, and there was concern about the elimination of memory and the altering of consciousness, so we again would meet with the scientists and elaborately create white papers with our advice, and sometimes, these more become regulatory. The regulations sit ready, like empty furnished mansions, while the scientists find out that biology is more difficult than theory. There are thousands of pages on human cloning and three decades of literature on gene editing, and now, when the tools changed from the use retroviruses to ferry the gene edits into place, to CRISPR-Cas systems, with guide RNA, more commissions, more meetings, and more literature, all of which repeated the same set of concerns and advice was assembled. All of this readiness occurred for technologies that have not yet been realized, and over the same decades, malaria cut a deadly swath through the children of the most vulnerable. About that lack, our field of bioethics still had little to say.[113]

Regulations create worlds—they are the architectural drawings for the homes in the city of research. Each report was written for a world in which the regulations were possible to implement, in which researchers were thought-ful and eager to transmit their work transparently, or in which elimination of a species so terrible for human health is not such a bad idea after all. But even the most correlative, insightful regulations have their limits. Remember, reader, that the grand plans for malaria eradication, a history that while not mentioned at all in the regulations, have failed dramatically—a fact that should attend our thinking about structures, plans, and promises for health-care interventions in the lives of others.

In the next chapter, we will look at the actual work of stakeholder engagements, where the people who are the "others" of the narrative and the regulations, the African villagers, think about the ethics of intervention and nonintervention in malaria, and paying full attention to the history of malaria control, I will describe briefly the context for the work itself.

4 The World as We Speak It: Stakeholder Engagement and African Discourses

This is a book about gene drives, but largely it is a book about the way the concept is imagined for a particular time and particular place for a particular disease. In this chapter, I am going to describe the fourth category of information that I argue one needs to understand in order think carefully about gene drives. Here, I will consider several things at once: the historical background of colonial medicine in Africa, the actual processes of stakeholder engagement that the scientists in Target Malaria consider so central to the work, and the questions of how a codevelopment project can take place ethically when the power relationships between the Western actors and the African actors is so historically fraught.

The work of Target Malaria has initially taken place within the African countries of Mali and Burkina Faso in West Africa and Uganda in East Africa. Ghana then joined as the location of the entomological studies of the insect and animal food networks. As the work progressed, other places joined. One village withdrew, and one country left when malaria was declared eliminated. All of these sites had particular reasons for participation or withdrawal, particular climates, and particular geographies. Yet, all are taking place within similar geographies, rural Africa, and the vector under consideration is an anopheline mosquito with an African range. To understand how the regulatory admonitions about community discourse that you read about in the last chapter are enacted, we need to turn to the particularities of the sub-Saharan African countries where this research is intended to be performed first. When we think about how stakeholder engagement plays such a key role in this project—in fact, why Target Malaria considers it as standing on an equal footing with the scientific research—we need first to understand more about the African context. This means the history of how science and medicine have taken place there, which inevitably means the history of colonial conquest as well.

But first let me add a brief caveat: How we think about science, and how we judge it morally, is deeply intertwined with how we think about this history. Thinking about the sort of thing that science is and inquiring about its purpose is a way of thinking about our time and our place within it. And in this moment of modernity, as anthropologists Stavrianakis, Bennett, and Fearnley suggest, there is a link between how one thinks about contemporary science and the "long genealogy of attention to science and medicine as a method of reflection and its critique, and that this is one of the defining features of modernity itself."[1] I will add that how one thinks about "Africa" and "the West" is also a factor in how one can come to judge the project of gene drives.[2]

But if our discourse about science as a phenomenon has become increasing critical, our evaluation of the scientific history in Africa is even more so as we become aware of radically different ideas about previously settled structure of permission and authority:

> For (scholars) of the contemporary world, this discursive proliferation has created a practical blockage: there are no longer any settled means, no set of settled term, theories or methods—for adjudicating or reconciling discordant claims about . . . the series of seemingly comprehensive and stable terms, such as Man, Culture, Nature, and Society. And although these terms are in disrepair today, it is worth keeping in mind that have been replaced by other, equally comprehensive terms, such as globalization, the environment, networks, and neoliberalism. . . . As historian of ideas Hans Blumenberg put it: with modernity, "Nature" can no longer be relied on to show "Man" the fixed limits of what "he" can and should make of "Himself."[3]

Of course, we have seen this in the discussion about the term "natural" in other chapters in this book, and I will explore that term again in the next chapter, where the term shifts in meaning and rhetorical power. And the linguistic instability of the term "nature" could be said about many of the terms in this debate. Attempts to make broad claims without the fine-grained detail of place and time have proven extraordinarily unhelpful in my field of bioethics. As Bennett and his colleagues remind us:

> The stakes of inquiry in the present and the question of our relations as "knowers" to a present that we both seek to understand and participate in are situated in a "paradox of the relations of capacity and power," a relationship that Foucault suggest is far more troubled and subtle that the eighteenth century may have believed. It is far more troubled and subtle because increased capacities made possible by technologies of different forms of production, reproduction, and self-formation has

had as their ends the intensification of certain forms of power relations, powers of regulation, or of normalization, which have frequently been at odds with the freedom that people have sought to exercise of the forms of their lives.[4]

One can be struck, reading the many position statements made long in advance of any actual trials of gene drives and long before gene drives are yet possible, by intricacy of effort and its distance from the practical realities of African rural life, or of African regulatory and academic networks. It is especially important to understand how the African conversation that is called "stakeholder engagement" is particular to the place where it is located.

This focus on the particularities of place and practices is not unique. In fact, I teach and do research at a university that is quite devoted to a pragmatic epistemology and to the methods of John Dewey, Charles Taylor Pierce, and Jane Adams. American pragmatist philosophers understood the problem of thinking within the contextual world and made it the basis of their philosophical systems. I am going to argue here for a bit of Dewey as a way to understand how the stakeholder conversation, so vital to the processes of community consent, operates and whether such discourses are adequate to the task. In other words, like a good pragmatist, I want to note that a theory can be derived from the practices I am going to describe. It is difficult to evaluate how something will work on the basis of theory alone, and ideology can end in intractable conflicts.[5] The American pragmatists of an earlier era believed that ideas were best produced by groups of individuals, that they were social, and that they were dependent on how they worked in the actual world and how they were adaptable and located in particular locations. Judgment on their moral worth could only be made as that happened, which is why knowing and testing were so closely linked. "John Dewey understood 'Education [is]an ethical and political phenomenon. It is one in which the questions of the sake for which a practice is done must always be held in view. . . . . The standard through which judgments could be made could only emerge through the process of what he called *inquiry*. Inquiry arises in problematic situations. The "only way out" from a problematic situation, that is, a situation that requires thinking. . . . in indeterminate situations.'"[6] Of course, the work of researching and implementing a gene drive is indeterminate in the way that the pragmatists mean. It takes place in indeterminate situations, which is to say the present—a present in Africa in which the past is everywhere apparent—which is to say, we are working in the history of the present, creating an ethics of the present, thinking about something new happening, and seeking new epistemic capabilities to understand it even has it unfolds. "Nothing less than the work . . . of forming, producing (in the literal sense of that word) the intellectual instrumentalities which will progressively direct inquiry into the deeply and inclusively human—that is to say, moral—fact of the present science and situation."[7]

It is in the rural villages that malaria is most impactful and most deadly, and it is here that the genetically altered mesquites will be released first. Therefore, it was to these villagers that the Western and nationally based scientists of Target Malaria turned to consider the moral inquiry of whether the act would be considered morally right and ethically worthwhile. It was, of course, not the first time that Western scientists had come to the villages, and I will spend a bit of time discussing that as well.

4.1 African Imaginaries

For the late Paul Farmer,[8] writing about the historical roots of what he calls the "clinical desert" of West Africa, the dynamics of the Atlantic slave trade set the stage for the broken economies, feuding tribal conflicts, and extraction markets that structure the relationships between Western and African peoples and lead to such catastrophic public health failures: deadly epidemics of Ebola, AIDS, and malaria.[9] If the16th century slave trade was the beginning of a deep and justifying logic of racial organization and hierarchy, the nineteenth century's rapid Western colonization deepened the problems. New technologies such as the telegraph and rail networks reified the position of colonial powers, allowed these power complete control of trade, and constructed a social order indebted to external expertise.

Farmer described the gilded hall of Radziwill Palace, where Britain, Germany, Belgian, and France met to carve up the vast territories of Africa, vast, largely uncharted, rich with resources—metals, oil, and precious stones—without waging a competitive war that might endanger their profits. They set in place the "Principle of Effective Occupation," which not only included trade agreements and the dividing up of land and taxes, but also the norms of hygiene and disease control. Farmer argues that the practices of hygiene, vaccination, and medical care that supplanted local knowledge were complex tools of global commerce and the justification for the control over vast areas of Africa.[10] The justification, he notes, was often done in the name of controlling deadly infectious disease."Many African communities had long practiced forms of variolation and self-imposed quarantine in the face of smallpox. As the century drew to a close, many Africans sought access to new vaccines. But the manner in which these and other preventatives were shared mattered, a great deal; much of that sharing was martial or imposed. The establishment of formal European rule saw the imposition of quarantine, isolation, and various schemes of social segregation as well as attempts to vaccinate by force."[11] Farmer focuses on the imposition of the "hut tax"—an unpopular tax imposed by the British, which was then fiercely resisted as the intensification and militarization of imperial rule in African colonies. In addition to increasing overt subjugation by armies, Farmer notes that hygiene rules were often enforced in punitive ways, promoted segregation, and structured to foreground the needs and health of the colonialists over the native populations.[12] This is what Farmer calls the legacy of the control over care paradigm. "While we can't blame colonialism for the most recent developments, we can blame its successor regimes. . . . The control over care paradigm is now caught up in a broader neoliberal one: when everything is for sale and public goods are few, both prevention and care are at risk of becoming commodities."[13] To understand West Africa, Farmer reminds us, it is important to foreground both the history ("for centuries, sickness and premature death have been commonplace in this part of West Africa, so too have forced labor, the extractive trades, conflict and outright war. That's why everyday here is saturated by discretion, concealment, and fear"[14]) and the possibility for change ("past afflictions are not the most striking thing about working in the region. What's more striking is just how much can be achieved"[15]).

Megan Vaughan also turns to the history of medicine in Africa, and she too locates the shaping of the medical subject and the larger medical project in the colonial efforts by first Portuguese, then British, French, Flemish, and German empires to control and exploit the vast territories in Africa. Her research in African colonies is in the service of understanding present-day Malawi and, in particular, the way that a changing biomedical discourse led to attitudes about "jungle doctors" and modern interventions that reappeared in the AIDS epidemic. Medicine, for Vaughan, constructed "the African":

> It is certainly true that many biomedical theories and interventions have failed in Africa because no account was taken of the social and political context . . . at the same time, what is striking about much of the medical knowledge produced in and about colonial Africa is its explicit concern with finding social and cultural "origins;" for disease patterns. Biomedicine drew for its authority both on science and

on social science. Biomedical knowledge on African was thus both itself socially constructed (in the sense that its concerns and its ways of viewing its object of study were born of a particular historical circumstance and particular social forces) and at the same time "social constructionist," in that it often sought social explanations for "natural" phenomena. Further and perhaps even more importantly. Biomedical knowledge played an important role in the wider creation of knowledge of "the African."[16]

How did the European colonists understand and address the diseases that were so much a part of the European experience of Africa? Vaughan's insight is that two concepts were employed. Here, we return to Ross and Manson, both members of a generation of medical graduates who were posted to the "tropical" empire, as were a full 20 percent of British medical graduates in the early twentieth century, eager to be a part of a new field of tropical medicine.[17] As David Arnold notes, "a geographical and perceptual space—'the tropics'—had to be constructed before the terms on which Western medicine could operate within this novel environment could be fully determined and before Europeans (and natives) could be effectively brought within its operational parameters."[18] Ross became associated with sanitation, relying on public health measure to eradicate malaria; Manson represented the medical research "campaign" that focused on the pathogen. Colonial medicine saw both the unfamiliar nature of Africa and the unfamiliar "primitive" culture as problematic.

> The rise of tropical medical research was an outcome not merely of the elevation of germ theory but of the continuing threat posed by epidemic disease to the entire colonial enterprise, As in India, so in Africa, early medical provision was entirely oriented toward protecting the lives of the continent's new European inhabitants, particularly soldiers . . . the nineteenth century European perception of the west coast of African was molded by the experience of very high European mortality. The representation of African as a place of disease, danger, and death was one which survived the reductions in European mortality effected by sanitarian policies of the mid-century.[19]

Africa was understood as different, wild, escaping the nineteenth-century obsession with order and control, with animals and native peoples needing "taming" or eradication. This has a long history. In the first chapter of this book, I reminded you, my reader, about how Shakespeare thought about Africans as carriers of this wildness. And for the nineteenth-century physician, who came to African or Asian colonies, horrifying illnesses, the malaria, the sleeping sickness, and the fevers all needed to be contained. At times, the colonial efforts made things worse. Of course, the slave trade itself, as Farmer notes, created huge human disruptions, potentiated local conflicts, and introduced new diseases into sub-Saharan Africa. We saw in my first chapter how in India, where irrigation ditches increased mosquito populations, in the use of armies of human porters to move goods from one place to another,[20] and other colonies, in the creation of vast enterprises, first plantations and then mines for extraction: metals, diamonds, and, finally, oil, all potentiated disease transmission. When populations become more mobile and more densely settled, diseases become epidemic more quickly. When diseases were epidemic, military campaigns were then waged against them and, often, against the culture of the native population, which was seen as a part of the environment. This biomedical gaze was complex. Sometimes it was the land itself that was problematic, sometimes the body of the African, and sometimes the culture of the group. Vaughan stresses the fact that Africans were seen not as individuals but rather as members of collectivities, "the features of which could be defined and delineated and which in large part accounted for the differential incidence of diseases on the continent."[21] Unlike India, where Western medicine and emerging science arrived in the seventeenth and eighteenth centuries, Africa was largely impenetrable until the nineteenth century, its fevers defeating colonialization until everything arrived at once, late in the century—railroads, medicine, science, and modernity.

If Farmer and Vaughan see the Berlin Conference of the International African Association in 1884 as the key moment when Western imperialist powers set in place the tragic history that would shape African health care, anthropologist Helen Tilley argues that it was British scientists, who saw Africa as a "living laboratory," who established the critical structures and norms for research some twenty years later. Tilley begins her narrative in 1929. In 1929, the British and South African Association for Science jointly met in South Africa.

> During his welcoming address to the assembly, the president of the South African Association Jan Hofmeyr, a rising liberal politician asked his audience, "What can Africa give to Science? . . . What can Science give to Africa?" Examining questions relating to astronomy geology, meteorology and medicine, he concluded, "For these investigations the diversity of conditions prevailing in the various regions of the African continent make it a "magnificent national laboratory. "Animals could be examined "not as stuffed museum species but in the laboratories of their native environment." Research into tropical diseases, "of which (Africa) may well

be described as the homeland" could provide "hope and healing for mankind." . . . "The development of Science in Africa, of Africa by Science—that is the Promised Land that beckons."[22]

The African Research Survey, of the "promised land," launched in 1929, was entangled in the larger project of intelligence gathering in the "Great Scramble" for power and control of resources.[23] Africa, especially the interior, was largely unknown to Western science. This was a familiar motif, of course—"Africa as terra incognita, which justified the European imperative of exploration and discovery."[24] Tilley reminds us of the complexity of this "Scramble": "there is no single explanation for the multiple territorial seizures that occurred across Africa between 1870 and 1914,"[25] but it was clear that a combination of factors—the Maxim gun, the telegraph, and the competition between European power for colonies elsewhere—made seizing and holding territories with armies increasingly possible, which then increased the importance of keeping these troops healthy. Without understanding how disease worked in "the tropics," it was impossible. But it was not only the instability of the epistemology that created dissent, there were fierce political debates as well on the nature, goal, and meaning of the project. How much was racialized science to be credited? How should the role of indigenous knowledge be credited? How should it be tested? What should be said about new fields of research in ecology and social anthropology, which stressed the primacy of local testimony? "Throughout the course of the project,[26] from its inception to the outbreak of World War II, a subtext of criticism, dissent, and debate flourished among the project's many advisors that at times challenge the very foundations of British colonial rule in Africa."[27] For crediting local experts, of course, would mean calling into question the concept that the Europeans ruled because of superior wisdom. "The juridical conquest of tropical Africa at the end of the nineteenth century was a watershed moment both for geopolitics and for knowledge. It transformed sub-Saharan African into an imperial laboratory where political, economic, and scientific experiments could be pursued with relative impunity."[28] Africa was a location to be used not only by the market but also by science and social science. Like many of the tropical colonies, it was a place of exploration and experimentation far from the constraints of the metropolis yet in service to it. Not all impulses were predatory of course. For many, the point was not only to learn but also to serve as a part of a larger goal of civilizing and Christianizing the native peoples. As Lord Hailey noted, "Africa presents itself as a living laboratory in which the reward of study may prove to be not merely the satisfaction of an intellectual impulse but an effective addition to the welfare of a people."[29]

Tilley argues that "knowledge may be situated but it is designed to travel. . . . to a great extent, theories of ethnoscience—folk, primitive traditional, local, and indigenous knowledge—owe their existence to imperial structures and sociopolitical asymmetries."[30] Populations are named in terms of their difference. But however different or primitive Africans were, they were to be a part of the empire, in a relationship of commerce and production, trade and exchange. "British states in tropical Africa were grounded in an economic logic from their inception. Imperial officials viewed the natives less as prospective political actors and more as potential producers. Colonial states in this sense were designed to be development states: their telos, from the start, was focused on resources, revenue, and production rather than political participation. . . . The fact that many British African states were unable to be economically self-reliant and that basic infrastructure projects could not be supported from within posed constant challenges for imperial administrators."[31]

After World War I, the administration of the colonies changed. Britain's newly acquired tropical dependencies in Africa were still considerably weaker than those elsewhere, when defined in terms of their revenue, staff size, and bureaucratic infrastructure compared to the population and geographies they were meant to rule.[32] However, over the next two decades, the scientific surveys continued. Health became a priority as populations themselves began to expect access to Western medicine and as physicians began to understand their duty to provide it. In 1924, the East Africa Commission noted the relationship between disease and economic decline. "No community can be healthy, unless its economic status is sufficiently high to provide at least reasonably effective housing and particularly a balanced and sufficient food ration throughout the year. It may therefore be said without fear of serious contradiction that the first task before the administrations of predominantly native territories of the raising of the economic status of the population, especially if it is subjected to periods of famine or semi-famine, the mere treatment of disease, no matter how effectively and widely carried out will achieve but negligible result."[33] The interwar period marked both a growing realization of the importance of more traditional medicine and native ecological management (e.g., of the tsetse fly by the use of controlled, late-season burns of wild grazing lands by Zulu leaders[34]) and the growth of what Tilley calls "vernacular science." Universally negative ideas about traditional medicine yielded to some mixed evaluations, and practitioners of traditional practices adapted aspects of Western science as their own.[35]

By the second decade of the twentieth century, tropical medicine was shifting gradually away from a linear understanding of disease causation, in which microbes alone were targeted as the culprit, toward a more integrated and comprehensive approach.[36] This led to the problem of cost and expediency, which we have discussed in previous chapters. One of the principal debates concerning malaria in 1930s was whether it should be controlled directly via short-term campaigns to eradicate specific mosquito species or indirectly through long-term social and sanitary measures, building clinics, eradicating habitats, or improving the general nutritional status of the people[37] at risk.[38] Cost and the size of the problem presented insurmountable barriers. This would require a "vast undertaking and would require financial provision which few African territories can at present afford from their own revenues,"[39] noted one administrator. Some worried about the problem of population instability—the rapid growth of populations should the disease burden suddenly change. Others worried that unless the change was permanent—very hard to achieve in rural Africa—some populations would simply lose their immunity, leaving them vulnerable when a new epidemic of malaria arrived.[40]

Moreover, the former confidence in the righteousness of the rationale for empire was fading. Charles Wilcocks, an epidemiologist who worked in Tanganyika between 1927 and 1937, offered in his memoirs a disarming statement to what he saw as colonialism's fatal flaws. "We the colonizers, dominated the indigenous people. This is difficult to justify, just as it is morally indefensible for one person to dominate another, to the extent of making him lose self-response through servitude." We must not make the mistake, he added, of confusing technical, mechanical knowledge with intelligence.[41]

By 1938, the British researchers came to understand the need for cooperation with the local population: "all initiatives . . . required the cooperation of the people themselves, and the complete sympathy and understanding of their own leaders."[42] Throughout the 1930s, durable scientific collaboration began, some formed from the original networks established by the survey. These included local projects sponsored by what would become the Scientific Council for Africa South of the Sahara, situated in the Belgian Congo, a nutritional study in Anchu, northern Nigeria, the Azande development scheme in southern Sudan, the Nyasaland Nutritional Survey, and Tanganyika's Bukaoba Nutritional Survey, all of which used new research on ecology, nutrition, and anthropology. Uganda and Northern Rhodesia had interterritorial development and training institutes, and a journal, *Farm and Forest*, was produced for West Africa.[43]

And while World War II radically changed Africa again, these institutions and collaborations endured. The Scientific Council members and other scientists participated actively in the emerging nation states and the new development plans. When the new nation states were formulated, the structures of a complex scientific research community, some of it bottom up, some of it top down, sometimes replicating exactly the structures before independence, were still in place. Scientific research was a complicated enterprise. To a large extent, it was directed at support for colonialist abolitions, but as Tilley notes, it always carried a subversive possibility, an instability based on the reality of unknown geographies, ones whose existence made it clear that European knowledge was not hegemonic.

The universities and Islamic schools, the teaching training programs, and the scientific institutes remained in many places throughout the long twentieth century. They were the basis for the robust research and regulatory systems in the countries that Target Malaria first approached for the codevelopment of the project. It is these institutions that are linked to the projects, co-sponsoring the newly built African insectaries and providing faculty and student advisors.

But the conditions in Africa created particular challenges. Fifteen countries in sub-Saharan Africa and only one country not there, India, carried almost 80 percent of the global malaria burden. Five countries accounted for nearly half of all malaria cases worldwide: Nigeria (25 percent), the Democratic Republic of the Congo (11 percent), Mozambique (5 percent), India (4 percent), and Uganda (4 percent). The ten highest burden countries in Africa reported increases in cases of malaria that started in 2017. Of these, Nigeria, Madagascar, and the Democratic Republic of the Congo had the highest estimated increases, all more than half a million cases. In contrast, India reported 3 million fewer cases in the same period—a 24 percent decrease compared with 2016. Malaria in these countries took a worsening toll.

Burkina Faso, for example, one of the first countries in which Target Malaria began its work, was part of the Upper Volta region of French West Africa where about 19 million people live. It is landlocked, with access to a major river, the Volta, which is a wide, slow, and marshy river used for trade and which is the major transportation artery in the region. It sits between the Sahel, the vast desert region of the Sahara of North Africa, and the states along what was called Africa's Gold Coast, where the Volta pours into the Atlantic in Ghana. It is at the very center of the malarial territory of West Africa, with infection rates of malaria responsible for 61.5 percent of hospitalizations and 30.5 percent of deaths. For children below the age of five, malaria is the leading cause of hospitalization (63.2 percent) and death (49.6 percent). Burkina Faso has become a frequent target for terrorist attacks, which have spilt over from a conflict in Mali. But while jihadist activity was previously confined to the north of the country, in 2017, it began moving to the east, a region already facing violence from organized crime. The median age of the population is seventeen. There are seventy separate language groups in the country, and even the country's name is a mixture of two of them. There are four major religious traditions, which represent colonist influence. From the Sahel, Muslim traders brought Islam in both the Sunni and Shi'a traditions. The Portuguese and, later, the French brought Catholic rites, and in the rural areas, a variety of traditional animist traditions were always practiced. This means that discussions about worth and merit of action, the meaning of knowledge and wisdom, all of which are a part of debates about gene drives, have to be understood in light of these complex religious systems in African tribal communities, which alter what Christianity or Islam means in each tribal system. Layered over this is the *longue durée* of French colonialism, which only ended in 1958 with independence, but there have been eleven coups since 1958, each one with a new change in government. Only 29 percent of school-age children actually attend school, even though it is free in theory—although schools are built, funding for teachers, books, or uniforms is not provided. The GDP per capita is $1,200. Even amid poor countries, Burkina Faso is one of the poorest.[44] In 2014, according to the National Institute of Statistics, some 40.1 percent of all Burkinabe lived in poverty—a rate that reached 70 percent in the arid north.[45] The struggles of independence are ongoing, but in 2017, after a long process of reform, elections were again held. A formal anti-corruption organization (ASCLE-LC), led by activists, brought corruption charges against the then President Compaoré, his brother François, the former finance minister, and a district health manager, all of whom were charged for corruption as well.[46] The example shows both the depth of the corruption that is possible and the sincerity and durability of the organization against it.

A National Commission on Reconciliation and Reform, created during the transition, summarized many of the most widely accepted proposals in a report released just before the elections: strengthening financial transparency in government institutions, political parties, civil society groups, and other entities; barring civil servants from establishing party "cells" at their place of work; reinforcing the independence and capacities of the judiciary and private media; bolstering parliamentary ad judicial controls over the executive; and ensuring that traditional chiefs, do not use their authority to sway voters or otherwise support particular parties. There were also a variety of economic and social recommendations, from general admonitions to reduce social inequalities and injustices to specific policies such as allocating set percentages to mining revenues to new investments, developing solar energy as a national priority, creating new mechanisms to resolve land-tenure disputes, and promoting the use of locally made cotton fabrics. Beginning in late March 2017, consultative sessions were held in all thirteen regions and among Burkinabe living in France and other countries. . . . Taking into account the views expressed in the public consultations, the Constitutional Commission was then to prepare a final draft for government review, before voters decided on it in a national election.[47]

Burkina Faso and Mali, like all of the countries where Target Malaria works, also face increasing challenges because of a changing climate. With 90 percent of the population engaging in subsistence agriculture, droughts can have a severe negative impact on daily life for both human and livestock populations, and the steadily increasing temperature also makes agriculture difficult, forcing many away from once-fertile areas to live in areas where they cannot grow enough crops to sustain their livelihoods. Deforestation is rampant because people rely on wood for trade when they cannot grow crops and for fuel. Every year, Burkina Faso loses an estimated 32,000 hectares of forests. This cycle of poverty, which means the people search out new areas of the land to use, impacts wildlife, resulting in some species becoming extinct due to habitat loss. In addition to all of these issues, Mali has been shaken by civil war, which, while not affecting the cities and areas nearby where the project works, has further destabilized the northern areas of the country. Meanwhile, in 2022, Burkina Faso experienced two military coups in a nine-month period, one in January and another in September, again, in the name of addressing significant levels of corruption, and an inability to address rising violence by Islamic militant groups—attacks had increased by 23 percent in the five months between the first coup and the second. The junta promised to improve the daily governance structures, and organize the security forces. As of this writing, the 34-year-old leader of the army regiment that took over, Ibrahim Traore has not held promised elections nor appointed a new interim leader yet, despite this, the scientific work continued.

The political climate is not the only concerns. For concern about how genetic research is conducted in Africa have a long history, dating back to efforts in the early 1970s to construct a genomic "map" of genetic variants on the continent. Bioethicists were concerned about the use of such samples. African researchers knew the work was important but wanted to have control over the databases that were created. The large data set was called H3Africa. H3Africa, which began in 2012, late in terms of genomic research but the first of its kind in Africa, presented a challenge. Most of the institutions, country regulators, and public health officials had not used genomic research before, and moreover, only a few research projects had engaged Africans. (There were three notable exceptions: MalariaGEN, the HapMap project, and the 1,000 Genomes Project.)

> In particular, the proposed storage and sharing of large amounts of African DNA samples and data—integral to genomic science and increasingly common in medical research—raised considerable concerns by African regulators and scientists. Amongst a range of concerns, what stood out most clearly were concerns about exploitation and harm. Concerns around exploitation were articulated mostly with regard to questions about the role that African researchers would play in H3Africa research. The worry was that they would simply be sample collectors and would not be empowered to lead study design, data analysis and write-up. On the issue of harm, concerns were raised about whether and how African research participants—who may have low research and health literacy—could be harmed by the research, for instance through an increase in stigma or reputational harm.[48]

It was against this background and these concerns that Target Malaria began its work. From the beginning, the project sought to create a participatory endeavor, with African scientists as collaborators in a process they called "codevelopment." Moreover, they intended to foreground the process called "community consent" in the literature of bioethics as a basis for their work in which the stakeholder in the rural villages would need to understand and authorize research.

Consent must take place in these contexts, not in an idealized relationship, in villages in Burkina Faso and Mali, under the trees of the outdoor assembly spaces, within tribal traditions, within gender relationships and extraordinary poverty, with these many different languages, with much of the population still very young, with ongoing struggles against corruption, with a long history of colonial taking, with a degraded terrain, with competing appeals for attention, and with no history of continuous democratic discourse as it is imagined in the documents drawn up in faraway places. I am aware of these challenges, to be sure, and the reader should keep them in mind as we consider the concepts of consent. Nevertheless, stakeholder engagement remains a key premise of the work, and it to this that I now turn.

4.2   The Stakeholder Discussion: The World as We Speak It

Consider Humphry Davy, poet and poor boy, made peer of the realm because of his extraordinary, nineteenth-century scientific mind, standing deep in the mines of northern England, holding a candle carefully in the dark, 600 feet deep, in the midst of winding tunnels. He has come up from an impoverished Cornish childhood because of his daring, his attention, and his relentless experimental zeal. He writes to his friend as he leaves for a position at the Royal Institution, its first professor of Chemistry, "I wish to do something for the public good." At the age of twenty-nine, he had already been the first to experiment with the anesthetizing power of nitrous oxide, recorded and theorized its use in surgery, and used the Institute's voltaic batteries to decompose potash to find the new elements sodium and potassium. He is a beautiful man, made wealthy by his science and his marriage to a dazzling, brilliant, and celebrated London widow. He does not need this work in the mines or the terrible danger of the great Northern collieries.

He is deep in the mine because the miners are dying. In the two years before, enormous mine explosions rocked the hard, iron hills and the dark mining towns with a new ferocity. The problem is straightforward but difficult: as the Industrial Revolution has quickened the drive for coal, mine shafts are sunk deeper. In the deeper mines, pockets of methane and other volatile gases that the miners call "firedamp" are exposed, and they gather, silently, waiting in pools at the bottom of the dark tunnels. The mines are lit only by fire, each miner with a wax candle stub on his helmet or in his hand. The open flame catches the draft, and the gases ignite, expanding and exploding in terrible explosions, flinging the bodies of men over the soft, green hills. The worst of the explosions was at the great Felling mine, seen as a clean and model pit, which killed ninety-two men, bringing the total of deaths from mining explosions to 300 in five years. Seven months later, a second explosion at the Felling mine shook the region, and twenty-two more men died. After the accident, a safety committee, led by the Duke of Northumberland, the Bishop of Durham, and virtually every leading vicar, business leader, and scholar of the region, was formed and put out a call for a solution, eventually calling for a national expert to turn their full attention to the lives of working men in danger. Fifty-seven more men were blown apart in Newbottles. The committee appealed directly to Davy, "of all the men of science . . . the one who could best bring his extensive stores of chemical knowledge to a practical bearing." Davy was abroad on his honeymoon, writing metaphysical science–inflected poetry ("Nothing is lost; the ethereal fire, which from the farthest star descents; though the immensity of space; its course by worlds attracted bends to reach the earth".)[49]

It was logical that the miners and their representatives turned to Davy, it was well known that Davy had volunteered five years earlier to oversee a ventilation scheme for Newgate Prison, the fetid, disease-racked last stop for England's most woebegone. He had fallen dangerously ill with typhus, nearly dying. He returned from Europe, decorated by several crown princes, and headed to Yorkshire. Davy was eager to prove the basic humanistic promise of science: to "serve humanity".[50] In 1840, he wrote that his goal was "to bring the lightning from the clouds and make it subservient to our experiments."[51] He studied the problem for three weeks in Durham, visiting mines, talking to miners, and watching the work. Then, he went to his laboratory in London for three months of intense work and "fearful explosions" until he had a working prototype of what would be known as the Davy lamp. It was science for the poor, and it was understood not only as an astonishing technical victory but also as a moral gesture of tremendous importance. Joseph Banks, head of the British Royal Academy, wrote: "Your discoveries will exalt the reputation of the Royal Society throughout the Scientific World . . . to have come forward when called upon because no one else could discover the means of defending Society from a Tremendous Scourge of Humanity; and to have by the application of Enlightened Philosophy found a means . . . to guard Mankind for the future against this alarming and increasing Evil, cannot fail to recommend the Discoverer to much Public Gratitude."[52] The lamps are simple and still, years later, cleanly beautiful, the gleaming copper handlings, the smoky glass, the fine mesh gauge that encloses the lit wick so that the gases cannot penetrate to the flame.

Davy then returned to the mines and spent hours underground, teaching the safety techniques and making little refinements to the design. Hundreds of miners wrote letters of gratitude. The lamps became the standard feature of international mining practice, saving thousands of lives. Urged to take out a patent, Davy refused, citing the need for the lamp to be widely distributed and well used. He never forgot who he served. In his formal manuscript describing his careful, inductive process, he began by writing about the terrible series of explosion accidents in the mines, the deep human loss they represented, and the horror that spread throughout the north. "The results of these labours will, I trust, be useful to the cause of science . . . but a much higher motive is offered . . . when that knowledge is felt to be practical power, and when that power may be applied to lessen the miseries or increase the comforts of our fellow-creatures."[53]

Why tell the nearly forgotten story of Humphry Davy in the middle of the book about mosquitoes and twenty-first-century cutting-edge genetic research?

He came to my mind, and now he will come to yours, when you consider how big science projects are typically initiated. Ideas for big science are drawn up at great expense, getting rooms full of experts to decide how funds will be allocated and what projects will be pursued. Sometimes, there are requests for proposals from billionaires with a special interest in a problem—aging research is often a favorite target for this sort of funding. Sometimes, politics at the federal level drives the science, when a leader or official has a particular interest in, say, cancer research. But while the decision will include the companies that will bank on the worth of the research, the local public conversations about where science should go next are typically not part of the plan. And increasingly, a nationally famous synthetic biologist told me that scientists have to tell a story that can be sold, promising investors that if successful, the research will make a large profit. Otherwise, the project cannot get off the ground. So, the choice of what to pursue is largely influenced by the desire of the market, not by the need of the most vulnerable. It is hard to imagine, say, a labor union or worker's council joined by leading clergy and political leaders sending letters to scientists asking for a solution to the issues that cause them such tragic loss. The worlds of ordinary people and scientists seem far more separated than in 1815. How many elite scientists today have been in the depths of mines, and how much of the world of the ordinary worker is a subject of research at elite laboratories? What would science look like if public need drove it as surely as financial concerns or if the "lightening from the clouds" really did serve humanity?

What makes Davy's work important for ethicists, and for anyone who wonders if science is "good," is that it recalls for us a time in which something other than market success rendered science important. The worth of the world was shared, insisted Davy, and the work of the scientist was to serve the needs of "all." And the idea about what science was important to pursue came from the unions and the clergy that supported them. It was not decided in boardrooms or at conferences of the elite. The point of science was the Davy lamp. Of course, if you remember, when I met Austin Burt, I was struck by how his concern for his project emerged from his attention to the problem of vector-borne diseases of the poorest, and that he initially sought to avoid the patenting and profit taking of so much of genetic medicine.

And it was this Northumberland story that came to mind on a March morning in a small room in Ghana, in 2019, where I had come to attend in a weeklong gathering of the entire Target Malaria team. I was watching the training session for a new set of leaders of stakeholder engagement teams. The young African trainees were new college graduates who were returning to their home regions to lead the discussions that are fundamental to Target Malaria's work. For the last decade, Target Malaria has tried to create different types of community conversations as a part of the larger project of stakeholder engagement. They organize meetings at the local, regional, national, and Pan-African level, and they organize meetings for the purpose of direct authorization of the work, or to empower particular groups, to co-develop the science with African partners. I was most interested in how the community engagement at the local level was done. And while global public opinion cannot be ignored, as we shall see in my next chapter, the project is clear that key stakeholders are the people in villages—rural families who have the most direct need for a different strategy for malaria and who would be most affected by the success or the failure of gene drives.

In document after document, in the ordering and linguistically defining sets of rules and norms published by the dozens who have sought to regulate gene drives, in think tank and ethics centers, in the halls of the WHO, National Academies, Royal Societies, and the groups of self-organized scientist, the final norm, rule, or paragraph is always the same: a call for stakeholder engagement. In part, this is a reflexive aspect of all bioethics, a ritual paragraph at the end of the ethical analysis of any new technology, new intervention, or new capacity: scholars call for democratic discourse and stakeholder engagement, often without explaining exactly how that is to happen.[54] However, it is by now canonical.[55] Stakeholder engagement is understood to be an essential part of all responsible public health research and, in particular, for responsible gene drive research.[56]

Since engagement is such a clear mandate in documents that propose regulatory schemes for gene drives, and since it is such a consistent part of Target Malaria's work, it can seem an entirely straightforward concept. Yet, understanding how it is supposed to work is far more complex. This is for two types of reasons: some technical, some conceptual. Vector-borne diseases raise an urgent problem, for they are, by definition, "public." Attempts to prevent or control them always involve more than the usual one-to-one consent process that is the hallmark of clinical research.

Of course, other stakeholder projects have long been in place, usually outside the remit of bioethics research. Multinational corporations have long understood the need to have local populations at least passively accepting their activities, and in more recent cases, a literature has developed to tell them how to do so:

> With the growing trend of globalization, multinational companies (MNCs) are entering developing countries at a rate faster than ever before. In this context, the behaviors of stakeholders, local or virtual, are having an increasing impact on any organization (Parmar et al., 2010). Stakeholder engagement, or the interactions and consequent relationships between an organization and its stakeholders (e.g., Noland & Phillips, 2010), is therefore critical to any MNC's survival and success. This research topic has gained increased attention in various research fields such as business strategy, business ethics, marketing (Parmar et al., 2010), and more recently, communication (Johnston, 2014). Stakeholder engagement is defined as "a type of interaction that Ni, Wang, De la Flor, & Peñaflor Ethical Community Stakeholder Engagement Public Relations Journal, Vol. 9, No. 1 (Spring 2015) 2 involves, at minimum, recognition and respect of common humanity and the ways in which the actions of each may affect the other" (Noland & Phillips, 2010, p. 40). In the global context, an MNC's use of ethical stakeholder engagement requires a focus on open information exchange and genuine care of its local communities, which facilitates effective communication and relationship building in the long term[57].

Originally proposed as "stakeholder governance," which was an economist term that argued that consumers, producers, and communities near extraction locations should participate in decisions that these companies made, for the both wealth that was generated and the risks that were accrued should be equally considered when the multinationals were making strategic decisions about their businesses. Stakeholder engagement promises something less ambitious than actual governance. Most of the original leadership in the stakeholder engagement projects in Africa have long experience with the corporate practice as former employees of extraction companies, which need to work with communities to secure relevant permits, organize labor, and create relationships with local agencies. Several of them came to Target Malaria, for example, after working with mining companies or oil companies in former French colonies of West or Central Africa, and sought now to do another sort of work—work in the service of affected populations. This, to some extent, explains some of the oddly corporate nomenclature of some of the language of stakeholder engagement.[58] Other researchers emerged from the public health sector, or academia, or development aid, and this cultural difference in origins of their expertise can often be seen in the different languages that describe the activities.

Let me describe what Target Malaria meant by stakeholder engagement. Please keep in mind that there is a significant literature on this topic and, of course, that this description is necessarily brief, in part because their activities took place over a decade and also because their project is but one version of possible types of such engagement.

The local stakeholder debates begin by what is called "problem mapping."[59] This allows the villagers to hear first what a gene drive consists of and why malaria prophylaxis has slowed in their region. For many areas, for example (as in 80 percent of all malarial areas), at least one of the insecticides is no longer effective because the mosquitoes have evolved resistance to it. The team listens to how the villagers understand the problem. Then, they explain the hypothesis that they would like to research to see if it is valid and if it might be helpful. After the science is explained, the villagers raise a long list of concerns, and questions and the team listens and then discusses each one. This process unfolds over many years, a long, progressive process intended to empower the community and allow it time to reflect and consider the research and its implications. New concerns are considered and brought to the scientific leadership. Sometimes, aspects of the endeavor are changed and the research is shaped by the villagers insights as well. Once, the team was asked to stop its activities in a particular village entirely, and they complied, which I will discuss in more detail later in this chapter. At different points, new issues emerged. How should established gender roles be understood? Is it fair to honor these roles in the name of tradition if the local women raise the issue that different sorts of work are paid differently and women are not traditionally able to hold those jobs? How should "outsiders" to the community (which might involve villagers who have lived together for years but not decades, for example) be part of the discussions? How should the voices of those with minority opinions be honored?

In meetings at the village level, the participants, as they began to trust their concerns would play an important role, learned to articulate their questions as a critical part of the process. For example, participants worried that the mosquitoes' new modification might enable them to carry new diseases or to spread AIDS, or that other more terrifying insects would inhabit the niches that the *A. gambiae* abandoned if their population numbers were suppressed, or that the gene construct would be spread by hybridization or horizontal gene transfer, or that the genes would somehow enter the food chain. Each one of these concerns had to be carefully unpacked and the science that made them extremely unlikely explained.

In 2016, four regional workshops organized by the African Union[60] were convened, largely of African biosafety regulators, policy experts, and science to learn from these practices and build capacity about the problem formulation process. Since this was to be a part of the first steps of legally required environmental risk assessments before in country releases of gene drives, it was critical to carefully evaluate the process of community engagement. The AU workshop participants were asked to evaluate hypothetical case studies involving gene drive research. From 2016 to 2018, well before gene drives had been tried in large cages, in anticipation of the first step of release, the AU asked the participants what they questioned about the research found results very similar to the Target Malaria village teams. Participants were concerned about a reduction in species diversity and about safety.[61]

Target Malaria teams learned that the language of the science needed to be translated into accessible words, and that each region had multiple languages and needed specific new words for many of the elements of genetic research. So, they then spent three years making a detailed dictionary or glossary of scientific terms translated into the several native languages, French, and English that are spoken in the regions where they operate.[62]

The project worked with linguists from other institutions (whether public research ones or private language centre) who developed a first potential glossary in the local language after better understanding the project scientific approach. This initial glossary was then tested during focus groups with community members, which significantly improved the proposed translations by making them more appropriate to the local context and cultural understanding. The stepwise process revealed the complexity and importance of elaborating a common language with communities as well as the imbrication of language with cultural aspects. This exercise demonstrated the strength of a co-development approach with communities and language experts as a way to develop knowledge together and to tailor communication to the audience even in the language used.[63]

They organized local groups to perform mime and plays to explain the science, and they created comic books that used images and local anime to show how the process worked in visual detail, so that children and people who could not read could also understand what they were being asked to decide. All of these—the dictionary, the comic, the plays—were co-developed and co-written by the African leadership in the villages and linguists and dramatists from the Target Malaria team. The teams thought carefully about how to define the "community." They considered who should be included in discussions in highly stratified societies. Thizy and her co-authors, a group of experts from Africa, American, and Europe noted:

> Once relevant communities have been identified at the theoretical level, there remains the often-challenging task of translating theory into practice. Participants agreed that the stakeholders from the relevant communities, whether the project activity that concerns them is direct research, monitoring, or something else, must be involved in decisions that delineate the bounds of their communities and in designating their own representatives. In doing this, project teams must strike a balance between consulting those recognised as having authority delegated to them by the community (elders, headmen, elected representatives etc.) and taking into account cultural or communal biases that may lead to the neglect of concerns expressed by some stakeholder groups (for example women, ethnic minorities, those with disabilities).[64]

In a project involving organisms that are likely to cross political boundaries—because mosquitoes, at times, had ranges far beyond the local village protectorates—the state, nation, and, eventually, large regional areas of the continent would need to approve the research. At the regional and the national levels, a different set of stakeholders were needed: regulators of biosafety and political leaders who would have to approve the importation of GM mosquitoes and the construction of local insectaries to raise them. "Relevant authorities who could play an advisory or decision-making role may eventually include national regulatory agencies and African ethics committees, health policy experts, formal and informal community leaders, representatives of marginalized groups and others."[65] Often, environmental interventions require the authorization and participation of several generations, and this, too, is a rate-limiting step. When the project began, there was no single established consensus on definitions or guidelines that would establish community consent or authorization in gene drive research or even on how research teams should establish such authorization discussions prior to initiating field studies. There is a long history of debate about "community consent" in bioethics, in other settings. Thus, the ongoing question—of what the broader project stakeholder engagement should look like in Africa—is also a part of the research.

In part to consider this, the Target Malaria team, along with the Kenya Medical Research Institute and the Pan African Mosquito Control Association, organized a series of workshops with people who were involved in stakeholder practices to take a careful and critical look at the Target Malaria model. The organizers then published a report of those critiques as part of their larger commitment to transparency. This process had already begun when I first wrote this chapter, and it has continued as I finished. In the summer of 2021, the group published a paper that summarized their work thus far and set in place ethical and research norms for continued engagement.

> Gene drive technology offers the promise for a high-impact, cost-effective, and durable method to control malaria transmission that would make a significant contribution to elimination and have the potential to spread beneficial traits through interbreeding populations of malaria mosquitoes. However, the characteristics of this technology have raised concerns that necessitate careful consideration of the product development pathway. A multidisciplinary working group considered the implications of low-threshold gene drive systems on the development pathway described in the World Health Organization *Guidance Framework for testing genetically modified (GM) mosquitoes*, focusing on reduction of malaria transmission by *Anopheles gambiae* s.l. mosquitoes in Africa as a case study. The group developed recommendations for the safe and ethical testing of gene drive mosquitoes, drawing on prior experience with other vector control tools, GM organisms, and biocontrol agents. These recommendations are organized according to a testing plan that seeks to maximize safety by incrementally increasing the degree of human and environmental exposure to the investigational product. As with biocontrol agents, emphasis is placed on safety evaluation at the end of physically confined laboratory testing as a major decision point for whether to enter field testing. Progression through the testing pathway is based on fulfillment of safety and efficacy criteria, and is subject to regulatory and ethical approvals, as well as social acceptance. The working group identified several resources that were considered important to support responsible field testing of gene drive mosquitoes.

Two more points were raised by these consultations. First, there had to be a mechanism for people who lived in the region and whose community approved the gene drive experimental process but who had personal objections to be able to express them. For example, one cannot easily opt out of the release of genetically altered mosquitoes in the way one can a drug trial. The groups thought it fair if the rules of the process could be mutually acceptable, even if the outcome was not. Objections had to be carefully heard, and the teams needed to respond to them. Over time, over years, because this project will take many years indeed, the teams worked to build a culture of mutual trust and transparency. Second, the teams identified a need for independent monitoring of the process of the experiment—both the science and entomology progress and the engagement process. The use of a third party to do this would reduce the problem of conflict of interests. Finally, the projects and teams, within Target this would mean the careful construction of an African community of discourse that allow them to say honestly that this project only proceeds within the limits of community approval and with considerable community leadership and this is a multiyear process, with collaboration across a wide range of local, civil society, and national groups.

Evaluation of the stakeholder engagement work by Target Malaria is difficult, although not impossible and it is central to my argument about the legitimacy of the project. Not everyone can go and observe in the villages oneself for very good reasons. White Westerners who are curious have no place in the villages, because most people living there wish to go about working and living their lives without being gazed upon by outsiders, and since the observation itself would, of course, change the dynamics and relationships. On one level, the ethics committee must trust in the integrity of the Target Malaria researchers who have carefully and consistently published their work. But that is not the only measure of the work, for the villages are visited and the work evaluated by the African institutional ethics committee of the partner universities as a part of the oversight plan. As a researcher, I had another advantage: I was able to meet the local leaders of the stakeholder engagement groups in four of the countries and speak privately to them about their experience. They were not without critique. However, they were also determined and thoughtful about their work, and most importantly, it was *their* work, and they were clearly deeply involved in its construction.

In the summer of 2019, the first genetically altered, self-limiting mosquitoes—sterile males—were released in Bana, a village located four miles from Souroukoudingan. It was a small release, intended to collect baseline data and to be a codevelopment project, after a seven-year dialogue there that had agreed on a set of principles—transparency, inclusiveness, and openness to different views—that would guide the decision about whether to allow the release. The acceptance was given in 2018. The team used a "mark-release-recapture" technique. The sterile males were dusted with colored powder and flew off, watched by the villagers and the team, including Abdoulaye Diabaté, the Burkina Faso PI who directed this phase of the work. Then, at intervals, after they had swarmed, the villagers monitored them to see how successful they were at being mosquitoes, mating, and surviving in the wild for a normal period of time. This was also overseen and approved by the National Biosafety Agency and the local ethics committee of the Institute de Recherche en Sciences de la Sante (IRSS).

Then, in 2021, the WHO published the second edition of its guidance for testing GM mosquitoes, reviewing the same guidelines noted in the NASEM and AU reports, and of concern in this chapter, for stakeholder engagement as the primary way to assure and inclusive research. In 2022, a member of the Target Malaria team, Delphine Thizy working with Claudia Emerson, from McMaster university, published analysis of their own that sought to articulate the ethical principles should guide the work, other papers from the Target Malaria team explained the rationale for selecting and making them operate in the field, and shared early lessons about the application of the principles. These principles included the selection and prioritization of the most ethically relevant groups, conduct engagement as a project that is codeveloped and with the full participation of the researchers as a part of the research itself, and "begin engagement early, engage continuously, and iterate often."[66]

The authors noted that formal "deliberate democracy" as imagined in the anticipatory documents may or may not be possible in different cultural settings—something that had become clear as they put the theories of consent into practice. They also noted the importance of principles of ongoing transparency in addition to consent, for the trustworthiness of the research rested on the idea that the team was dedicated both to the science and to the villagers.[67] The stakeholder process clearly involves a great deal of talk, time to discuss, and time for the teaching and learning to be exchanged from both directions in a horizontal rather than vertical fashion. Again, the process takes years, which is why the paper stressed the iterative nature of the discussion—something that in philosophy might be called reciprocal deliberation or responsive discourse, in which the insights gained from the community then change the research direction of the work. Humphrey Davy would find it familiar.

In 2022, alert to the criticism raised by, among others, one of the reviewers of this book that the stakeholder project—which is, of course, an intervention itself, in addition to the actual release of insects—should be evaluated externally, in a process called a "scoping study" that would also look at the social, economic and health impacts of the work. Target Malaria contracted with an independent assessment consulting group from three private consulting and research organizations (Insuco, Swiss Tropical and Public Health Institute, and Oryx Expertise) who formed a team that would visit the regions and communities affected by the project. The plan was for an independent group to review the impact of the planned release on the people in the villages and on the environment around the village communities, interviewing selected individuals who were key informants and workers at local health-care centers as well as regional officials. Additionally, they planned to have focus group discussions with small groups of local women and men separately. The idea was to have a review of the process by which the community would agree or refuse the next step in the research: the release of the non-gene drive male bias mosquitoes. This was not only an idea generated by the internal dynamics of the Project, for an ESHIA review "is a legal prerequisite prior to release of the next phase of the work in Burkina Faso and is intended to propose measures to avoid, reduce or mitigate negative impacts or to optimize positive ones."[68]

Just to review from chapter 2, this next phase is the release of the non-gene drive male bias mosquitoes that were created by using a nuclease gene that, when activated during sperm production, fragments the X chromosome of the sperm, resulting in a mosquito that mainly has Y-bearing sperm and thus produces predominantly male offspring. The nuclease gene is inserted into a mosquito autosome. An autosome is any chromosome that is not a sex chromosome. *A. gambiae* mosquitoes have two pairs of autosomes and one pair of sex chromosomes. Non-driving genes on autosomes are inherited by 50 percent of offspring.[69] Thus, moving from sterile males to biased but fertile male mosquitoes is a fundamentally important step, and it was important to have a thorough understanding and assessment of the success of the engagement process, the science, and the environmental effects before each stage. Gathering more information about the dispersal, survival, and competitiveness of the genetically altered male bias mosquitoes, is part of the staged process that would move in an iterative fashion toward the actual release of a gene drives in the coming years.[70]

All in all, as I considered the care with which the work has been done in Mali, Burkina Faso, and Uganda, despite long odds, COVID-19 precautions, and all the realities of Africa that I have described, I thought about how much more robust and thoughtful the work was, even compared to the "notification" given to me as my county sprayed for West Nile virus and sent texts telling me to "look out for" mosquito larvae, but not offering any meetings, discussion, or description of what was involved.[71]

Turning to Theory

On her seminal work "Governing the Commons," about how common pool resources can be organized, Elinor Ostrom considers the issue of how to govern natural resources used by many individuals in common.[72] She argues that "one can observe in the world, however, is that neither the state nor the market is uniformly successful in enabling individuals to sustain long-term, productive use of natural resources systems," but that community based, newly created institutions that are unlike both the state and the market have worked over long periods.[73]

Are we incapable of this work? Many models have suggested this to be so. In 1968, writing in *Science*, Garrett Hardin spoke of the "tragedy of the commons" to describe this failure. If everyone sought only to advance their own interests, resources needed by all would fail: "Therein is the tragedy. Each man is locked into a system that compels him to increase his herd without limit—in a world that is limited. Ruin is the destination toward which all men rush, each pursuing his own best interest in a society that believes in the freedom of the commons."[74] Hardin's model of the failure of rational market forces was used throughout the environmental movement to describe acid rain, climate change, and more: urban crime, and even international relations. Other models—game theory, collective action theory—concurred. All were pessimistic about the possibility of cooperation. But Ostrom had another idea in mind. She began by considering the success of many small enterprises she had studied and considered why people did work together. She found that it was possible to create agreements, self-generated and self-enforced, that must be agreed on by all parties. In this situation, the only feasible agreement—and the equilibrium of the entire project—is for everyone to agree that prior sharing of resources and profit must be equitable and that the worst alternative is to abandon the collective. These systems work, she argues, because the local participants have better local knowledge about conditions and limits than a distant state authority, but they are also able to enforce the rules they decide in advance for themselves.

The capacity for self-organization is critical. In part, this is the rational theory behind the rhetorical call for community engagement that end so many of the codes and norms I analyzed in earlier sections of this book. There is optimism about stakeholder engagement, and this is due, in part, to the determination that historical practices of colonial medicine can be changed.

The deeper moral question is the ethical issue in all research on human populations, which is the use of the bodies and lives of the other, done, at least in part, instrumentally. The interesting paradox, as the reader will see, is the juxtaposition of the profound utilitarianism of the justifying argument with the need for the liberty of consent.[75] I will return to this issue in the last two chapters of this book as we think about the justice consideration raised by the research. Gene drive research has two different end points to be considered successful, entomological, which can be proven in the laboratory and observational field studies, counting mosquitoes and mapping population crashes of insects. But it also must have a clinical endpoint, and work to reduce and hopefully eliminate malaria in the lives of the Africans who are the subject of the research. What this means is that although computer models can predict outcomes and although small-cage and then large-cage experiments can clarify these outcomes in model environments, there is nothing that can prove the hypothesis that a gene drive will actually work to reduce malaria except enacting the thing itself, tested against the human bodies that will or will not become infected, just as bed nets and spraying were proven effective. The only response to the dilemma of human experiments has been the informed consent process. This is true for any medical research innovation. Every single drug, every vaccine, and every device that is used in a modern hospital is only made possible because some human beings allowed it to be tested on their bodies. Some things are tested in healthy volunteers, some only on people with the disease that is the target of the innovation, but in all cases, it is an ethical question, made decent because we agreed that human beings are moral actors who can decide this question for themselves.

Bioethicists try to ensure that vulnerable populations are not targeted, that no undue pressure or inducements that are offered, so that the choice to participate is made freely. The sort of research done in the nineteenth and mid-twentieth centuries on prisoners at Statesville is no longer ethically acceptable of course, but communities still need to agree to participate in human landing catches and whole-house spray catches as they have indeed done for more than 100 years, as I noted in an earlier chapter and finally, to the releases of the GM mosquitos.

Stakeholder engagement and scientific codevelopment have long been a part of Target Malaria's work as a concrete response to this very problem. For the last decade, in article after article and in presentation after presentation, the consortium published, promoted, and practiced this work. Authorship, scientific leadership, and lay leadership, I could see at the conference, had all been given careful attention. Committees in the project on which I participate, for example, the ethics advisory committee, and grant projects such as the religious scholars project are structured so that no more than half of the members are Westerners and half are Africans. Their publications describe years of thoughtful local work and long meetings under trees in small villages over a period of years. The training I was witnessing would take several days, and Jonathan, Patrice, and Buki[76] would then go back to the villages to talk about the project and learn about their places, the families, and the work of the people who they would meet.

Later that week, I would attend a meeting of the leaders of the village stakeholder engagement groups from Uganda, Mali, and Burkina Faso as they discussed what they saw as the ethical issues in their work. For several women, it was the problem of gender roles. The higher-paying jobs, such as nighttime capture of mosquito swarms, were ones that only men were doing, in part out of respect for a widespread cultural and very real concern for women being out at night alone. But these traditions meant women were paid less for participation in the work of the project. So, how to arrange equity? How about in villages where the real tradition was that the women did go out at night for water for the children but not officially? The villagers want the researchers to be there and want the release of the first stage of the project, another participant said, but not everyone is happy, and is it permissible to move ahead without complete agreement? What if the person making the complaints makes complaints all the time about every aspect of village life? Does that weaken his case? Someone else asks about the villagers from the next place over and whether they get to participate, and the team considers this as well.

These are complicated debates. How one knows what is true, what is trusted testimony, is different in different villages. Even though Target Malaria teams are very careful about who goes to the villages from their team, the decision about other visitors are decided by the village itself. At times, reporters appeared there with cameras and interviewed people. Sometimes, these were people from NGOs, sometimes, advocacy groups from other regions or countries. Sometimes, they would ask, and be invited to give their perspective, and sometimes, according to reports, they would tell the villagers not to trust the stakeholder engagement teams from Target Malaria. This did usually not interrupt the work, for the community engagement has been well established. "Then they leave, and we are still there," said the community engagement leaders when I asked about this.

In 2019, the stakeholder engagement teams finalized the new glossary project, creating a dictionary of terms about genetics, GMOs, and mosquitoes that translated the science into local languages. They wanted to be certain that the problem that vexed golden rice—that villagers did not understand genetics or that the rice was genetically modified GM—was not repeated here.[77] They showed one another visual aids that they had used: cartoons that explained malaria and genetic modification and a video of a play in a local language with village kids acting out the ideas.

Even this is a process that will take many more years, quietly unfolding as the research project is developed, long, long before the technology itself, always chancy, might be rolled out in these villagers, and the stakeholder leaders have been working for years in the villages already, year after year of thoughtful discussions. The WHO and AU guidelines require that the work be in phases, and at that meeting in Ghana in 2018, they were getting ready for the first part of the release plan: the release of sterile males. After the data were collected and analyzed, the next steps would follow as described in earlier chapters, and as I write, the plans for the male-biased release are being formulated. But always, reader, remember that this is a research project primarily, and it will be years even before the details of how to create a successful and durable gene drive are worked out, and more years before the first impact of a gene drive will alter the disease, even if everything goes to plan, even if the political climate is stable, even if the opposition stops the global pressure to halt the research that you are about to hear about in the next chapter. And of course, it simply may not work, which is always a possibility.

One the final day of the Ghana meeting, everyone—the stakeholder leaders, the scientists, the entomologists—met in one huge auditorium, and Burt opened with a discussion about what to call the gene drive. In 2018, it was called Product 1, and it was the product described in the Kyrou and Hammonds paper. People voted on ideas and images, and because different words sounded different in different languages, it took a long time. I was struck by the deeply democratic nature of every small aspect of this project.

At the beginning of this book, I told readers that I was not writing a straightforward ethical assessment of a new technology but rather a meditation—or doing what Hannah Arendt describes as "thinking"—that process of considering, reasoning, discernment and judgment of the ethical issues that are considered with new technology, with our changing mastery, with our reflections on the idea of nature, and illness, and befallenness, with what is real respect for the cleverness of the science, and real reservations about whether it imperils the fragile ecology of a place such as Africa. But judgment is important, and throughout this book, I ask again and ask about judgment: What is the right act? What makes it so?

To these topics I will add the question of Africa, and the moral complexities of thinking about a technology that is created to address the hundreds of thousands of children who are sickening and dying in Africa. In some sense, this is an absurd claim. Like so many in my field of bioethics, I write and reflect on genetic technology without really being touched by the problems it seeks to address. Moral philosophy is an abstraction, and bioethics prides itself on being more "applied," but in fact, in many cases, it is really not. For the last several years, considering the issues in this book, I have heard people confidently opine on the ethical issues of a technology that is planned for a place they have never visited, do not know a great deal about, or will never be touched by. The great moral panic that is so often tragically on display in the discussion is often without any humility or any sense that one needs to be responsible to know enough about rural Africa to have a coherent opinion. And I am only slightly better: I have visited Ghana, I have read extensively, I have spoken with scholars and participants, and I know that is inadequate. Still, seeing Africa, even on a short visit, matters, for it is so very different than the "Africa" that appears in the bioethics literature. For one thing, when you get off the plane in the airport, you are immediately greeted by enormous signs about malaria and huge advertising posters selling anti-malaria pesticide. It is, quite literally, front and center of the discourse. For another, Accra is a place of extraordinary contrasts between modernity in the form of fancy office buildings, nineteenth-century poverty, and a great many new projects that announce in Chinese and English the intention to build the "belt and the road" projects in Ghana.

Those March days in Accra, as I remember them to write about them now, four years later, were sepia toned, the dust in the air from the Sahara coloring everything. We did not visit the villages because the project did not think it was a good idea to have visitors in and out as if the villagers were zoo animals. Ordinary humans going about their work did not like to be observed and photographed in that way—something we saw when we walked out of our hotel to go to the open-air street market, for example. I understood the impulse to record the novel that impulse that Tilley identifies in her book. Everywhere we looked on our walks and drives, we saw something compelling: extraordinary animals, colors, and activities. We could see the discarded edifices of the waves of empire: the slave prisons of the British. And in the small alcoves of the fortress, near the barred window, we saw the bones of chickens and other evidence of religious sacrifices: black smoke smears, bright bits of clothes, and wrapped candies, offerings to the souls of the slaves that died there, because they are still remembered, and they still matter. In a small grassy area by the sea, we saw a wrecked nineteenth-century "folly" built for the long-ago wife of the long-ago merchant who walked on the cliffs in her garden overlooking the slave fort. In the city center, we saw the abandoned, endless, blank parade grounds and the monument to the heroes of the national liberation, with a large carved stone fist.

And we saw Jamestown, as bleak a slum city as I had ever seen, an enormous shantytown that had grown up in the shadow of the abandoned British fort. We were shown around by "Big Men" who were indeed very tall, thin men who, when seeing a group of foreigners, ascertained we were doctors (I wondered if my PhD counted) and told us that we needed bodyguards, for a fee, which seemed prudent. They led us down the dirt path toward the harbor, past huge smoking open ovens for burning wood into charcoal, something I had read about in the Talmud but had never seen, to the warren of paths between the shanties. There were goats wondering about, and beautiful hand-shaped wooden fishing long boats painted blue, yellow, and deep red, with the words of the Hebrew Bible painted on them, "God will protect his people." The distinctive blue mosquito nets were everywhere. They were coiled into boats; they were full of tiny sardines as the fish were emptied and spread onto the dirt to dry in the sun; they were held in the surf by the older children, the turquoise blue of the nets, the gray-green foamy water, to catch fish. There were red cloth flags in the harbor and discarded cloth bags that said, "Play in Ghana" in the trash. There were open sewers, and there were ditches full of trash—many, many trash-filled ditches, with water glistening in the cracks. And there was a perfectly dressed baby girl, with white lace and pink little shoes, sleeping in a basket in the middle of a stone patio. I could see her grandmother watching from the deep shade of a hut, and I nodded, "She is beautiful." There was a large pile of yellow flowers that the men said were for mosquitoes, and a lovely yellow-painted school for children, right in the middle of the town, with high ceilings, books, a painted mural ("God is love, love God"), and a picture of a girl with a book on the red painted wall. "I teach here," said the Big Man closest to me. "This is what we do with the Big Man money." There was a little store, with a Big Joe popcorn machine that had a sticker of Santa Claus and another sticker for the Fire House Prayer Ministry. The store also had a poster for the Total Freedom Convention, which seemed to feature an assortment of ministers; another poster that was an obituary for Madam Lydia, age 53, and a list of all of her relatives and official mourners; posters for Sasso mosquito spray, featuring a mosquito with a huge, phallic probiscis; and another, a Hindu meditation poster, for Sri Chinmoy, Peace, Love, Joy, yoga and "the inner awakening." There was a faded campaign poster for Peter Boamah Otokunor, "#my victory Our victory." Otokuor, I knew, was a leading figure in the Ghana political scene—an academic and professionally trained agronomist who was also the president's chief aid and running for election in 2020. Part of James Fort Prison was now the customs collection house, the old institutional brick-and-mortar building, still asserting some sort of power, but around it, on the broken bricks, lay the brightly colored cotton clothes, freshly washed, drying in the bright sun. Africa: defying easy descriptions, all the religious ideas, politics, competing for attention.

The next day, we drove out to the university to see the beginning of the new project on developing a map of ecological "food networks" to understand better the role that *A. gambiae* played in the ecosystem, a new part of the Target Malaria project, initiated because the question of the impact on the environment was so consistently raised. The research would focus on what ate mosquitoes and what mosquitoes ate. It is a complex question. Would a fish species collapse if the mosquitoes disappeared, or would another mosquito species—one that was not adapted over thousands of years to harbor the *P. falciparum* parasite—fill in the gap? What about bats? How dependent on the species were they?

We went outside to look at the entomology project. There were insect collection sites, which were simple, low-tech strings and tarps, called malaise traps, looking like small sails for grounded boats, for flying things to fly into, or small round holes in the ground with a plastic cup to catch the crawling bugs. There was a net lifted against the wind and a collection of long-handled butterfly nets with tightly woven white muslin to catch the mosquitoes when they swarmed. The beautiful low-slung buildings had open courtyards and had no screens. There was a lovely little museum, packed with enormous skeletons of bats that careened over the rafters; a beautiful, intricate chart of the *P. falciparum* parasite life cycle; huge, coiled snakes in large glass vats; crouching scaled animals I could not identify; and samples of the huge land snails that we had seen in the street market, as big as a dinner plate, labeled in someone's elegant, looping Latin scrip; drawers and drawers of butterflies and night flying moths; dozens of skulls with astonishingly long horns, with antelope and species of deer lining the hall walls; and of course, mosquitoes, of all different shades and sizes, carefully pinned and mounted. This was the living laboratory that Tilley describes: people from the West, dazzled by all of the variety, collected, named, and catalogued. The project had a tiny wet laboratory and a few very good microscopes, but there was barely enough space to turn around. "Fieldwork can be challenging," one of the scientists said quietly. It is a complex product of social values, circumstances, and experience.[78]

Indeed, even years of careful stakeholder engagement can falter. In 2019, villagers in Uganda, in a village that had engaged for years with the project, became concerned when Project subcontractor in charge of doing a geospatial information system (GIS) mapping, which would supplement the way computer modeling data could capture features of the geography and vegetation to make the mathematical models more accurate, began to photograph the area,[79] and a rumor swept through the village that they were really from an oil company that had come to survey the land for exploitive purposes. It was not true—they were studying habitat, but they had not properly asked for permission and had not contacted the right people, and the damage was done. Some of the villagers felt distrustful. The meeting tree in the center of the village was cut down as a symbol of the loss of trust, and the entire team withdrew, first from that village and then from a wider area until they could take stock of how the error had been made after many years of engagement. The project as a whole stopped all of its field activities and brought in external consultants to undertake a very thorough review after this happened and studied a variety of other concerns, some around gender and culture, others that participants also raised, before the work went forward, under the new 2022 guidelines that incorporates the lessons learned from that experience, and defined ethical guidelines for ongoing stakeholder engagement.

Taking stakeholder engagement seriously and taking as absolute the willing participation of the villagers is central—the beginning of the scientific enterprise. If it is not available, no matter how important other aspects of the work, the project will not go forward in that region. Approvals for all the work are done at the local and then the national level. In Mali, obtaining approval for importing the GM eggs and rearing them took two years and needed National Ethics Committee approval in addition to approvals at each local level. Speaking a new idea into existence is a long and complex process.

Of course, all of this beauty, tragedy, complexity, and poverty, and all of the African solutions to the challenges I saw, are rarely part of the discourse in the bioethics literature on gene drives for malaria. In the place of the actual African context, bioethics constructs a fictive imaginary, in which the specifics of place, time, and people do not matter. Bioethicists are quite comfortable debating abstractions about nature and its violation or science and its hubris. I do this as well, for abstraction from the particular to make normative claims is a part of how one is taught to think logically when one is taught philosophy. But the specifics turn out to matter a great deal. There is a specific, actual baby girl in pink shoes in the middle of Jamestown, and her beloved existence ought to matter, at least to a field such as ethics, which is dedicated to goodness. The problem arises when only the abstraction matters, such as when we discuss "the ethics of gene drives" as if some global claim against technology or mastery is more important than the baby girl in pink baby shoes, who, of course, never knows about the panels of experts in Western universities whose lives, whose very speeches, are enabled by all sorts of technology. Her odds of being one of the 600,000 who will die of malaria this year are far too high, and that is, actually, the ethical issue. Jamestown's entire existence is not ethical. It is the result of 500 years of the most wicked sort of mastery of nature, from the Portuguese, who first built the fort, to the British, who made it impenetrable, to the global economies that allow—perhaps create—places such as Jamestown, this broken world that we have made.

The intention of this chapter was twofold. First, I wanted to remind readers of the context in which gene drives are being considered: the discursive world of African rural villages and the reality of African political organization and the robust and country specific regulatory systems, both of which are too often thematized or ignored in the bioethics literature of the West. Second, I wanted to explore the final aspect of the project of gene drives: the stakeholder organization that takes place in these villages and which has, for more than a decade, created an ongoing conversation about genetic alteration and human disease. In the next chapter, I will turn to the work of the people and groups that oppose gene drives, for that speech too has become part of the discourse about gene drives, and I will carefully consider their arguments as they, and we now, with all the pieces of the narrative to hand, begin to ask what the right act is, and what makes it so—the question of ethics.

5 The World of Dissent: Listening to Opposition

In the work this far, I have presented the history of the desperate and difficult problem of malaria; one of the innovations intended to address it, a gene drive in mosquitoes; and some of the private and public proposals for doing the work within the structures of public policy. I have also reviewed the context—Africa—and the stakeholder engagement that is part of the project. The structure of the presentation in this book—problem, solution—should alert you as reader to one danger in thinking about new technology. It is that one can be overwhelmed by the tragedy of the problem and then dazzled by the elegance of the science, and thus one can come to believe in its redemptive power. The problem of human suffering is so tragic and the prophetic power of science so important to modernity that it is nearly impossible to turn away. The work of ethics should, in theory, protect the scholar against this temptation, but alas, the scholar, like the reader, is appalled by the suffering of children and fascinated by the tricky intricacy of the gene drive. Of course, this is the case, for one cannot hold a "view from nowhere"[1] when one is always someplace particular—in my case, in a university where the intense charm of the scientific holds such importance and, not tangentially, so many resources. It is the task of the ethicist to raise doubt, or at least to ask difficult questions that, if we are any good at the task, shake the assumptions enough to test the load of all that is carried by the promises of science. It is my intent to do this with generosity, for after all, while of course I have my critiques readily to hand, the scientists in Target Malaria are doing the very things that I spent an academic lifetime urging scientists to do: focusing their genius on the problems of the poor, not taking profits, and engaging the community.[2] Thus, reader, we have now come to the part of the book where I will begin to discuss how I assess research as ethical and morally justifiable, and you will see the sorts of arguments I use to think. However, there are some who oppose the research and development of gene drives entirely and are wary of proposals to evaluate and structure their use for any purpose. These include members of organizations whose work it is to oppose all GMO technology.

When I brought the first draft of this book to colleagues at the WHO, in Geneva,[3] they urged me to be certain to listen carefully to the arguments of people in NGOs who opposed gene drives as well as to the scientist and the regulators, and this was entirely correct. So, let me give the first chance at ethical assessment to those groups. In this chapter, I am going to ask that we listen carefully to the array of people who have mounted this opposition and indeed are working assiduously and persistently to oppose gene drives, often in organizations, often as a full-time enterprise, often in ones that are structured and funded to oppose genetic research in general. I will invite you first to read, without my comments or critiques, their own public statements about gene drives so they can put forward their arguments against it.

Let me turn directly to the groups and their arguments. Reader, I am going to cite long sections here, rather than summarizing their arguments, because I wish to allow you to see the arguments in some detail and the exact words of the groups cited.[4]

5.1 Arguments and Documents

One of the leading NGO groups is ETC, which has, for twenty-five years, first as the Rural Advancement Foundation International (RAFI) a Canadian group, opposed genetic alterations first in seeds, then in all food crops, and then for the entire range of genetic technologies in agriculture and beyond. ETC stands for "action on Erosion, Technology, and Concentration," which was intended to mean all "corporate concentration and related issues for civil society."[5] They explain in their mission statement what they see as wrong: "The world has grown infinitely more complex: new technologies have developed, economies have globalized, multinational companies have expanded their reach, wealth and capital are concentrated in the hands of fewer and fewer giant corporations. Life itself has been manipulated, picked apart, re-assembled—and then patented."[6] The ETC Group has often been first to investigate new technologies: "In the 1990s, our work expanded to encompass social and environmental concerns related to biotechnology, biopiracy, human genomics and, in the late 1990s, nanotechnology. [As RAFI] We were the first civil society organization (nationally or internationally) to draw attention to the socio-economic and scientific issues related to the conservation and use of plant genetic resources, intellectual property and biotechnology." ETC was one of the first groups, and the most organized one, to attend to the development of synthetic biology as a new field and, in fact, was invited to participate in the community engagement panels held at SynBio 2.0, 3.0, and 4.0, the annual academic conference for the presentation of work in that field. Jim Thomas, the co-director, who, like all the other members of ETC, including its board of directors, works as a full-time activist in the organization, was interviewed about gene drives in 2017. Here is the interview, published in an organic farming journal, in which he describes his concerns with gene drive technology.

What's significant about gene drives is their ability to relentlessly spread a genetically engineered trait through a population until ultimately you change or destroy an entire species. A lot of gene drive research aims to render a species of mosquito or parasite extinct.

ACRES USA: Sounds like deliberate extermination.

THOMAS: That's right. The application that gets talked about most involves eradicating mosquitoes that carry malaria, Zika or dengue fever. Or maybe it would be possible to engineer a mosquito so that it couldn't carry a particular parasite. They could also be used though in many other areas. Gene drive developers say that this technology will end up in agriculture.

ACRES USA: Many people would be thrilled to get rid of a mosquito species that carries the Zika virus. What are some of the problems to anticipate before releasing a gene drive?

THOMAS: First, there are the ecological implications of taking out or changing an entire species. While mosquitoes are problematic for a number of reasons, they also are important as pollinators and as elements in the food chain. Bats, birds, fish and other animals eat them. The disease might well move to other vectors. Initially only one species of mosquito seemed to carry Zika, but it turns out other mosquito species can carry it, too. Ultimately, it's also likely that organisms will develop resistance to gene drives and then gene drives will have a limited effectiveness. What you're doing is launching these weapons into the wild against the mosquito or the parasite and fighting its evolution. Evolution will win every time with who knows what side effects. Then there are a bunch of social and ethical questions. If a northern hemisphere organization decides to release gene-drive mosquitoes across Africa, they'd be carrying out a very controversial experiment with a potentially ecologically disruptive technology over a whole continent. Since it's a health application and mosquitoes bite humans, you would need the consent of all the subjects in that experiment—i.e. all Africans. That's a very big political decision. But the debate about gene drives won't just be about mosquitoes and malaria or Zika. That's just the case that the developers want to talk about.

ACRES USA: Who stands to gain from gene-drive technology?

THOMAS: It's interesting to look at where the funding comes from. Currently there seem to be three big players. The Gates Foundation is putting $75 million into developing gene drives because of malaria. A big Indian industrialist's philanthropy just threw in $70 million. And the Pentagon would say they're funding gene drives because they're potentially a terrible biological weapon and they want to know how to remove gene drives from the environment should they end up being released with belligerent intentions. In the process, of course, the Pentagon is learning exactly how to create and optimize these bio-weapons. One could imagine a number of hostile uses, from engineering a parasite to decimate a human population to releasing a gene drive to destroy a food crop on an island nation. Agricultural biotech companies are extremely interested in gene drives. There's been much talk about a gene drive to overcome glyphosate resistance in weeds, like Palmer amaranth (pigweed), which would give Monsanto's market for Roundup a very healthy bounce. Another agricultural application getting attention involves putting a gene drive in pests like fruit flies that attack soft fruit, the objective being their eradication. The idea of gene drives is very attractive to agricultural input companies. Gene drive developers are now talking about developing "local" gene drives that would spread for a certain number of generations and then stop. That would enable corporations to sell gene drives as a service, for instance to eradicate pests or make the weeds on your farm susceptible to herbicides.

ACRES USA: So that explains some ways that gene drives could generate a profit.

THOMAS: Gene drives are very new. The first proof of principle—the first working gene drive—wasn't announced until late 2014 or early 2015. Since then, there has been a frenzy to get on top of the implications of gene drives and a steady increase in the numbers of labs developing them. Gene drives are also being developed for supposed conservation uses. For example, a consortium of five universities, government agencies and an NGO are building a gene drive mouse that could be released to eradicate mice on islands.

ACRES USA: And those mice are not going to stow away in someone's luggage?

THOMAS: We don't even know whether gene drives can jump species! Yet an NGO called Island Conservation that works internationally and is based in Santa Cruz already has gene-drive organisms ready for field trials. They want to be ready to release gene-drive mice by 2020, but no agency could possibly have regulations ready by then, and we won't have a good understanding of the implications.

ACRES USA: I really enjoyed the ETC Group article about the conference in Britain at which conservation biologists and biotech geeks were courting each other. It was appalling and hysterical.

THOMAS: At the UN Convention on Biological Diversity, the issue of synthetic biology has become a topic for international discussion among 198 countries. Given the level of concern, synthetic biologists want to attract some allies in that forum, so they've made a deliberate effort to come up with ways in which synbio could be used to conserve biodiversity. That explains this crazy idea of using gene drives in conservation. Thirty leading conservationists like Jane Goodall and David Suzuki have signed a letter declaring that gene drives have no place in conservation. When the International Union of Conservation and Nature recently held its big World Conservation Congress, the developers of gene drives and other synbio promoters tried very hard to get a statement supporting the use of synthetic biology in conservation. Instead the IUCN approved a moratorium statement on gene drives. The pro-synbio countries and the organizations associated with that were horrified.

ACRES USA: ETC Group's report "Reckless Driving" asserts that gene drives pose a grave threat to the environment, food security, peace and security on par with nuclear power.

THOMAS: I really think so. Gene drives are probably the highest leverage technology I've ever seen except maybe for nuclear power. The idea that releasing a single mosquito or fly could thereby change an entire species and by extension entire ecosystems—that kind of leverage is unparalleled. The ability to release something small and change something big offers a tremendous amount of power. That's why militaries and corporations are so excited about it.

ACRES USA: This is very sobering.

THOMAS: It's hard to know how it will go. Developers are saying that CRISPR is so easy to do (gene drives basically work on CRISPR) that any fairly smart high school or undergraduate biotech student could do this. It would be difficult to detect in the first instance. That makes for very serious challenges. We're calling for the United Nations through its biodiversity convention to enact a moratorium on gene drives, but even knowing how to do that is going to be very difficult.[7]

The ETC Group has published two position papers about gene drives. The first, "Reckless Driving: Gene Drives and the End of Nature," published in 2017, raised concerns about unintended consequences, the creation of new ecological niches left unfilled by species lost to gene drives, the jumping of drives from species to species, and market monopolies and bioweapons, and it called for the immediate end to all research on gene drives. (The ETC Group was also the main organizer for the call for a moratorium on all synthetic biology research in 2015.) "These 'technofixes' continue to be over-sold to the public through deceptive media campaigns, corruption of regulatory agencies, and by inflaming the public's fears and anxieties about disease, climate change, and species extinction. 'Silver bullet' technologies distract from, rather than contribute to, the work that needs to be done to root out the systemic causes of these problems—such as providing sanitation, defending human rights, addressing poverty and upholding community land rights and stewardship over nature."[8] By October 2020, the ETC Group released a second report, "Driven to Extinction: Bill Gates and Gene Drive Extinction Technology," which was "part of our contribution to a new Global Citizen's Report 'Gates to a Global Empire.'" In this report, the BMGF is linked to the US government's Defense Advanced Research Projects Agency (DARPA) program as the "main funders of gene drive technology." The main thrusts of this report are to describe the project funded by Gates ("bankrolled" in the language of the report) and to raise concerns about influence. Target Malaria, Austin Burt, and Andrea Crisanti are among the scientists listed as subjects of the funding. "From bankrolling the technology development and creating the underlying tools, to shaping the narrative, picking the policy negotiators, and even paying the lobbyists, Bill Gates and his Foundation have so far been tightly interwoven into every part of the story of gene drive extinction technology."[9] The Group reads the support of African leaders and politicians as problematic—to the extent that the regulator of the AU opposes moratoria, it is because they are "influenced by Gates funding."

> The African Union's technical arm, the New Partnership for Africa's Development (NEPAD) released a report in support of gene drive mosquitoes for malaria eradication. A year prior to the report, NEPAD was awarded $2,350,000 from the Open Philanthropy Project, a major co-funder of Target Malaria alongside BMGF, to support the evaluation, preparation and possible deployment of gene drives. Open Philanthropy's funding priorities often move in lockstep with BMGFF priorities and they are part of the same "effective altruism" movement of technocratic billionaires. Additionally, a new crop of African negotiators, new to the CBD, arrived at the Sharm-el-Sheikh negotiations vocally arguing in favour of gene drives. Many of this new cohort were drawn from ABNE, the African Network on Biosafety Expertise—a Gates funded biotech policy network on the African continent that is at the heart of BGMF influence on African biotech policy. It was no surprise then when, at the CBD, the consensus position of the African group of delegates was one that was in favour of gene drives.[10]

The 2020 report was written by Zahra Moloo and Jim Thomas, both members of staff at ETC. The 2017 report was written by the "Civil Society Working Group" (this consists of the following groups: Biofuelwatch, Econexus, ETC Group, Friends of the Earth US, Hawai'i SEED, Navdanya, and an independent author and lawyer Claire Hope Cummings, MA, JD).[11] There is no indication of how the group was selected or the criteria for selection.

ETC noted that the "Driven to Extinction" paper was written for a conference organized by the Navdanya Foundation. This group is the NGO that is perhaps the most vehemently opposed to gene drives. It is headed by Vandana Shiva,[12] who has opposed GM technology of all kinds: golden rice, Bt cotton, fertilizer, and now gene drives. Her organization also signed the moratorium on all synthetic biology research. Perhaps the clearest written statement about her views was made in an essay "Biodiversity, GMOs, Gene Drives and the Militarised Mind."[13]

Here are excerpts from her argument, in which she cites her own Twitter comments. (she has 119.7K followers on Twitter)

> We see how the patterns of technocratic solutionism, powered by an unholy alliance between big-capital, science and technology institutions and states, are embodied by the Bill and Melinda Gates Foundation #Gates2GlobalEmpire Close & direct relationship with nature contributes to non violent ways of knowing & #coocreation. Mechanistic reductionism attempts to know fragments of nature as an outsider & master Creates violent epistemologies & violent economies that cause harm to nature & people@UNGeneva

> Globalization is corporate rule, it is recolonization. We recognize it because
> these are the laws of #freetrade through which the British colonized us, left
> our peasants destitute, created famines. WB /WTO rules promote corporate
> hijack of food & agriculture #FarmersProtests
>
> Philanthropy has become the instrument for diverting democracy and colo-
> nising people's lives, in order to extract money from them. It is not 'giving'.
> It is sophisticated appropriation[14]

To make her points, in another article, she compares gene drives to Nazi
extermination camps: "The project of deliberately exterminating species is a
crime against nature and humanity. It was a crime when Bayer and others,
of IG Farben, exterminated Jews in concentration camps, and is a crime still.
The very idea of extermination is a crime. Developing tools of extermination
in the garb of saving the world is a crime. A crime that must not be allowed
to continue any further."[15] She continues, pointing to funding from DARPA,
which has also provided seed funding for a wide range of medical research,
immunology, stem-cell research, neuroscience, as well as the internet itself:

The DARPA-Mind is obsolete

> We are members of an Earth Family. Every species, every race is a member of
> one Earth Community. We cannot allow some members of our Earth Family to
> allocate to themselves the power and hubris to decide who will live, and who will
> be exterminated.[16]
>
> The aforementioned study on ghost-tech was sponsored by DARPA (The Pen-
> tagon's Research Ghost) and The Bill and Melinda Gates Foundation (The ghost
> of the Microsoft Monopoly). DARPA has been busy.[17]

Shiva is concerned about DARPA funding for any technology: "Interestingly,
Microsoft BASIC was developed on a DARPA Supercomputer across the street
from MIT, at Harvard. Where does DARPA end and MIT start? Where does
Microsoft end and The Bill and Melinda Gates Foundation start. The orientation of our technologies has been dictated by the DARPA-Mind, a Mechanical Mind trained in War, and Gates continues to colonise meaning, just as
gates [sic] had done to our lands, and the Green Revolution has done to our
food."[18] Shiva opposes the Green Revolution altogether, along with the use
of fertilizer, pesticides, or mechanization of plowing, planting, weeding, or
sowing (because of the use of petroleum to fuel them). Advocating a return
to the land and the "care of the soil" and a return to earlier eras of farming is
imperative, she argues.

> Our planet has evolved, in balance, creating balance, for 4.6 billion years. *Homo
> sapiens* emerged around 200,000 years ago. About 10,000 years ago, Peasants devel-
> oped the selection and breeding of seeds and domesticated agriculture began.

Human creativity combined with nature to provide the abundance that allowed the evolution of societies and species. Humanity and Nature renewed each other, sustaining civilisation and providing the potential for the Industrial Revolution.

75 years ago DARPA-Mind began its Extermination Experiment, and sent humanity off-axis. The Chemicals, Materials, and Technologies acquired during "The War", and patented (interestingly, the Internal Combustion Engine Patent belongs to Texaco), were forced on Amaranthus Culturis—The Cultures of Living Cycles.

DARPA-Mind called it "The Green Revolution", colonised the meanings of those two words, and began Stockpiling Chemicals of War in Our Fields; there is nothing "green" or "revolutionary" about Extermination, it must be a secret service code name for the assault that now has the names "Gene Drives", "CRISPR", or more accurately, Genetic Engineering.[19]

Gene Drives have been called "mutagenic chain reactions", and are to the biological world what chain reactions are to the nuclear world. The Guardian describes Gene Drives as the "gene bomb".[20]

Turning toward indigenous farming and health care is valorized in her work. In fact, her recent column on the coronavirus on her blog "Jivad," a pun on the term Jihad,[21] blames the worldwide pandemic on modern agriculture, arguing that "good food," and not, for example, the vaccines of the pharmaceutical industry, is the key to the response.

We need to shift from a mechanistic, militaristic paradigm of agriculture based on war chemicals to Regenerative Agroecology, an agriculture for life based Biodiversity and on working with a living nature, not engaging in war against the earth and her diverse species. Central to a living agriculture is care and gratitude, of giving back to the earth, law of return or the law of giving, creating circular economies which heal the earth and our bodies . . . Indigenous systems of health care have been criminalised by colonisation and the pharmaceutical industry.

We need to shift from a reductionist, mechanistic, militaristic paradigm based on separation from and colonization of the Earth, other species and our bodies, that have contributed to the health crisis to systems like Ayurveda, the science of life, which recognize that we are part of the earth's living web of life, our bodies are complex self organised living systems, that we have a potential to be healthy or sick depending on our environment and the food we grow and eat. Health depends on healthy food (Annam Sarva Aushadhi—Good food is the medicine for all diseases). A healthy gut is an ecosystem and is the basis of health. Health is harmony and balance.[22] Indigenous health systems and knowledge systems that are based on interconnectedness need to be recognized and rejuvenated in times of the health emergency we face . . . All species have their right to ecological space and freedom to evolve, and all humans as part of the Earth have a right to access to chemical free biodiverse food.[23]

In 2018, several NGOs (including ETC, Navdanya, as well as what was said in their literature to be 200 others—a number that could not be verified) put forward a similarly worded resolution about gene drives that called for a general moratorium on the research, calling it "genetic pollution":

> Gene drives are new tools that force genetically engineered traits through entire populations of insects, plants, animals and other organisms. This invasive technology represents a deliberate attempt to create a new form of genetic pollution. Gene Drives may drive species to extinction and undermine sustainable and equitable food and agriculture. Gene drives threaten natural systems. If released experimentally into the environment they may spread engineered genes uncontrollably through wild and domesticated species. This could alter ecological systems and food webs, harm biodiversity and eradicate beneficial organisms such as pollinators. Gene drives could disrupt lands, waters, food and fiber economies and harm Indigenous and peasant agroecological practices and cultures. Gene drives are being developed for use in agriculture. If applied, they may make farms even more genetically uniform and foreclose farmers' rights, as enshrined, among others, in the International Treaty on Plant Genetic Resources for Food and Agriculture and in the UN Declaration on the Rights of Peasants and other People Working in Rural Areas. Use of gene drives may further entrench a system of genetically-engineered industrial agriculture, extend agro-toxin use and concentrate corporate control over global food systems, undermining the food sovereignty of farmers, food workers and consumers. Gene drives hinder the realization of human rights including rights to healthy, ecologically-produced and culturally appropriate food and nutrition. We, the undersigned, call for a global moratorium on any release of engineered gene drives. This moratorium is necessary to affirm the precautionary principle, which is enshrined in international law, and to protect life on Earth as well as our food supply.[24]

Shiva is also a member of the International Forum on Globalization, another group that has opposed synthetic biology and which endorsed the moratorium. The group has historically focused on antimilitary and anti-war activism, and describes itself as "A research, advocacy and action organization, founded in 1994, focused on the impacts of dominant economic and geo-political policies. Led by an international board of scholars and citizen-movement leaders from ten countries, IFG collaborates with environmental, social justice, and anti-militarism activists, seeking secure models of democracy and sustainability, locally and globally."[25] However, they too turned their attention to synthetic biology and a generalized sense of alarm, not about malaria but about the rapid changes in consciousness about technology. At a conference they held on "techno-utopianism and the fate of the earth," they noted:

> Many in our society see the ecological crisis as a grand new economic opportunity for growth and profit. If nature is being destroyed, we can create new nature.

Technologies are rolling out to introduce *substitute nature*. For example: GEO-
ENGINEERING (to "solve" the climate crisis by "re-seeding" the heavens and
inventing techno-climate); GMOs (to re-arrange the genetics of food, animals, and
trees, making them more profitable); SYNTHETIC BIOLOGY (creating new artificial life forms, including genetically redesigned humans–*taller? smarter? better looking?*); and NANOTECHNOLOGY (to replace the planet's billion-years-old molecular
structures for greater efficiency.) *We prefer the old planet.* [emphasis in original][26]

There are several other groups who oppose gene drives, and other NGOs have
come to the fore to join in these arguments, but these three represent the
scope and intensity of the opposition to gene drives. Several of the members of the groups overlap, serve on one another's boards, or work closely
together. Now we have reviewed the literature that the groups provide publicly, let us turn to some analysis of these claims.

How should we consider these concerns?

5.2   Some Notes about Core Arguments

Now that we have listened to the critiques with some generosity, let us now
consider what I argue lies behind such intense opposition to gene drives. I will
note here that while the target about which the groups are alarmed changes
(nanotech, synbio, genetic modification, gene drives), the language of the
opposition is remarkably stable. The objections of the critics to new technology are largely based on classic arguments, many of which have been a part of
larger debates about relationships at the borders of many discourses and are
deeply embedded in foundational cultural narratives. Let me delineate three
overriding concerns that define the logic of the argumentative terrain for any
novel innovation.

First, for example, as a culture, we struggle to define the borders of democracy: Whose voice should count, and how are decisions made? Here, many of
the objections to gene drives reflect a sense of powerlessness—a sense of being
left out of the decisions about science policy or public policy in general—and
this is an objection that makes a great deal of sense. Yet, it is striking that
although all of the NGOs call for more democracy and transparency, it is
actually quite difficult to learn how the leaders were elected—by what process
of selection they were chosen to lead what they describe as "large groups of
farmers" or of "civil society" itself. Some of their position papers opposing
gene drives call for a worldwide oversight of science, but it is unclear who

would do the oversight. Some tell us that "all people are one," but they are wary of funding that flows from the wealthy to the projects of the poor. Yet, a review of the photos and biographies on the public websites of the NGOs seems to indicate that the people on the staff and board are predominantly white people who live in the cities of the West and North. Many are lawyers, people with doctorates, or wealthy people from or with foundations. None seemed to be, for example, members of trade unions, or local elected leaders, leaders of granges, or farm coops, or farmers, or actual peasants, for that matter. Moreover, there do not seem to be patient advocacy group members or health professionals fighting the disease that gene drives might address on the boards. Perhaps most striking for groups so critical of external funding for science, especially the BMGF, is that it is extremely hard to work out how the NGOs themselves are funded. Sometimes, board members appear as private funders. Sometimes, it is large law firms or banks. These issues of process are only one important critique, but they are the frame around the content of the opposition that these groups raise. Let us turn to this content now.

Second, several of the debates are focused on the definition and borders of "nature." Nature (often, portrayed in a gendered way, the imagery is of a virginal woman) is not precisely defined. Was nature temporally fixed? If so, during what time period? Are farmed fields "nature"? Or only wilderness? Shiva opposes the Green Revolution reforms of the 1950s. The ETC Group has as its logo a young woman in peasant clothing, bent nearly double, hand sowing seeds—a task that if actually done by a woman for hours on end would be exceptionally oppressive and not at all romantic. Is this the moment when we are still "in nature"?

One characteristic of the literature of the anti–gene drive NGOs is the view that "nature" is something that is separate from human beings, who are its enemies. Nature, meaning sometimes the rare areas on Earth without any signs of humans and sometimes hunter-gatherer societies and sometimes the elegiac vistas of early modern farms, is to be protected, and curiously enough it has a temporal order. "Nature" is an event in the past, circled and surrounded (menacingly) by humans, who go "to" it "from" modernity. Nature is "then." And to return to "nature" is a powerful return to the past, to what is seen as a simple time. This odd confusion about time is an epistemic construct, for it inverts the usual idea of our modern expertise with the "deep wisdom" of the primitive Other, as if we live in asynchronous eras.

This idea, first discussed by Johannes Fabian in his book *Time and the Other*, is predicated on the notion that actually living in the same century would mean living precisely alike in the century, or being "coeval," in his words, with the same ideas about the value of technology, the place of the natural world, the worth of science, and the most sensible way to produce food. Thus, the Other is not only different from us, they are "primitive," and this designation means that the peasants are both somehow closer to the really real of the natural world and free from the consumptive desperation that drives contemporary society, with all that this implies about good sense, understanding of limits, and, perhaps, morality itself. "Civilization, evolution, development, acculturation, modernization (and their cousins, industrialization, urbanization) are all terms whose conceptual content derives, in way that can be specified, from evolutionary Time. They all have an epistemical dimension apart from whatever ethical or unethical intentions they may express. A discourse employing terms such as primitive, savage (but also tribal, traditional, Third World, or whatever euphemism is current) does not think, or observe, or critically study, the "primitive" . . . it thinks, observes, studies in terms of the primitive."[27] For Fabian, anthropology takes up the idea of time from French *philosophes* and the eighteenth-century "elan," which sought and found a universalist language of time in the creation of "epochs" in geology and in history. Anthropology is schizoid, he argues, for it denies "coevalness," which is the denial that anthropologist and interlocutor exist at the same time or, in other words, because it locates its subject in a different time, the field itself is allochronic, and the discourse always asynchronous. Structurally, a field such as research genetics is allied with the present, a sign of modernity, and then the natural world becomes allied with the past, a romantic past in which happy, healthy peasants lived in a benign nature, which is about as far from the real fifteenth century as it is possible to be. But Fabian has pointed to a more fundamental aspect about the Romantic conception of nature that is found in the writings of many of the anti–gene drive groups. There is a yearning for a fictional past. And not only is this past fictional, but it also holds durable tropes about "natural" orders of power and judgment.

In her thoughtful essay on issues about "nature writing,"[28] Kathryn Schultz reflects on what she sees as the "old familiar strain of fascism in nature writing, the strain that despises cities as breeding grounds for the foreign and impoverished while promising to restore to a purer people glory and lands . . . Humankind as destructive, culture as corrosive, progress as decline: these are old saw, dull from use, dull from their stalemate combination of truth and falsity . . . (they see) a world that would be wonderful if it weren't for all the people in it."[29] Schultz picks up on the deeper tropes in the anti-GMO, anti-science thrust of the arguments, which are that these groups see nature as it was seen by the Romantics, and as the American Transcendentalists did, its wildness and innocence and virginal purity as a spiritual phenomenon, always at risk, always threatened. But she also notes that the anti-immigrant, anti-urban rhetoric and the return to the better, more Volkisch way that has been used by authoritarians and fascists repeatedly.

Third, the arguments are familiar, classically so. This is yet another aspect of the opposition's arguments. Some of the objections are based on the classic fears of the ancient world, in particular the tropes of Greek drama or Central Asian origin narratives. In such a world, all of nature is terrifyingly mutable and unfixed in its borders and caprices. Here is the origin of the fear: that the god–person boundary is always at stake, and that humans tempt disaster by "playing" at being gods. Here is where Pandora releases trouble, where there is punishment for figuring out how humans use fire. I want to note at this point that the concept that it is inappropriate to act as God would act does not emerge in traditional texts of Jewish, Christian, or Islamic thought. In fact, in these traditions, the congregant is often told to act in God's stead, doing the work (healing, teaching, care of the poor, etc.) that God or Jesus would do. In fact, unlike Greek mythology's worry about power, or mastery, technology is not seen as a violation of divine order. The first "invention" is the use of fire and this understood in classic midrash—Jewish rabbinic legal and narrative texts—as humanity's first independent act. Creative and useful tools make human life less grim or painful. The anxiety about technology reoccurs in Socratic thought, where in the Phaedrus, the first technology of "writing" is seen as less authentic than the spoken word. And thus, writing is the first technology to be opposed. From 370 BCE to modernity, the worry reappears at the threshold of each innovation. It is a long argument!

However, gene drives—like stem cells, CRISPR, or synthetic biology—also stand in as signs for larger contemporary anxieties of the modern world, not only the anxieties of the Greeks of the 5th century BCE, for they are a synecdoche for modernity itself and thus carry all the weight of the 200 years of anxiety since the Industrial Revolution. That is, by the way, the reason behind a text—*Frankenstein*, written just as the Industrial Revolution was unfolding and science was gaining new explanatory power—having such resonance.

Fourth, if arguments from deep within the Western tradition are one source of objection, arguments about the anxieties of modernity itself are another. One can see that much of the opposition to gene drives has been repurposed from earlier documents used to oppose GM foods, and this is not simply a matter of expediency—it is because the fears are the main point, no matter what precise technology is at issue. The upsetting sense that the world has changed for the worse ("we liked the old planet") and the nostalgia for a past imaginary in which things were cleaner, safer, and, well, nicer is pervasive in these essays, when the actual past was far more dangerous, far dirtier, with wood and coal smoke that choked even small towns, and wildly unsafe working conditions, farms lost and torn apart by sectarian violence, unregulated barons, the bleak poverty and mortality of peasant life, the terror of the pagan gods, and the pervasive hunger just at the border of every single year. Floods from undammed rivers inundated millions in China and India, a feature of the "old planet," for example, and plagues swept through entire regions with regularity. Yet, it is modernity, industrialization, and genetic research that seems to trigger a yearning for simplicity and, ironically, for control—a world that is simple and easier to understand, local, with local custom and folk wisdom in the place of expertise. Yet, let us look more closely at that world. The actual world, nearly every place, is imperiled, to be sure, but also made more habitable by technology. The peasant girl pictured bent over in ETC's logo is now more likely to have been vaccinated for polio and tetanus, she is more like to have had at least an elementary education, and she will likely be far better able to marry later and control her fertility than her seventeenth-century peers. It is a mixed bag, this modernity, which is why we need to spend time thinking carefully about its use, not immediately condemning any technology as a cover for the military or an expansion of a terrible social discipline.

5.3   We Break for Small Metaphorical Comparisons

Consider the cassava wasp, *Epidinocarsis lopezi*. In fact, consider the cassava plant itself. In chapter 2 of this book, when I described Austin Burt's talk to the NAS, I mentioned that he argued that using insects to control disease is not a novel strategy and that this manipulation of nature has long been a part of human agricultural practices. And while critics often point only to the disasters, like rabbits in Australia, it is at least worth noting the successful use of this concept, as Burt reminded the committee. Let me expand on his reference.

Cassava, or manioc (*Manihot esculenta*), is a root crop native to tropical America that is now consumed by millions of people throughout the tropics, where it is largely grown by women. It is used in food preparation in many industrialized processes where it works as a filler. Although it is not well known outside the tropics, cassava now accounts for about 30 percent of the world's production of roots and tubers. It is an exceptional producer of carbohydrates and better able to tolerate seasonal drought than other major food crops. But it is not a source of plant protein, and it is not especially nutritious in other ways. Moreover, while there are two types of cassava, sweet and bitter, both contain toxic cyanide, more so in the bitter version. So, it has to be carefully prepared to remove traces of cyanide. Sweet cassava is the one generally used as food, and growing and preparing it is nearly always done exclusively by women.[30]

For the last several years, scientists have been interested in seeing if a genetic set of instructions can be inserted into the DNA of plants used for food in the world's poorest countries to make them more useful in addressing issues of food scarcity. One of the most interesting projects is BioCassava Plus, a multidisciplinary team of international researchers in science, sociology, and anthropology working both to create a nutritious crop for sub-Saharan Africa and to try to anticipate the impact of a GM food in that culture. Inadequate nutrition is the single greatest cause of the steadily rising mortality, morbidity and suffering in sub-Saharan Africa, which is facing a rapidly changing climate. So, enter cassava—the root crop harvested by the world's poorest women. Two hundred and fifty million Africans rely on this starchy root crop as their staple food, which is itself an irony.

Interestingly enough for our story, cassava roots are not native to Africa. They were brought there by soldiers and missionaries from South America in a first effort to provide food. But they were not a fortuitous choice, for while they are easy to grow, they have the lowest protein-to-energy ratio of all the staple crops, with a typical cassava-based diet providing less than 30 percent of the minimum daily requirement for protein and only 10–20 percent of the required amounts of iron, zinc, vitamin A, and vitamin E. Worse still, they have high levels of harmful sugars. The goal was to alter the cassava genetically, so that people who can only afford to grow this one crop would get everything they needed from it, without the harmful effects. That would not be all: researchers would work with African traditional farmers to make sure the crop actually tasted good and was still easy to grow.[31] Cassava was an interesting choice. It is the crop most commonly grown in Africa—a crop whose production is nearly entirely in the control of women in the villages. Where starvation is a constant threat, making cassava a high-protein, highly useful food would be of inestimable value.

The cassava plant is hardy and better able to tolerate drought and poor soil conditions than most other food plants, unequalled in its ability to recover when foliage is lost or damaged by diseases or pests or stamped on by animals. Cassava was the staple crop of the Amerindians of South America when the Portuguese arrived in 1500, just south of what is known as Bahia, Brazil. The Amerindians living in the area relied on cassava as a dietary staple, processing it into bread and meal.

When the Portuguese began to import slaves from Africa around 1550, they used cassava in the form of meal to provision their ships and began cultivating cassava at their stations along the coast of West Africa soon afterward. From their stations near the mouth of the Congo River, cassava diffused to all of Central Africa,[32] in the same area where malaria rages most intensively today. As historian Richard Norgaard describes it:

> But in the early 1970s two pests of the cassava were also, inadvertently, introduced from South America, cassava mealybug and cassava green spider mite. These pests are relatively minor nuisances in South America where predators and parasites have coevolved to keep them in check. In Africa, however, these pests spread rapidly and devastated cassava fields in the absence of their natural enemies. In the mid-1970s, biologists began to search in South America for natural enemies of the cassava mealybug and the cassava green mite that would control their population outbreak. A classical biological control solution, in particular the reuniting of predators and parasites with their previously dislocated prey and hosts, was deemed the best solution because subsistence farmers in Africa do not use chemicals. *Epidinocarsis lopezi*, a small wasp, was found to be a parasite of, as well as a hostfeeder on, cassava mealybug.[33]

The predatory wasp from South America was released in a several countries to eat the pests from South America that were eating the cassava from South America. All the species reunited in their new habitat, Africa, and this rather ingenious solution reduced the existence of the mealybugs by

95 percent—something that Burt notes in his research talks. Not only has there been no reemergence of the pests in the last fifteen years, but the wasp has now been released throughout Asia in countries where the West brought first the crop, then the pests, and now the biological control. This complex story is worth thinking about carefully, which is why it is mentioned here. It provides a bit of complex side history that creates an interesting example of human responsibility and the previous uses of field releases in Africa. Consider this somewhat circuitous narrative, reader, as part of how to think about this issue. But also consider how rarely this success story has been told—it is just not a part of the narrative. Nor is anyone protesting the very non-natural use of cassava, or its mealybugs, or the killing of all the mealybugs by the wasp, flown in on planes for the purpose of eradication. If this is not curious enough, let me turn to a second example.

Consider the New World screwworm, *Cochliomyia hominivorax*, the larvae of a species of blowfly. They are a particularly horrific parasite, living largely within the wounded flesh of birds and small warm-blooded animals, but they will live on—and destroy—larger mammals, domesticated animals, and, occasionally, human beings. The female flies, after mating once, like mosquitoes, are attracted to any torn flesh to lay their eggs. They prefer larger and bloodier wounds, but any break in the skin will do, including the small pricks of insect bites or scratches from a twig. They favor the fresh surfaces of newly born animals, the small soft spot where the umbilical cord detaches, or the abraded vaginal area of a female just after she gives birth. In twelve to twenty-four hours, the eggs hatch into masses of larvae, which use the open flesh of the wounded body for food, burrowing or "screwing" into the torn tissue, enlarging the wound and causing it to bleed and suppurate,[34] which attracts more female flies, who lay more eggs. A fully infected animal will die, exhausted and frantic with the pain, in five to ten days, usually of overwhelming sepsis.[35] Afterward, the larvae will crawl out of the wound and drop to the ground, where they will burrow into the soil, pupate, and emerge again as flies, seeking the bloodied flesh, beginning the cycle again.

Long feared as a pest, the larvae's cycle was fully characterized by the 1930s, when screwworms, native to North America, were destroying thousands of cattle, sheep, and goats in the agricultural Southwest and then were spreading into the Southeast. The great herds of Texas cattle, rustled together, horns and hoofs, a threat in close quarters, were a particular target. There was no effective prevention, and cures were labor intensive, involving checking the entire herd one at a time, looking for infected wounds, and culling the animals. The first treatments were pine tar and then thick, smelly, sticky insecticide ointments smeared on the hide of the cattle. In 1935, screwworms resulted in 180,000 livestock deaths in just under half the counties in Texas, in spite of the manpower and constant effort invested in keeping the insects at bay.[36]

Army entomologist Edward Knipling and Army physician Alfred Lindquist, newly returned from a war that had interrupted the research they were doing on the screwworm, were both Texans. Lindquist had recently studied the work of fruit fly geneticist Hermann Mueller. Mueller had been reaching heritable mutations in flies, which he would induce by using a radiation gun to shoot fly eggs or adult flies. He developed linages with crooked wings or white eyes or that were sterile—the radiation created stochastic effects. Knipling is credited with writing to Mueller to learn more. It was the sterile flies that interested Knipling and Lindquist. They realized that they could radiate flies, sterilizing them, and release the sterile males into the wild, and since each female fly only mated once, if the field was saturated with sterile males, it would eliminate new populations of larvae entirely. They proposed a field test. There was no opposition, only enormous enthusiasm from ranchers.

Funded by the powerful Cattle Growers' Association, the sterile males were then flown off the coast of Florida to Sanibel Island and released from low flying planes, in long clouds over the jungle. This was tested in next in Curacao, Venezuela, where the screwworm was completely eradicated in only ten weeks. By 1958, the federal government was producing 50 million sterile flies per week and releasing them over Florida that winter. By 1959, screwworms were eradicated from Florida and the Southeast, and by 1966, the USDA declared the USA free of all indigenous screwworms.[37] Every year, since 1955, despite some setbacks, larger and larger areas of endemic screwworm populations are eliminated from the environment.

Mexico eliminated screwworms by 1993, as did Guatemala, then Belize, then El Salvador in 1994, then Honduras by 1996, then Nicaragua in 1999, and Costa Rica in 2000. The barrier between ecologies without screwworms and ecologies with them now is between Panama, free of screwworms, and Columbia, infested. The line is at the Darien Gap, exactly at the spot the alert reader will remember from the disastrous and fatal collapse of the Scottish colony at Darien because of the overwhelming malaria epidemic. And every week, "planes drop 14.7 million sterilized screwworms over the rainforest that divides the two countries. A screwworm-rearing plant operates 24/7 in Panama. Inspectors cover thousands of square miles by motorcycle, boat, and horseback, searching for stray screwworm infections north of the border. The slightest oversight could undo all the work that came before."[38] All of this—a billion sterile male flies reared on trays of festering beef, radiated, altering their little fly genomes, and then released to fall from the sky by busily thrumming prop planes—is run by a joint commission of Panama's agricultural department and the USDA known as COPEG or the Comisión Panamá–Estados Unidos para la Erradicación y Prevención del Gusano Barrenador del Ganado.[39]

I raise this narrative about flies in some detail in the middle of a chapter of a book on mosquitoes not because it is the only or even the very best example of the use of sterile insect technique (SIT) using genetic mutations, but rather because it is one of the oddest and most invasive interventions in the nature world that I can describe, with every single element that would, one would imagine, raise deep and fundamental concerns with the NGOs that oppose gene drives because they interfere with nature's order or because they eliminate the parasite.

Consider: it is a techno-fix that originated in the work of Army-trained researchers; it uses radiation; it uses radiation to create a vast array of genetic and biological changes in a species that renders them sterile; it was funded and supported by big Agricultural ("Big Agri") interests, indeed by ranchers raising vast herds of cattle for meat production, in the otherwise uninhabited rainforests and plains of Latin America; it drops the GMOs, whose genetic sequences have been blasted by radiation x-ray beams to render them sterile, from low-flying airplanes, and the inhabitants do not seem to have been asked about this; it eliminates an entire species from an eco-system; and the range of extermination grows annually and here again, there was no painstaking community consent process, and no outcry about its absence. Does it interfere with the natural order? Absolutely. Does it destroy a species without really knowing that delicate food network it disturbs? Yes. It does this in the name not of a significant human disease, but of one that largely affects the cattle that so upset the activist organizations. What other effects might the radiation that renders the males sterile have, and how might these affect the rest of the ecosystem? That is unclear. Can some males sterilize incompletely but survive mutated to wreak some sort of vague havoc? Could mutated females inadvertently, in the mix of released flies, survive and be released? We know that even under very careful conditions, this sort of mistake is very difficult to prevent—they are not checking fly by fly, of course.

None of these objections have been raised. In fact, none of the NGOs that are so careful to protest, well, much of new technology, have lodged protests about any aspect of the screwworm SIT project, despite the fact that it has been written about in the popular press—two articles in the Atlantic and coverage on National Public Radio.

In 2016, a new screwworm infestation began suddenly, first in the Florida Keys and then on the Florida mainland in Homestead, Florida. Wild fawns began dropping dead on suburban lawns and wooded areas. Then, pets began to sicken, and the state moved in swiftly. Checkpoints were set up to examine every car for animals; 80 million sterile male flies were swiftly introduced in the area.[40] The epidemic was halted. Again, there were no community meetings, no outrage, and no petitions from any NGO. None of the fears we have noted in the literature about gene drives, in which "all it takes is one mosquito" were raised. No one raised concerns about the human mastery of nature or of the techno-optimism of the project. Radiation is a fairly primitive tool to use to make genes turn off, as they do in the flies, or to induce mutagenic effects, hard to control—a technology of the 1950s. But there was no comment on this, even though the project (minus the checkpoints to examine your cat or dog) was nearly identical to the Oxitec SIR that caused an outcry against "Franken mosquitoes." As a scholar, it is critical to understand why this is the case.

5.4 Typography of Canonical Arguments about Genetics

Why is the reaction to gene drives so fierce, when the entire Guinea Worm Eradication Project goes unremarked upon? In part, this reaction can be understood in light of several objections that can only be called canonical, in addition to the three overriding ones I noted above. We do not have a moral panic about wasps or screwworms, in part because the story of the screwworm is not well known, despite being covered by reporters from *The Atlantic* and *National Geographic*, and in part because flesh-eating worms are so appalling. In addition, unlike malaria, outbreaks have occurred close to home in Homestead, not in African rural areas. But it remains a puzzle why such a dramatic genetic technology, featuring low-flying planes dropping irradiated insects in the millions, does not cause an outcry. To understand why, I will turn to the special role that genetics has in the modern imaginary. Gene drives, even in their nomenclature, stress the genetic manipulation aspect of the project, and as I have pointed out, genetic science evokes a particular, ontological concern.

Let us review these specific concerns about genetic technology in more detail, since they reoccur with such frequency.

First, many groups oppose any manipulation or alteration of the DNA of an organism, any organism. They oppose all genetic modification, no matter what its goal or intent, and have done so since the first use of recombinant DNA technology. "GMOs (to re-arrange the genetics of food, animals, and trees, making them more profitable); SYNTHETIC BIOLOGY (creating new artificial life forms, including genetically redesigned humans—*taller? smarter? better looking?*)."[41] "DNA" in this argument represents the inviolate and essential reality of a being, fixing species as if static, and perfect, in an Aristotelian order. The moral worth of a living being, which is to say its embodied form, lies increasingly in the "DNA," an entity as elusive but as present as the soul was for medieval thinkers. So, to alter the "DNA" of a species is impermissible. The dignity of the being, be it a cotton plant, a redwood tree, or an insect, requires this intactness. This ipseity is this identity. This ipseity is integrity itself. It means that any deliberate, invasive proximity to the "DNA" is wrong. Since the term "DNA" had come to mean identity or values in common language ("It's in our DNA!" is the phrase used by politicians, university presidents, and marketing executives, which they use in our secular age instead of "It's in our soul!"), then the stakes for alteration represent an ontological threat to being itself.

Of course, humans, or, as Shiva calls, them "Peasants," have been altering the DNA of species for millennia, for that, of course, is what breeding consists of. "Our planet has evolved, in balance, creating balance, for 4.6 billion years. *Homo sapiens* emerged around 200,000 years ago. About 10,000 years ago, Peasants developed the selection and breeding of seeds and domesticated agriculture began. Human creativity combined with nature to provide the abundance that allowed the evolution of societies and species."[42] Thus, evolution of species, selection of traits, and alteration of plants and animals is permissible in principle, just not if this breeding is done by scientists not Peasants, not permissible if it is done in a laboratory, with precision, and oddly permissible if it is done by repeating the chance of a genetic change by forced mating for traits thought useful. Notice the use of the term "nature" in this account and the absence of the word "genetic changes," although, of course, that is exactly what is at stake in selection and breeding, practice no less humanly constructed.

Second, the claim is made that Nature—the concept, not exactly the place, because as I noted above, it is unclear if Nature is a category that refers to organic farms, or wilderness, or if any such place of untouched habitation exists. In this account, Nature—is itself normative, good, and ought to be permanent. Nature—human nature and the nature of the green and living world—is fixed, for it has borders that cannot be broached without violation and species that are fixed in an Aristotelian way, each one perfect (despite the millennia of agriculture as noted above). Nature is also normative, meaning it directs us toward certain actions, and, finally, morally good, if left free; and it will express itself in a primal harmony that our use, and our machines, threatens. Because Nature's aspects are said to be normative, or directive, altering nature "breaks rules." This argument sometimes appears in right-wing conservative literature as a reason to oppose, for example, gay marriage or extramarital sex, but it also appears in left-wing progressive arguments about disrespecting Gaia in various ways. In both cases, Nature will assert herself in a sort of vengeance.

Third, sometimes, movements in opposition to genetic research make a complicated argument about our need for suffering, and it is that human beings are shaped by suffering in ennobling ways. Suffering is the main thing that defines our species being, goes this argument. Suffering and its noble acceptance is the great teacher of our need and of our love. Without suffering, we would become soulless. In this argument, suffering, morbidity, and mortality create the moral structures that define our humanity. Without suffering, the world would be a poorer place, Leon Kass notes: "We are concerned that our society might be harmed and that we ourselves might be diminished, indeed, in ways that could undermine the highest and richest possibilities of human life. The last and most seductive of these disquieting prospects—the use of biotechnical powers to pursue 'perfection,' both of body and of mind."[43] Of course, seeking to end malaria in Africa is hardly seeking "perfection." African villages, even if free of malaria, will still be challenging places to live and to raise a family, of course. Seeking to end diseases as our collective understanding grows has never meant that human beings became diminished. It has just meant we did not die of smallpox or weren't paralyzed by polio.

There are a few versions of this argument that are particularly troubling. One is that there is a need for human diversity, just as there is for creaturely diversity in general, and that addressing illness or disability threatens this goal. Largely, this is never put forward as wanting to be ill or disabled oneself, but illness or disability is a general event that occurs to others, of which one is tolerant and welcoming.

Another part of this troubling argument is that eliminating suffering, in particular eliminating malaria, would allow the survival and growth of "too many" African children and that this would be disruptive. Sometimes this problem uses the language of nature-speak to make the point, as in "we should allow nature to take its course," or "this would create a burden on the environment," and sometimes it uses the language of social policy, as in arguments that talk about economic disruption. This bad argument has a long history in colonialist concerns when it was raised repeatedly in the nineteenth century by British authorities, who were anxious about the growth of native populations in general.

Fourth, some groups, as we have seen, turn to the "slippery slope" argument—that we need to oppose even salutary uses of gene drives because once the technology is used for malaria, it will be used recklessly for other sorts of vector control. Indeed, the history of DDT would seem to validate this fear. DDT was intended to be used only to kill the flies and mosquitoes that carried dangerous diseases, and then, when it was shown to be so tantalizingly effective it was used widely in agriculture to boost food production, and even in home gardens without restriction. Slopes were slippery then—and if we use a technology for good, there will be no way to stop it from being used for larger and progressively more evil or more trivial purposes, argue some, until there is no longer species diversity. In this argument, human beings will not be able to stop themselves or regulate their use of a powerful technology. (But of course, I would argue, we have been perfectly capable of limiting many technologies in the past. This is an argument to which I will return in the next chapter.)

Fifth, not only are slopes slippery, some worry that the temptation to use a gene drive for harm—so-called dual use—is also inevitable. Gene drives, goes this argument, will be used as a weapon of the world. Imagine you could destroy the food crops of your enemy by unleashing an organism that would be powerful, hungry, and immune to all pesticides, or one that could spread a disease to which your side had a preventive vaccine. I will return to this in the next chapter as well.

Sixth, yet another concern raised in this literature is about mistakes. I understand this concern, having co-edited a book about mistakes in bioethics and medicine.[44] Research, like any other human activity, is riddled with errors. In this objection, error is inevitable, and here, the objectors focus on the long history of nineteenth-century errors in science that had world-changing implications: importing mongooses into Hawaii to kill rats in the newly established sugarcane plantations, which ended up killing native birds but not rats, since rats are nocturnal and mongooses are not; or the introduction of cane toads for the same purpose in Australia, which ended up overrunning the habitat, along with the rabbits that new Australian settlers brought for food and company; or the sparrows let loose in Central Park in New York that crowded out native species.

Seventh, opposition to new research is also based on a healthy disdain for the marketplace. The marketplace will corrupt science, in this argument, or it perhaps already has. The researchers are said to receive millions in profit, or perhaps they are on the take from the billionaires who control the marketplace. The deeply felt opposition to the Bill and Melinda Gates Foundation seems to be based on this concern, or the fear that scientists, driven by monetary concerns, are not to be trusted at all. The mix of marketplace and medicine is troubling, and the very success implied by genetic medicine—its widespread applications—should alert us to its danger.

And the marketplace is indeed chancy—it could, as in the imagination of many who oppose gene drives, greatly reward, even unfairly reward, some actors. But it can also collapse, and as a project for social good, the market forces can make a project fail. Indeed, this has occurred once before, in the first attempt by the new field of synthetic biology to address malaria.

Consider this story: One of the first problems taken on by the new field of synthetic biology was the problem of malaria. The most effective drug used in the last ten years is, as you have seen, made from Chinese wormwood, called artemisinin. But Chinese wormwood is rare and hard to process. Crop yields go up and down, creating huge market swings. Could there be a different solution? This was an early, visionary project in synthetic biology I considered, and you can see why—because it was for the sort of research that I was always most interested in: research on the diseases of the poor.

Jay Keasling invited me into his laboratory at the University of California at Berkeley on a cool March morning to explain his project to me: a way to make a desperately needed drug that countered malaria but whose ingredients were rare and hard to obtain, making the drug costly. Keasling had turned his attention to the problem of malaria for all the reasons of social justice, but also because the disease relies on an interesting host–carrier mechanism with a high rate of mutation. This means that a multidrug-resistant form was becoming dominant. Keasling had developed:

> a technique for transplanting yeast and plant genes to construct an entirely new metabolic pathway inside bacteria can be used generally to produce a broad family of so-called isoprenoids—chemical precursors to many plant-derived drugs and chemicals of interest to industry, including the anticancer drug taxol and various food additives. Isoprenoids, found widely in microbes, plants and marine organisms, currently are very expensive for the chemical industry to synthesize from scratch and nearly as expensive to extract from plant material. (Unlike standard pharmaceutical rDNA techniques) where protein drugs are produced primarily through fermentation by recombinant yeast that seldom have more than one gene inserted in them, Keasling assembled 10 genes, including control elements, from three different organisms—bacteria, yeast and wormwood—and got them to work together successfully.[45]

Chinese wormwood has genes that produce artemisinin, which, when placed in yeast, can replicate the plant process, and this "cassette" of genes is placed into E. coli, which can divide rapidly enough to allow for commercial production. Further, such a system could allow this new "product" to evolve in response to any resistance that is developed, for it is a biological system.[46] It is important to note that the rights to the project were donated to Amyris Biotechnology, which will sell the drug at no cost (25¢ for the needed three-day dose) instead of the $2.40 for the traditional drug. The testing would be overseen by the Bill and Melinda Gates Foundation via the nonprofit OneWorld Health Organization.[47] On a visit I made to his lab, in 2006, Keasling held out his hand and showed me the prototypes. "Three of these, just a quarter, and you are cured of that bout with malaria," he said. By 2014, his company would sell the rights to Sanofi, which announced that a new laboratory in Italy would make up to a third of all artemisinin. However, by 2016, it turned out that while the science worked, the market economics did not.[48] The plant closed; the project has still not started.

Eighth, this sort of story led to another point: the issue of justice and resource allocation. For many genetic interventions, objections are raised about justice. This comes into play when we think about genetic interventions linked to human enhancements. The world is already unfair, and life's lottery already distributes physical attributes and genetic diseases unfairly, with physical health linked to social and economic status. So, the concern is that in the future, genetic advantages will rebound to the wealthy, leaving the poor, marginalized groups, and racial minorities out, and this will worsen injustice. Reading the literature of the anti–gene drive groups, and you will see a consistent concern about potentials for injustice, although unlike most genetic experiments, which do in fact focus on one or two patients, gene drives are specifically designed to meet the needs of the world's poorest people.

Finally, ninth, some of the literature reveals an unease beneath arguments about dual use, error, or injustice—a general sense that the world is already inauthentic and *umhiemlich* enough, alternated and manipulated enough, and that more intervention and more mastery is simply wrong. We are defined by our finitude and our contingency, goes this argument, and control—"mastery"—is a mistakenness that is wrong, not only because mastery is considered wrong but because it is inauthentic, Disneyfied.

The term "synthetic biology" or "engineering biology" or "molecular engineering," which are all names for the larger category of genetic research in which projects such as gene drives lie, is itself is confusing. What the scientists who coined each term meant was to parallel their field with "synthetic chemistry," which is how chemists describes chemistry that synthesizes different molecular structures to make new compounds, or to communicate the field as one that is a merger of biology, chemistry, and engineering, using the tools of many disciplines. One idea was to synthesize new biological "parts" that could be standardized and used in imaginative ways to make new biological possibilities, and other ideas were based on the concept of reengineering the world at a very small scale, just as it had been reengineered at the macro level with civic engineering—bridges and dams, for example. But what the public heard was the lay use of the term "synthetic" and thought "fake," "rayon pants," and "pleather." Synthetic biology sounded like scientists would replace the authenticity of the natural world, all the green and mossy parts of it, with plastic, and of course, because words matter a great deal, this nomenclature made the opposition even stronger. And while engineering the world sounded great to some people, to others, it smacked of nineteenth-century hubris and overweening prideful mastery.

5.5   What We Talk about When We Talk about Gene Drives

What can be said about these types of objections, which the groups I followed raised not only about gene drives, to be sure, but also about GM foods,
"designer babies," synthetic biology in general, nanotechnology, stem-cell
biology, and gene therapy. Not everyone makes every claim; some emerge
politically from the left, some from the right in an increasingly divided polity. I will make two observations about these arguments. First, all of them are
more than trivially correct, and any sensible person could agree with many
of these statements. The trouble begins here in their extremity when taken to
their logical conclusion. (Yes, slopes are slippery, but they are not impossibly
slippery, and we can erect fences and barriers to stop a slide to the bottom,
to give just one example. Yes, dual use is a real problem, and that is why we
need a great deal of care about the issue, to give another example.)

Second, all of these are profoundly religious statements. They are statements of faith, worldview and eschatology, not of moral arguments. As such,
they will not—cannot—be entirely agreed upon in pluralistic democracies.
Like many faith claims in our world, they are claims about the world to come,
but of course, we cannot yet know that. Some claim that the world to come
will yield great advances using genetics, but that this social good will not be
fair; others claim that the world to come will be a disaster, like many other
interventions, but this too is a matter of disputed judgment. Faith claims
are extraordinarily difficult to refute or change, for coming to a compromise
can feel like a betrayal of sincerely held beliefs. So, arguing about who is correct is oftentimes futile because disagreement about the nature, goal, and
meaning of science is so deeply contended and so profoundly a part of one's
worldview. The fact that the people who make the arguments do not identify
them as faith based is not the point, certainly not for a scholar of religion
like me who cannot be help but see the eschatological nature of the visions
of the future, either hellish or redemptive. Western culture often "bootlegs"
ideas from theological sources and texts to make an argument. Consider,
for example, the "brotherhood" of Man, which derives its power from the
implied fatherhood of God, or the notion of society's special obligation to
the widow, orphan, or stranger. These examples are derived from Hebrew,
Christian, and Islamic scriptural texts. And, by the same token, some of the
ideas about trees having a spirit or ecosystems having a deep goodness or the
order of species having a moral valence are ideas about divinity—a sincere

belief in polytheism or animism or paganism, not science. Modernity seems secular, to be sure, but the passion of these claims reminds us that they have older sources.

What responses can be given to the NGO member who raises this mix of complex claims against the project of gene drives? Let us take as sincere that the intuitive concerns that the groups raise are important, and let me then suggest a way to respond.

1. Living under the Fallen Sky

First, is the sky really falling? Do gene drives mean that nature, as defined in this literature, is threatened by their use? Is the world about to be fundamentally changed by genetic medicine? Let me note here that it is very understandable that many NGOs believe this is the case because all too often, scientists themselves, or their university publicity offices or the companies that fund them, promise it to be so. Both the scientists and the opposers honestly believe that the future is a certainty—that we are at an eschatological moment in human history. But this is an error. The contemporary literature about biotechnology reflects a rather touching sense that the future can be named, known, and spectacular. But it cannot be fully known. I will discuss this further in my final chapter.

We cannot know the social impact of technologies that will occur against a changing horizon of other temporal and technological changes. It was not long ago that living as a healthy eighty-year-old was unprecedented, and this has, in one generation, swiftly become obtainable for many. It is also the case that the defining suffering for all of human history—infectious disease—can be addressed in nearly every case, even in COVID-19, but there is no empirical evidence that we are living without our souls. Is the world empirically cheapened by IVF babies, gene therapy for sickle cell disease, or any other scientific advance—odder perhaps, complex maybe, but it is hardly the reason for any of our social or familial problems.

May we make the world? On some level, how can we not? What would it mean to turn away from the research I describe in this book because it might be used for evil intent, or because we believe it to be unnatural, especially compared to the fight against the Guinea worm, or the previous eradications of malaria mosquitoes in the early twentieth-century campaigns? We live, nearly all of us, surely everyone on the boards of the NGOs, in a world that is highly engineered, and there is something disingenuous when people who can afford to live in safety in that world protest interventions that might make it better for the poor who do not, all in the name of "naturalness."

This is perhaps a religious matter, as is all sort of discussion about the end of time. For many in religious traditions, the sky was a chancy thing long ago. The idea of the sacred canopy, in the sense that Peter Berger intends it, has surely fallen to pieces after the Shoah or the Irish Potato Famine or the fires of global warming—all examples of humanity's capacity for evil, surely—and it lies like shattered glass, everywhere. People walk around a world that is difficult, not Eden, and not even a natural wilderness.[49]

The "world to come," the future that is so much at stake in this literature, is, in a sense, one that we must make. In the words of the French Jewish philosopher Emmanuel Levinas, Utopia is that one can be chosen to be called upon by the needs of the other people. For Levinas, authenticity has little to do with some aspect of being—rather "the authenticity of the I. . . . is this listening on the part of the first one called, this attention to the other without subrogation. . . . the possibility of sacrifice as the meaning of the human endeavor. It is this sort of authenticity that. . . . is the very meaning of Utopia—justice and transcendence, love for the other, and willingness to live within a code of law that still contains within it the possibilities of mercy."[50]

It is no accident that Levinas argues that the free person is one who "before all loans, ha[s] debts," meaning that duties are prior to rights and are specific (I owe something to the neighbor, I am responsible), chosen, and unique and, in this responsibility, we want peace, justice, and reason. For Levinas, this is the way to think about the meaning of being human. If one thinks that the world, as it is, is morally correct, with fixed orders, and that change is not only dangerous but a seduction, a destabilizing one—threatening to alter our species being—that must be, in this account, protected, singular, a thing entirely belonging to us, then the sort of thing that genetic research represents is terrifying—for it deconstructs the world into pieces and suggests that it can be reimagined, and reimagined largely for the need of the other. In a sense, it is a close account of the moral gesture of all medical research.

I would argue that it is not suffering that defines us, it is healing—the moral gesture of healing is the precise non-animal thing. It is not our pain, which we share with every mouse, it is the fact that in the medical school in which we teach ethics, we teach doctors and nurses to work in blood and feces and bone for the need of the other alone, that the dying man and the laboring woman command our complete attention. It is not achieving my fine aspiration that makes me human, or even reading the Iliad, rather it is my willingness to sacrifice my very breath to resuscitate, if need be, or to wash the back of the indigent stranger if that is who I am given to care for, that allows me to become human. Without our duties and without our love, we are just words on paper.

We are turned to by the neighbor for the world is not yet good, and we can change it because scientific research is powerful. It can be reckless, but it can also be wise, and our neighbor understands that. We—and by this, I mean especially but not exclusively science as a profession—must be interrupted in our story line to answer to our debt to her. If the literature of opposition to gene drives suggests that we do not have a duty to address the suffering of malarial illness or the death of a child every two minutes, then it is more than troubling. It is failing in its essential moral task.

2. A Familiar Discussion

Second, is this a unique time in human history? Is our world-making ability unprecedented? Hardly. At many times in human history, the sense that large forces clash over the power to control the world is apparent. One critical time is the ninth through the twelfth centuries, but the conflict appears in the Renaissance, in early modernity as well. Let us turn to the medieval period and to the work of medievalists. Jonathan Cohen and Richard Landes and others have argued mysticism, millennialism, and calls for a return to natural order often emerge just at the moment that science forces new relationships of knowledge and power. Landes, who studies millennialism, notes the comparison between our period and the ninth century. We can see that the literature of opposition to science is largely based on resonant tropes— tropes particularly but not uniquely shaped in the early medieval period.

Hence, the debates, every where given force by secular arguments, are deeply driven by faith commitments and arguments of religion as I have noted. We are faced, globally, with a deep yearning for the past, for the present can be a terribly uncertain place. There is a sense that medieval tropes are true or essential ones—that we live in a spirit-haunted world, with an affection for clarity in good and evil, aliens, or pure natural beings that are linked to nature, like in the *Lord of the Rings* or *Harry Potter*. Old prejudices reemerge, and fundamentalism is a powerful force politically and religiously. In such a period, there is a struggle with phenomenological knowledge—science, observation, empirical wisdom, and received knowledge from religious leaders. In the West, such fears are often the subject of intellectual discourse, but merely discourse, but in the developing world, such theories have had dramatic consequences. In Nigeria, the polio vaccine was refused in fear that it would cause female sterility, and in Zimbabwe, grain was refused in a famine in fear of genetic engineering. In the USA, questions based on a notion that an instinctual moral repugnance, or the deep-seated knowledge of faiths, ought to guide moral discernment—but what are we to think of moral repugnance when it means that babies are not given polio vaccinations or women are not allowed to read or five-year-olds go to bed malnourished? In bioethics, the basic Heideggerian ideas—that truth can be recovered from a pre-literal past, that authenticity is formulated by one strong "I," and that suffering and death are the fulcrum points of essential humanity—have made a strong argument. But it is a problematic argument. The calls in the USA for resistance to vaccination or the wearing of masks emerge along with the old argument about simple wisdom, or frontier independence as more authentic, and better than science.

But rationality, science, and what has come to be understood as modernity have always been in collision with such ideas. Modernity is uneasy with received knowledge and seeks to learn from a process of trial and error, of open knowledge and phenomenology in which the observation of the world, its description, and its failure to comply with theory was long noted by Galileo and by Vesalius. Linked to open knowledge and to a positive legal code is an equality before a positive law. Science performs with an idea of progressive optimism, with its intervention to change fate, with an affection for machines, and with an attention to units of time. Natural philosophy—science—is based on cause and effect and direct experience. This is why medical research was always radically violative of both the natural order and of the naturalness of suffering and death—think of the theft of bodies so that cadavers could be studied, the anger that greeted Darwin.

How can such claims of the critics of gene drive research be best evaluated? What normative course is suggested by this understanding of science? Many agree fully with the arguments I have listed above, and they argue that the future is something that should worry us. The fear of technology, its potential catastrophe, plots directly with the general sense of fear that permeates our lives, that animates every science fiction, and that drives the anxieties that are instantiated and reified by movements of opposition.

The careful reader may at this point be considering why all of these claims and counterarguments are even important. If, I agree, these groups seem somewhat marginal to the larger discourses of states and nations, that they seem not to represent a democratic process or to represent any particular population that holds such views, and that this really matters, then why spend an entire chapter reflecting on their claims? Why should a minority of groups largely dominated by Westerners[51] be so central to the debate? But the NGOs described here do matter a great deal, for they have been able to play very serious roles in the development of other technologies, most famously the use of genetic engineering[52] to create a species of rice that contains carotene, the substance in food that produces vitamin A. I want to turn to this example because it is instructive for our considerations of gene drive technology. Vitamin A deficiency is extremely rare in developed countries, where the majority of the members of anti-GMO groups are based. It is a disease of extreme poverty. According to the WHO, an estimated 250,000–500,000 children who are vitamin A deficient become blind every year, and half of them die within twelve months of losing their sight. Vitamin A deficiency is associated with significant morbidity and mortality from common childhood infections, and it is the world's leading preventable cause of childhood blindness. It also contributes to maternal mortality and other poor outcomes during pregnancy and lactation, and it also diminishes the ability to fight infections. Even mild, subclinical deficiency can be a problem because it may increase children's risk for respiratory and diarrheal infections, decrease growth rates, slow bone development, and decrease the likelihood of survival from serious illness.[53]

Like malaria, it is an ancient problem. The Ebers Papyrus, an Egyptian medical papyrus from 1550 BCE, describes the symptom of night blindness, and a cure—eating animal liver, which contains vitamin A.[54] It took centuries to learn. But as gene editing became a reality in the late 1990s, attention turned to genetic solutions and to altering the food that, unlike animals' livers, was the cheapest-to-hand source of nutrition for almost half the world's peoples, the world's poor: rice.[55]

Rice breeding has been a part of human civilization for centuries. Indeed, there are more than 40,000 varieties of the most cultivated species, *Oryza sativa*. In the 1960s, a scientific rice breeding program began, located in the Philippines, to focus on the development of rice bred for traditional reasons, yield increases, and durability, called the International Rice Research Institute. In 1984, at an international meeting of rice scientists, the concept was raised of using the new gene transfer technologies to breed a variety with beta carotene in the endosperm—the part of the rice that humans use for

food. Not only are rice plants ubiquitous, but they already produce beta carotene in other parts of the plant, and so this seemed possible because other
plants—maize in particular—do produce beta carotene in the endosperm.
Thus began a long road, fraught with intensely difficult scientific challenges
and mistakes, which would have made the project difficult in any case, complicated by questions about consent documents in a human trial, but also
attacked passionately and consistently by a large group of NGOs, especially
one of the largest and most successful, Greenpeace.

In 2020, Greenpeace spearheaded the drive to prohibit the use of gene
drives under EU rules, charging that altering the mosquito sex ratio was
equivalent to eliminating the species.

> Gene Drive technology aims at the eradication of populations and even entire spe-
> cies by means of genetic engineering. Currently, reversal of its effects is not possi-
> ble. The environmental release of Gene Drive Organisms poses serious and novel
> threats to biodiversity and the environment at an unprecedented scale and depth,
> since any Gene Drive Organism carries a serious risk of uncontrollable spread of
> genetically modified genes and genetic mechanisms into wild and domesticated
> populations. While the new Corona virus is a very different phenomenon, it stands
> as a stark warning for the need of precaution regarding the potential effects of
> the uncontrollable spread of a new organism. Any environmental release of Gene
> Drive Organisms would violate the EU's GMO directive 2001/18/EC, which states:
> "Member States shall, in accordance with the precautionary principle, ensure that
> all appropriate measures are taken to avoid adverse effects on human health and
> the environment which might arise from the deliberate release or the placing on
> the market of GMOs."[56]

The alert reader will also note the absence of clarity about precisely which
species is being eliminated, perhaps *A. gambiae*, although that is of course
both extremely unlikely and very easily overcome with the simplest precautions, such as saving colonies and releasing them after the parasite is no longer viable in a population. Perhaps they are referring to the loss of *Plasmodium*
diversity if the *P. falciparum* species is eliminated. In any case, they make no
mention of the current adverse health effects on some 400,000 children annually because of malaria, its uncontrolled spread, and its potential for more
uncontrolled spread if more mechanisms to control it, such as anti-malaria
drugs, fail. Perhaps they refer to the non-native house mice that threaten
Pacific Islands, for they are another target of gene drive research, urgently
needed to save the diverse but threatened native birds on those islands in
what is called the GBiRd Project and which, ironically, is devoted to preventing the loss of species.

Greenpeace turned its attention from protecting whales and baby seals from hunters to opposing all GMOs in any form and for any reason, long before gene drives and concern about species elimination. They are opposed to altering rice to make it carry vitamin A. Their concerns range from fears about contamination of non-GM rice to fears that people will not "grow home vegetables," and that "it is irresponsible to impose GE 'golden' rice on people if it goes against their religious beliefs, cultural heritage and sense of identity or simply because they do not want it." Instead, Greenpeace wants us all to "end poverty."[57]

This is, of course, a laudable goal. In fact, ending poverty would also go a long way toward fighting many diseases, including malaria. However, the concept that the solution is to have the poor grow organic leafy green vegetables is nearly impossible for the urban poor, for the poor who do not have land, or live where the land is unsuitable for that sort of farming, or would compete with crops that the farmer could sell, farmer who does own or rent land they control. Greenpeace does not specify exactly which religions and cultures would rather their members, especially women and children, go blind and die so that they can oppose GM food. In fact, the turn from brown rice to white rice as a cultural preference is problematic in terms of nutrition. Sometimes, cultures are not the best source of wisdom. Their website urges the use of "several difference types of organic rice" that they think will "naturally" contain "important nutrients," but it is not clear what those are or how they would suddenly start to address a centuries-old and heretofore intractable problem in these very cultures. There is language in the Greenpeace documents to suggest that the "more natural" past, as we have seen in the literature of so many groups was a better place for the poor, somehow, yet, every measure of infant mortality, childhood vaccination rates, the end of so many infectious diseases, brooding of education, and the expansion of human life span tell us that modernity has improved the lives of so many. But despite this, the opposition has successfully erected a thicket of regulatory barriers that make approval of any GM product extraordinarily difficult (as opposed, to, for example, unregulated products with homeopathic health claims). Golden Rice as an experiment indeed have many flaws—there was a lack of transparency and confusion during some of the informed consent discussions with parents, the concentration of beta carotene was initially not adequate, and there were troubling scientific problems getting the construct to work properly. And while the technical barriers to the rice's development have been slowly overcome, the concentration of beta carotene made adequate, the informed consent process changed, the reparations made, and the career of the scientist who is at fault ended, the opposition has not altered since it was first launched, even in the face these significant changes, and of course, in the face of the continuing loss of sight and death in children.

In this chapter, I have attempted to give this literature its fair due, allowing the groups' own arguments to direct my reflections. I would argue that it is important to look beyond the inflammatory rhetoric of the NGOs, discount the symbolic and hyperbolic claims, and concentrate on core ethical problems, some of which are embedded in the opposition literature, some of which are not.

There is also a final consideration, one that I mentioned in the chapter on regulation, which is the ethical problem raised when an intervention is judged by people who will not be affected by that judgment. Moral standing, in this view, is held by the people who are most directly affected by malaria—by the rural villages in sub-Saharan Africa in the case of gene drives for malaria. There is something troubling, and it should be troubling, about international recommendations that mothers in the world's poorest villages need to use somewhat ineffective bed nets rather than gene drives, lest the ecological order of nature be threatened should gene drives be proven effective. It is for this reason that Target Malaria has spent over a decade in those villages to do the stakeholder engagement, I described in an effort to codevelop the new technology in line with the languages, narratives, and values of the members of those communities. This is because the villagers and stakeholders, just like you, reader, and just like me, see the complexity of the problem. We all care about preserving the beautiful, fragile, and now imperiled world, but we all also care deeply about ending malaria, and one can hold both ideas at the same time. As we saw in the last chapter, this is what has happened, and the stakeholder engagement has proceeded durably and steadily, despite the international and largely external opposition.

In the next chapter, I turn from the concerns of these groups to consider what I argue are the key ethical and philosophical questions. I will ask you to think along with me as I describe the concerns that can be made legible by a thoughtful reflection on these questions. Let me return to the four questions I asked in the Introduction, which can be asked about the ethics of any new technology:

(1) Are there reasons in *principle* why using this technology should be impermissible?

(2) What contextual factors should be taken into account, and do any of these prevent development and use of the technology?

(3) What purposes, techniques or applications would be permissible and under what circumstances?

(4) What procedures, structures, involving what policies, should be used to decide on appropriate techniques and uses?[58]

We will consider these questions in light of gene drive research for malaria and see if this way of thinking about nature and power will be important for your judgment about gene drives.

6 The World as We Judge It: Ethical Issues Considered

If I am making the argument in my last chapter that the concerns raised by external groups, largely based in the Global North, do not capture the ethical issues properly, then what are the ethical concerns that are critical and might prevent the development of gene drives? Or to ask the optimistically positive question: What would make the development and deployment of a gene drive ethical? How does one know? How does one judge? Thus far, I have assembled all the pieces of the argument—the history, science, the regulations, and the context—and thought carefully with you about the opposition to the technology. In this chapter, let us think together about the complex questions that are being raised by gene drive technology, and consider how to judge its implications and its worth. This chapter will be a taxonomy of the ethical issues and a discussion about how I have come to think about them.

Ethicists within the tradition called principlism begin their consideration of issues by thinking about standard principles of bioethics: standards of beneficence and non-maleficence, seeking to do good and avoiding harm; justice, allowing equal chances for all without regard to sex, age, race, or social class; and autonomy, allowing individuals to decide the fate for their own bodies. Others use what is called narrative theory and turn to common narratives to discern ethical values. Historically, the principle of the autonomy of an individual moral agent has been the core consideration in research ethics. This is also important within the narrative theory, for there is the historical narrative that I described earlier about the Nazi Doctors' Trial after World War II, which was understood as a catastrophic moral failure in the heart of the civilized world of science. Much of what we think of as modern research codes of ethics are direct heirs of the traditions of judgment that were made at the Doctors' Trial at Nuremberg. There were codes for research ethics prior to that of course—ones that German scientists were well aware of, and ignored—but the Nuremberg Code and the Declaration of Helsinki emerged after the worst ethical violations of the Shoah: the use of human subjects for torture and death in the name of scientific research, that was largely sadistic torture. Science and medicine are powerful and, when wielded in the name of the state, nearly inescapable as logics. Bioethicists tell this story and others to remind our students that the only defense of the individual is the power of consent or refusal to participate, a hard-won human right that is a part of the norms and rules of research. But it is clear that principles of autonomy or narratives of its abuse alone are not sufficient for the evaluation of much of public health research, which takes as its subject entire populations, regions, or nations, or research that affects not only humans but also other species and environments.

Here, different considerations come into play.

I am going structure our thinking in this chapter in three sections. First, I will consider the ethical issues in the existing research and treatment of malaria, which affect the ethical evaluation of any intervention. Then, I will consider the existing ethical issues that arise within genetic engineering and synthetic biology, and in the context of our times, with all its limits and facticity. Finally, I will discuss the particular ethical issue within research and deployment gene drives and in using gene drives for malaria—the specific application about which I focused in this book. Before I begin, I have some caveats.

6.1 Malaria as Moral Indictment

In the fall of 2021, at the UN Annual General Assembly meeting, the secretary-general, António Guterres, spoke about the wildly unequal distribution of COVID-19 vaccines. He was commenting on the fact that while the Global North and most industrialized countries had received vaccinations, Africa was once again left out of the public health interventions: "This is a moral indictment of the state of our world. It is an obscenity. We passed the science test. But we are getting an F in ethics."[1]

Indeed. But Mr. Guterres should have added that the world's ethical failure is really a long-standing one. And pre-dated COVID-19. I want to begin a discussion on the ethics of gene drives for malaria by reminding you, as reader that scholars have long known that research on and treatment of malaria itself presents ethical challenges, regardless of the existence of gene drives. This set of important ethical issues, which have emerged along with the disease and the treatment and prevention modalities, has changed relative to changing concepts of disease, bioethical standards, and environmental awareness.

Perhaps the most important ethical issue with which to begin is that the disease of malaria is largely preventable and is prevented in all of the developed world, even in countries—Singapore, South Africa, Cuba, China—where malaria had existed for centuries and which are surrounded by neighboring countries with similar geographies, population demographics, and ecologies, that stagger under the burden of disease. Most of the tools that humans use against malaria were well developed by the late nineteenth century. Malaria could have been controlled then by spraying and applying larvicide, funding basic hygiene, and providing bed nets, which were all tools that were in play and could have been widely used. But there needed to be money to hire workers to do the hygiene and upkeep. There needed to be money to buy, distribute, and ensure the use of bed nets. There needed to be money to hire enough workers to do effectively what the Tennessee Valley Authority did in the 1940s and 1950s in the American South or even to do what the Elizabethans did in the Fens in the 1500s, for that matter: build dams, divert streams, drain swamps, and build on high ground.

Additionally, over the last centuries, it would have been possible—and still could be possible—to regulate insecticides such as DDT so that they are used only to kill disease vectors and not pests on agricultural crops, and to use these insecticides in a concerted and organized campaign. Finally, there have always been treatments for malaria—from quinine to combination artemisinin—and these were given to Westerners as soon as they were judged efficacious. Drugs that were carefully regulated could of course also be given to people in the tropical world as well. That the prevention and treatment of malaria is completely dependent on whether one is a child in a wealthy country or in a poor one is, in a word, not fair. It is certainly not ethically acceptable. And this issue of justice has also long been noted. Celli's report in the 1920s made the same point. Malaria is a disease of poverty, particularly rural poverty. Jeffrey Sachs and Pia Malaney, careful economists, have calculated the massive loss of income and human resources lost to malaria annually: "Where malaria prospers most, human societies have prospered least. Vulnerability to malaria, like many other infectious diseases is largely a product of social determinants of health—such as poverty, malnutrition, and insufficient access to health care."[2] In the countries in which we will see that Target Malaria is intending intervention, the GDP is quite low. They are among the poorest countries in the world. In fact, the GDP is inversely related to the prevalence of malaria. Other ratios exist as well. High levels of migration, land erosion, floods, unjust labor practice, and unjust land distribution schemes all correlate with high levels of malaria. Thus, that fact that malaria can be prevented and the fact that it is not is the central ethical problem.

For bioethicists such as myself, this financial inadequacy and policy inattention is mirrored in our scholarly inattention. While we seek grants for projects such as whether consciousness resides in the in vitro neuronal cells lumped together in a Petri dish (organoids), or whether reanimated pig's brains are really "alive," or whether skin cells can be reverse engineered into male and female gametes and then used to create human embryos, to mention just three recent preoccupations in my field,[3] we barely consider the long, fatal, and unjust history of malaria. Except for a glancing interest when malaria intersects with something our field really cares about—the Nuremberg Doctors' Trial, and whether the desperate search for a cure in 1943 harmed the prisoner research subjects (it did not)—there is no mention of the issue or of the extraordinary, staggering death count of a child every two minutes from the disease. Our energy, our attention, and our money go to things we consider important, interesting, and urgent. And that inattention, too, is an ethical issue.

What makes the justice issue most tragic is that the history of the countries most at risk—the Congo, Burkina Faso, Mali, the Gold Coast—are the places were colonial takings were the most acute. West Africa was stripped not only of gold and other minerals—hence the name—but of generations of slaves, whose labor, instead of being used to build infrastructure, railways, schools, and farms in their home country was used to build them in the West. America grew wealthy in part because it did not pay the slaves, whose labor created value—in Marxist terms, surplus value—for the class that owned them. One does not need to be a Marxist to understand that it is not only poor management or graft or corruption (although it is also surely that) that affects the economies of African states where malaria is so personally and economically costly, it is also a history of exploitation of resources taken to enrich others that is part of the structure of economic and thus health-care disparities. This global disparity of wealth is mirrored in how deeply the population is burdened with disease and how little money is available for vector control.

A fraction of this created wealth for the West is returned as charity, and largely thanks to this and to aid from governments that are directed to control efforts, malaria began yielding to new efforts by donor-funded initiatives in the 1960s. But the donations are, at best, inadequate. As a WHO report notes: "A minimum investment of 6.5 US Billion will be required annually by 2020 in order to meet the 2030 targets of the WHO global malaria strategy. The US 2.7 billion represents less than half of the amount. Of particular concern is since 2014, investments in malaria control have, on average, declined in many high-vector burden countries."[4] This was all prior to the havoc wreaked by COVID-19 on the world economy and on the health of the poor. This gap means that many people cannot even have access to simple interventions. As Euzebuisz Jamrozik, one of the few bioethicists writing on the ethical issues of malaria, notes: "Many people do not even benefit from the simple protection of inexpensive and cost-effective bed nets. Furthermore, access to such interventions is often inversely proportional to wealth and proximity to major urban centers and can be especially poor for mobile populations at high risk for malaria. . . . international efforts toward malaria control thus represent a major opportunity to remedy some of the past and present injustices manifested by global disparities in wealth and freedom from preventable disease."[5] The ethical obligation to care for the suffering stranger, whose situation is in some part due to your unjust taking, is a stable principle of human societies, particularly societies in which notions of human solidarity[6] or a preferential option for the poor is at work. This is the basis of most theological and philosophical social ethics. And in the case of the burden of malaria, it is surely at play. As Jamrozik argues: "Issues of justice and moral obligation are at the center of the problem. The prevalence of malaria is inversely proportional to GDP per capita. Sachs and Malaney aptly note that "where malaria prospers most, human societies have prospered least." Vulnerability to malaria, like many other infectious diseases is largely a product of social determinants of health—such as poverty, malnutrition, and insufficient access to health care. . . . International efforts toward malaria control thus represent a major opportunity to remedy some of the past and present injustices manifested by global disparities in wealth and freedom from preventable disease."[7]

6.2 Malaria and the Politics of Public Health

A second ethical issue in malaria was—and is—the turn from a public health model to a disease model in addressing it. For this part of the chapter, let me return to the historical account of malaria and its treatment to consider the ethical issues. Malaria is one of a number of health-care crises for the rural poor, and often what turns a treatable illness into a death sentence is the simple lack of a local clinic, staffed by nurses and doctors. This is the case throughout much of the developing world, but it is not a fact of natural order: this lack, this absence is also a decision. The decision by public health agencies to focus on the aspects of malaria control that most resembled a war—killing mosquitoes—is historically understandable, and the single-minded focus on drugs to kill pathogens similarly is within the logics of the study of infectious disease—since Pasteur, the search for what Paul Ehrlich called "the magic bullet" (yet another war metaphor) shaped medical science. But for many scholars, it is this single-disease focus that is also a moral decision, and it has meant turning away from the provision of basic health services as each disease is tackled one by one—thus, the search for the silver bullet that could address malaria.

Malariologist Paul Russell, argued for a grander vision: "Russell argued that having physicians, malariologists, and sanitarians integrate their activities with those of agriculturalists, demographers, social scientists, economists, educator, and political and religious leaders is of utmost importance. For only thus can there be joint planning of social reorientation that will result not in bigger populations but in healthier communities."[8] For historian Randall Packard, the struggle to define the scope of the work of public health, particularly global public health, was at the core of international agencies and their approach to malaria.[9] Early efforts as the Children's Bureau, a Progressive Era institution that was created prior to World War II as a part of the US Department of Labor by economic philosopher Jessica Peixotto and others, were based on the idea that the health of children and women depended on a just economy that addressed the totality of their well-being, just what the Italians were arguing for in the same historical period. This was also the first impulse of the UNRRA, which addressed malaria in its first years. And it was still at stake in 1955 when the UN founded the WHO:

The Expert Committee on Public Health (1955)—cited Article 25 of the UN UDHR. "Everyone has the right to a standard of living adequate for the health and well-being of himself and his family, including food, clothing, housing, and medical care and necessary social services and the right to security in the event of unemployment, sickness, disability, widowhood, old age, or other lack of livelihood beyond his control. . . . The potentialities of world health are great if WHO can become the spearhead of a movement for the social and economic betterment of the under-developed countries while serving as a channel . . . for the exchange of ideas on health administration in all countries. Public health defined as the development of social machinery to ensure to every individual a standard of living adequate to the maintenance of health . . . social welfare, social security measures, education, food production and distribution, reservation of land, labor standards, recreation, transportation and communication, irrigation, environmental sanitation, conservations, family planning.[10]

But the vision was always in danger of being narrowed: "The Bengal famine of 1943 which killed an estimated 3 million people raised the specter of a world wide food catastrophe. . . . This worked against efforts to build comprehensive, integrated programs that combined advances in health with broader social and economic transformations, Instead it favored short term, immediate solutions. The perception of crisis would shape global health planning over the next half century."[11] Packard, citing the view of American health officers in the Philippines who thought that Filipinos were not able to carry out control by themselves and could not be trusted to take quinine properly, and felt could not take responsibility for the villages for which they were responsible, sought other ways to cope with malaria. "Colonial contexts shaped the attitudes and practices of a generation of American public health authorities who would go on to lead future international-health efforts. These authorities would continue the tradition of attacking disease by applying biotechnologies, while largely ignoring the need to develop basic health services or addressing the underlying causes of ill health." It was not only in the Philippines.

> Changes were the benefits of colonial rule, and Aykroyd and his coauthors (of a report on The Rice Problem in India—about famine) did not ascribe the poverty and indebtedness of Indian villagers to British colonial policies. Like many colonial authorities of his day, he viewed the economic conditions he was seeing as characteristic of an Asian economic system that had operated largely unchanged since the distant past. The prevailing attitude was that colonial rule had introduced modern technologies, but not the oppressive economic forces that had encouraged changes in food-consumption patterns. Viewed in this way, the more destructive impacts of colonial policies were often unseen or unappreciated . . . in making recommendations . . . Aykroyd at no point suggested changes in land use, food production, labor patterns or the commodification of rice.[12]

The turn from basic health-care needs to a fascination with the idea of a one-shot cure was linked to a growing wonder about the new tools brought to fruition in World War II, making it possible—for the first time—to reduce the global burden of disease greatly through the application of these new biomedical technologies. The war had also brought advances in many other areas of technology, all of which contributed to a new faith in the ability of technology and science to transform the world. Whether it was nuclear weapons, atomic energy, drought-resistant plants, or penicillin and DDT, the postwar world was one that technology promised, (or threatened, depending on one's perspective) to transform.

The WHO preamble states: "Health is a state of complete physical, mental, and social well-being and not merely the absence of disease. The enjoyment of the highest standard of health is one of the fundamental rights of every human being, without distinction of race, religion, political belief, economic or social conditions. Governments have a responsibility for the health of their peoples which can only be fulfilled by the provision of adequate health and social measures." By 1950, the WHO was moving rapidly toward a set of strategies and interventions that focused narrowly on the application of newly developed biomedical technologies to eliminate diseases one at a time. As before, they were designed by experts who met in cities in Europe and the USA to discuss and make plans for improving the health of peoples living in Africa, Asia, and Latin America. They shared a confidence in the superiority of Western knowledge and a disregard for both the ideas and the practices of those for whom the campaigns were created. They also paid little attention to the underlying social and economic determinants of health or the need to develop basic health services.[13]

Along with the "magic bullets" (literally and figuratively) would come a persistent problem—the power of the outsider who controlled the technology: "Faith in technology and the optimism it inspired about the ability of the United States to transform the world carried with it certain assumptions about the peoples and societies that were to receive this technology and be transformed. . . . Truman described the underdeveloped world as "primitive and stagnant" . . . reports privileged the skills and knowledge of the outside expert while placing local populations in a position of dependency, in need of guidance and assistance."[14] Even the formulation of the issue was phrased in the language of technological expertise of George MacDonald. The sixth WHO Expert Committee on Malaria designed the malaria eradication strategy in 1956 based on a mathematical formula ($-R = RateRo > 1$ = transmission $Ro = ma\,2\,bpR\,\log 10\,p$ (where M = man biting rate, A = abundance of vectors, B = vector competence, P = life span).

The problem with MacDonald's elegant formula was that it reduced a multitude of complexities associated with each element of the formula to a single value. For example, the man biting rate was a product of the feeding habits of the malaria vector, the housing conditions and density of the human population, and the clothing and sleeping habits of the host population. These, in turn, were shaped by the local social, cultural, and economic conditions, which varied greatly over space and time. The formula produced a false sense of uniformity, which belied the complexity of malaria transmissions . . . Which quickly became apparent.[15]

But the struggle for malaria was always also a struggle to create a system of health care for the rural poor. This was an argument championed by the French and Italian researchers and even by Ross. It was a tradition carried into the later twentieth century.

By 1961, however, it was becoming clear that many programs were running into problems, particularly in the attack and consolidation phase. Time and time again, the procedures carefully worked out in Geneva came up against the social and economic realities of life in developing countries. . . . Mud wall absorbed DDT and reduced its killing power (sorption) . . . the eradication protocols also assumed populations were stable. Yet in many places, households were mobile, or people resided in different places at different times of year. In South Africa, spray teams working in the Eastern Transvaal Lowveld had to cope with the massive influx of displaced persons, expelled from the highlands as a part of the apartheid governments grand plan for racially segregating the country. This resulted in the overnight creation of large new settlements in areas that were thought to have been effectively protected. Moreover, these and other social or cultural practices were viewed as isolated problems that could be overcome. They were not seen as significant enough to undermine eradication campaigns. This turned out to be a serious miscalculation. Spray teams also ran into resistance from house owners who found the activities of the eradication teams disruptive, particularly after two or three rounds of spraying.[16]

Doctors from the WHO sent into villages tended to view the resistance as a product of ignorance or irrational, traditional native beliefs—just as the colonial authorities understood resistance to eradication campaigns for yellow fever. Without community discussion, they believed that armies and authorities could enforce a campaign. But this was no longer the case.

In the fall of 1979, the WHO held a conference to define and then advocate for basic health-care services that focused on primary health care that was accessible to local communities worldwide. A total of 3,000 delegates from 134 countries, sixty-seven international organizations, and a handful of NGOs were able to reach a consensus on what was needed in a package of basic health care. The resulting document was called the "Declaration of Alma-Ata" after the name of the place in the Soviet Union—now Kazakhstan—where the meeting was held. It argued for seven concepts:

(1) The formation of primary health care "around the life patterns of the population."

(2) The involvement of the local population.

(3) The "maximum reliance" on available community resources while remaining within cost limitations.

(4) An integrated approach of preventative, curative, and promotive services for both the community and the individual.

(5) Interventions to all be undertaken at the most peripheral practical level of the health services by the worker most simply trained for this activity.

(6) The design of the other echelons of services in support of the needs of the peripheral level.

(7) PHC services to be fully integrated with the services of the other sectors involved in community development.[17]

It reaffixed the UN and WHO definition of health as a broad account of human flourishing, "a state of complete physical, mental and social well-being and not merely the absence of disease or infirmity,"[18] and it added the provision that health was both a human right and an obligation of governments. It stood firmly in the school of thought advocated since the early days of the twentieth century—that social and economic factors were critical in the attainment of health. It stressed the need for community participation in building health-service infrastructure[19] and, in a burst of extreme optimism, announced it anticipated that this sort of health care should be available or all by 2000. This sort of health care "turned away from technical solutions, top-down programs, and curative medical care provided by physicians—that had dominated international health efforts since the 1950's. It also implied a major shift in the allocation of health and financial resources toward peripheral populations and away from large urban centers."[20]

But this idealism was not sustained, for a variety of reasons, and instead, and a few years later, a different meeting was held, in one of the world's fanciest resort towns, Bellagio, attended by chairmen of the World Bank, Robert McNamara (who had just retired from his post as the US Secretary of Defense and who had been the architect of the Vietnam War), the Rockefeller Foundation, and the Ford Foundation. The head of the US Agency for International

Development and the head of the Canadian International Development and Research Center also attended. As they sat by Lake Como in the sun of the Italian Alps, they decided that the Alma-Ata vision was too expensive. It would be better for poor countries, if they were to be aided by wealthy ones, to have access to only a less robust package of benefits, called Selective Primary Health Care (SPHC). These were to include "Vaccination for measles, and diphtheria, tetanus, and pertussis, for children under 6 months old; tetanus toxoid injections for pregnant women; the encouragement of breastfeeding; chloroquine for children under 3 years old in malarious areas, to ingest during febrile episodes, and oral rehydration packets for and instruction on the treatment of diarrhea."[21] There was no need to actually build hospitals and clinics or to train doctors for villages, argued the planners of SPHC—mobile vans could come by every six months to provide the "selective basic" care. It was a purely utilitarian scheme—the greatest lives saved for the (limited) dollar. It was called "selective primary care," and it was only for the poor, since the wealthy sitting on the shores of Lake Como would be assured of ICUs, dental care, and rehabilitation for any of their children's ills. Thus, the second ethical issue is why the health-care infrastructure was never built, even after the period specified in the SPHC plan. We will return to this question in our consideration of how malaria should best be treated, but let us not forget that this ethical issue long preceded gene drives.

The failure of the vision of Alma-Ata was in part because of its links to the socialist theories and practices of the countries that most robustly supported it, but it revealed a fundamental ethical problem: Which system of justice would undergird the world's efforts to eradicate malaria? The ethical conundrum was that relationships of power, global and local, were still designed to limit the scope of public health's widest vision, but that only the largest public health vision had ever eliminated malaria successfully.

> At the heart of PHC was the commitment to popular participation. Communities needed to be actively involved in planning for their own health needs. These requirements could not be dictated from above. . . . The reality was often quite different. Inequalities in wealth and authority meant that decisions were seldom made in a democratic fashion. The time constraints of daily labor often prevented some members of the community from participitation in planning discussions. Women, in particular, who often played a major role in meeting the health needs of communities commonly experience a high demand on their labor which limited their participation in community planning activities.[22]

In addition to the overarching ethical issues of social and economic inequality as determinants of health, the justice issues inherent in climate change, and the deep etiologies of malaria, there are other ethical issues that are specific in the prevention and treatment of malaria, long before new technology plays a role. The climate itself was beginning to shift. Jamrozik argues: "Anthropogenic climate change affects human health . . . by changing the habitats of *Anopheles* mosquitoes and potentially by displacing human populations . . . an increase in malaria burden due to climate change is also a matter of justice since those who would suffer the most are usually those who are already among the worst off groups of global society and themselves contribute the least to climate change."[23] In earlier chapters, we have considered the problems associated with mosquito nets—the simplest and theoretically the least invasive concept in malaria prevention. But there are ethical issues even here as well: even ITNs are only successful in preventing malaria in 20 percent of cases in children below the age of five. Faced with the choice of using the net to protect one child while they sleep—difficult to keep on a sleeping, kicking baby in the best of conditions—versus using the nets to fish for all your children, it is rational to use the net for fishing.

Insecticides present significant ethical choices as well. They are often poorly regulated, and insecticides banned in the USA can be used in Africa.[24] As Rachel Carson pointed out about DDT, insecticides insinuated themselves into the environment in profound and permanent ways. Poured on waterways, painted on the walls of habitation, and sprayed all over villages, insecticides kill without the discrimination of a targeted solution, every insect, every habitat, every food web. The use of pesticides was growing, not only for malaria but also for agriculture. "In recent years the widespread adoption of agricultural pesticides has paved the way for pesticide manufacturers and merchants to enter the growing African market. "As agricultural pesticides have become more common, the most harmful aspects include (i) weak or non-existent regulation and (ii) poor knowledge of pesticide hazards among users. Africa's widespread adoption of pesticides is troubling because it suggests there is an abundance of new users who are typically unaware of the consequences of pesticide use, even when used properly. Without regulation and adequate training/capacity building of farmers, Africa is at risk of widespread pesticide poisoning."[25] In general, it is accepted by many scholars that most African governments do not have adequate resources to prevent environmental contamination from pesticide use or to clean up after accidental spills. Consequently, increased reliance on pesticides has led to the contamination of African freshwater sources and has threatened wildlife, including many endangered species.[26]

In 2005, the WHO reapproved the use of DDT, and twelve other synthetic chemicals, to continue to combat malaria, banning its use in agriculture but permitting it for malaria control. "DDT is one of 12 pesticides recommended by the WHO for indoor residual spray programs. It is up to individual countries to decide whether or not to use DDT. EPA works with other agencies and countries to advise them on how DDT programs are developed and monitored, with the goal that DDT be used only within the context of programs referred to as Integrated Vector Management. IVM is a decision-making process for use of resources to yield the best possible results in vector control, and that it be kept out of agricultural sectors."[27] To regulate these chemicals, international conventions were established. For example, the Stockholm Convention on Persistent Organic Pollutants was adopted in 2001 and entered into force in 2004. It is a global treaty requiring all parties to eliminate or reduce these chemicals:

> to protect human health and the environment from chemicals that remain intact for long periods, become widely distributed geographically, accumulate in the fatty tissue of humans and wildlife, and have harmful impacts on human health or on the environment. Exposure to POPs can lead to serious adverse health effects including certain cancers, birth defects, dysfunctional immune and reproductive systems, greater susceptibility to disease and damage to the central and peripheral nervous systems. Given that these chemicals can be transported over long distances, no one government acting alone can protect its population or its environment from POPs. For more information on the Stockholm Convention and POPs, The Secretariat of the Basel, Rotterdam, and Stockholm Conventions, or BRS Secretariat, supports Parties implement the three leading multilateral environment agreements governing chemicals and waste management, in order to protect human health and the environment.[28]

The existence of such a Secretariat attests to the deadly significance of pesticides and the full import of the ethical conundrum that they clearly present.

Am I making the argument that since pesticides are so dangerous, any alternative would be permissible? No—for that would be bad philosophy. The harm of pesticides stands on its own for our judgment, and the use of innovative technologies cannot just be morally good or ethically better in that by being better than a truly terrible alternative, for it must also be judged on its own merits. Yet, the context matters a great deal, and the deep insufficiency of the pesticides is the background of our consideration of the landscape of interventions. There is more. This is a fraught landscape of ethics concerns in the existing paradigm![29]

For example, there is the issue of counterfeit drugs and our inability to stop them from being sold. Linked to this is the issue of the reluctance on the part of drug companies to create and sell drugs cheaply enough for states to afford, so that people in desperation turn elsewhere, to the fake ones. Chemopraxis is a critical part of malaria eradication—but it does no good if only the wealthy or foreign travelers can afford the drugs that are actually effective. It is simply not ethical that the newest and best drugs of the twenty-first century are out of reach for so many, but it is far worse that the tools of the nineteenth century—bed nets, house screens, and swamp draining—are not universally available at a cost that can be afforded by all who need them and of course, it is wildly shortsighted. However, in addition to one-off vertical interventions, five-year plans, and proclamations, if basic public health in Africa is going to improve, then counties must commit to a robust determination to build local clinics.

Let me give one example. As I was writing this book, a colleague sent me a news item about a new drug that could be given via a suppository to young children who often died while waiting to be transported—often in a rough carriage, often hand carried—to clinics for care for their severe *P. falciparum* malaria, which had left them febrile or comatose. The researchers were pleased that the suppositories meant that the children could survive the bicycle ride of four hours or more, carried in a little pull cot to a regional clinic. The project gave the villagers the bicycles for the duration of the trial. But there was no discussion of why there was no clinic in the village in the first place, or why no doctors and nurses had been trained to care for the children there. The lack of health-care infrastructure was as profound as when the Wilsons, wife and husband, wrote about the villages in Africa in 1939.[30] When this sort of isolation exists, it becomes nearly impossible to take a sick child to the hospital miles and miles away—there are other children, there is no bus or truck—and the child simply dies.

When nothing is done to deal with underlying conditions, and drugs and insecticide flood an area, as was done in 1955, resistance to lifesaving drugs and repellents is swift, within six months in some cases. Poor or inappropriate, incomplete, or inadequate courses of treatment often occur when families can afford only half the course of treatment or split medicine between several children, or when poorly trained or completely untrained shopkeepers

sell black-market drugs. As we have seen in the previous section, antimalarial resistance to combination drugs is a deadly problem: "Anti-malarial
resistance, especially to artemisinin based combination therapy (ACT) is a
major threat . . . generally results for . . . (and) most often occurs in the context of poverty, counterfeit medications and weak healthcare infrastructure."[31]

6.3 Climate Change and the Intensification of Disease

The third and final overarching ethical issue that surrounds all discussions
about malaria interventions is the deepening problem of increasingly irreversible climate change and its disproportionate impact on the most marginalized, especially the poor in the tropics, and on diseases such as malaria
and dengue that pursue them so relentlessly. When the world is warmer and
wetter, it becomes a far more hospitable place for insect vectors of all kinds,
makes the tropics a far worse place for human habitation, and makes more
of the world tropical. Mosquitoes, which are advantaged by every puddle
left after every rainfall, will be a particular problem. Not only is it likely that
the mosquito habitats will be increased, anopheline species in areas free of
Plasmodium that once carried it quite happily can, of course, carry it again.
Now, when a traveler comes from Thailand with the parasite in his blood
and goes home, to say, East Anglia or Scotland,[32] the mosquitoes are unlikely
to bite him and transmit the illness, but if the climate was warmer and the
mosquito habitat more welcoming, it might become more likely. Not only
do mosquitoes expand their range, but they also bite more frequently in
hot weather, and the *Plasmodium* reproduces at a faster rate, making the bite
more likely to carry parasites (as in the MacDonald formula). Human habits
will change too. More people will need to sleep outdoors or open windows
for air, and more people will begin to think that mosquito nets are too hot.
Already, climate change has made some regions unable to be farmed. Long-
term droughts push farmers off their land, as do devastating floods and
hurricanes, all of which are more likely as the world's average temperature
increases. And when people migrate, they do not sleep in snug homes rather
but in tents on the road or in outdoor refugee camps.

Just as Samuel Christophers saw as a British army doctor in colonial India,
who we met in Chapter 1, when there is scarcity, there is poverty, and then
there is epidemic disease. All of this is horrible, to be sure, but what makes
climate change an ethical issue is that the people who have largely driven the
temperature up by filling the air with carbon emissions are not the people

who are affected first and most—it will be the poor. In fact, it already is the poor, who stream out of Northern Africa, Honduras, and the Eastern Mediterranean as the pepper fields and cotton fields dry up.[33] The farmers of Bangladesh, who do not have cars, eat meat at every meal, or fly to Bellagio for vacation, or to discuss policy, all of which are profligate uses of carbon, will be the first to have their homes flooded by rising sea levels. People who have done little to change the climate will need to leave their homes, to migrate. When I first wrote this, a caravan of desperate Central Americans was on the move, trying to flee north. Its occupants were met by violent opposition, and it is unlikely that in their poverty they have caused much of the shift in climate that made growing food impossible in their village. As I review the chapter, it is Haiti refugees who are fleeing a climate change driven disaster. It is this asymmetry that creates the ethical and moral dimensions of the problem, and it will first be displayed through the grim calculus of our oldest diseases: cholera, typhus, plague, tuberculosis, and, of course, malaria.

Poverty and statelessness create deeper complexities. Many histories of malaria point to the emergence of new strains from South Asia, in the borderlands. In the Mekong subregion, populations have never been quite stable, and stateless people go back and forth over borders, looking for work, often leaving the highlands to go to lower, malarial lowlands, becoming infected and then returning home, taking the parasites with them. This practice is characteristic of many other places—South Africa, Burkina Faso—any place where there are many people who need work next to countries or region where there is enough wealth to hire them, at least seasonally. When drug resistance is a factor as well, and when larger numbers of stateless people leave their lands seeking work, the potential for the parasite to spread among them as they travel presents a special problem, especially if they are unwanted or resented and thus have no health-care services. The presence of impoverished, mobile, and politically marginalized populations, including large numbers of refugees, could allow the spread of drug-resistant strains beyond the borders of the Mekong, where it is likely that this pattern of human migration created the initial drug resistance to chloroquine that first arose in 1957.

6.4   Ethical Issues in the Existing Treatment of Malaria

The unique aspects of malaria present other long-standing ethical issues. Peculiar to some illnesses, and malaria is one of them, is that some people, while ill, and in this case who have gametocytes ready to be picked up by a mosquito and transmitted to the next stage in the life cycle of the *Plasmodium*, show no overt signs of illness. They are afebrile, they have no headache, and they appear for all intents and purposes as immune. In fact, in most medical literature, they are described as immune when in fact what they have is a low-level infection that seems to block acute new infections. There are some true immunities: Duffy-negative people are indeed immune to *P. vivax*, although not *P. falciparum*. Here was the standard account that described this immunity:

> In humans, various types of acquired or adaptive immunity against plasmodia have been: (i) antidisease immunity, conferring protection against clinical disease, which affects the risk and extent of morbidity associated with a given parasite density; (ii) antiparasite immunity, conferring protection against parasitemia, which affects the density of parasites; and (iii) premunition, providing protection against new infections by maintaining a low-grade and generally asymptomatic parasitemia Here, protection is defined as objective evidence of a lower risk of clinical disease, as indicated by both the absence of fever (axillary temperature of >37.5°C) with parasitemia and lower densities of parasitemia. Across sub-Saharan Africa where the disease is holoendemic, most people are almost continuously infected by *falciparum*, and the majority of infected adults rarely experience overt disease. They go about their daily routines of school, work, and household chores feeling essentially healthy despite a population of parasites in their blood that would almost universally prove lethal to a malaria-naive visitor.[34]

However, the theory that people are in a state of "premunition" and thus are protected from malaria in a way that is somehow beneficial has been recently challenged.[35] "An important question is whether "asymptomatic" malaria infections are truly benign and, if not, whether the advantages of premunition are outweighed by the harm that arises from persistent blood-stage parasites . . . not just to the individual's well-being but to elimination and eradication."[36] But should these cases be treated? Again, it is a question of worth and duty. This raises several ethical issues. First, in resource-scarce areas, suddenly treating not only active cases but also every single case is an enormous challenge. Would it impact on the severe cases to have some of the resource diverted to people who are not "sick?" Of course. Second, how would the identification proceed? Would everyone need to be screened—mandatory or voluntarily? If so, at what intervals? If premunition is renamed "chronic malaria," then our obligations are altered. The usual issues of privacy and confidentiality need thoughtful reflection, for concealing one's infective status creates serious risks to a community that is attempting to eradicate malaria using this method. Given the fecundity of mosquitoes and of parasites, even small amounts of *Plasmodium* are dangerous and will keep the infection in play. So, logically, every infected person should be found and treated. It poses major scientific, operational, and ethical challenges if communities are serious about treating every person. The problem becomes particularly troubling when nonimmune migrants are unwittingly exposed to parasites from seemingly well people or when blood donation is at stake, when ordinary transfusion can carry the risk of silent malaria infection. And in many cases, it is very hard to detect cases in the subacute phase because low levels may not show up, even on serology tests. Should public health authorities treat all cases of asymptomatic malaria, in people who may not know that they are ill, but who carry the parasite and will spread it? Consider the complexities about testing in that case, which we reviewed in Chapter 1:

> Recent findings suggest the task of elimination will be even harder than expected. Health workers diagnose malaria using a simple rapid diagnostic test (RDT): a pinprick of blood is added to a test strip which quickly turns it red if it detects proteins from *P falciparum* . . . But Mallika Imwong, a molecular biologist at Mahidol University in Bangkok wondered whether some people might carry too few parasites to make them ill—or to not show up on a RDT. To find out she fished for parasite in vials of blood shipped from Cambodia, Myanmar and Vietnam, using a sensitive method called PCR (polymerase chain reaction. In 2015 she reported that only 25% of *Plasmodium* infection were detected by the usual RDT on average. The disparity was at times remarkable. "I was really surprised" says Imwong. "In one village, only 4 or 5% were positive with RDTs but 68% were infected."[37]

On the other hand, not treating asymptomatic cases raises significant ethical issues as well. Children are especially at risk when low-level disease causes poor school performance, when cognition is affected, and when they have chronic anemia. Low-level disease causes significant risks in pregnancies, often fatal risks, and the risks of opportunistic bacteria that are potentiated by malaria are serious and have long-term effects on populations as a whole. Adults are affected as well as children. One study in Uganda found that "asymptomatic" malaria parasitemia is associated with poor performance in tests of sustained attention and abstract reasoning.[38]

There is also the issue of equity. No other chronic disease, especially in children or in pregnant women, is typically ignored, which raises the issue of why, in this one instance, it is seen as somehow helpful to ignore the existence of these prodromal or chronic low-level infections.

If the decision to test everyone is too complex, malaria does not have to be simply ignored—it could still be treated. One strategic response to the problem is to use MDA, which is a method that simply treats everyone at once without testing. However, in addition to the obvious problem of increasing the probability of resistance, MDA will mean that some will be treated, at some risk, and get no benefits at all. As bioethicist Jamrozik noted: "Ethically, it is important to consider the fair distribution of benefits and burdens, noting that infective individuals will receive the greatest immediate benefits while all may share the risks and burdens of treatment, including increased resistance where MDA does not achieve elimination."[39] If the drug used for MDA is primaquine, or if it contains primaquine, it will cause high-risk side effects, but only in people who have the *G6PD* gene, an adaptive variant for malaria. But ironically, doses above a certain limit (which is different for different people) can trigger catastrophic illness. Pregnant women cannot take primaquine either because of the underlying anemia of pregnancy. "When used in low doses as a gametocidal agent for *P. falciparum*, primaquine is safe and largely effective yet higher doses used in anti-relapse therapy carry high risks. While treatment related risk from hemolysis are rare . . . different genotypes and phenotypes in different populations has not been well defined and there is no point of care test for *G6PD*."[40] The issue of vaccines for malaria raises another ethical question. Some vaccines (tuberculosis vaccines are an example) are what are called "transmission blocking vaccines," blocking not disease but the capacity to spread the disease agent. This means, in the case of malaria, that some vaccines could be designed only to be active against gametocytes, meaning that the vaccine interferes with the ability of the parasitic cycle, blocking the formation of gametocytes. But many of the current vaccine projects are not intended to block sporozoites, meaning it does not help the infected person. The red blood cells can continue to be attacked before they then burst and release parasites, continually sickening the subject. Since they do not protect the individual from becoming infected, instead only protect others, the point of the use of such vaccines is to get a certain population to have a version of a herd immunity, and for this, one would need close to universal vaccination. Using human subjects for this genre of vaccine deepens the ethical stakes. One can see how volunteering to take such a vaccine would be difficult and would require a sense that one's neighbor will also be taking a vaccine—something that is possible only in a deeply and mutually altruistic community.

A final strategy, which raises other ethical issues, newly suggested, is the use of the drug ivermectin (which was having its moment in the public gaze as I wrote this, when right-wing commentators urged followers to use it for COVID-19 despite the fact that it did nothing to change the course of the disease used in filariasis at a low dose. It does not affect the person, keep the red blood cells intact, lessen the fevers, or block transmission. Rather, it works to sicken the vector, poisoning and weakening the mosquito when it bites someone who is taking ivermectin: "Ivermectin is being considered for mass drug administration for malaria due to its ability to kill mosquitos feeding on recently treated individuals. However, standard, single doses of 150–200 mcg/kg use for onchocerciasis and lymphatic filariasis have a short-lived mosquitocidal effect (<7 days) Because ivermectin is tolerated up to 2000 mcq/kg, we aimed to establish the safety, tolerability and mosquitocidal efficacy of a three day course of high-dose ivermectin, co-administered with a standard malaria treatment."[41] Since the drug seems to kill mosquitoes in the low doses used in filariasis, where the effect lasts about a week, the theory was to see if it is well tolerated in higher does. The study mentioned above has concluded that it does, and that it reduced mosquito survival for at least twenty-eight days after treatment. Thus, for about a month, treated people would walk around as mosquito killers but could still have malaria themselves. Here, too, the strategy is altruistic in nature, the point being yet another way to reduce biting by using people in the place of insecticide sprays—an odd but possibly effective, if roundabout, plan.

Of course, an effective vaccine continues to be the best way to combat infectious disease. Vaccines have been theorized since Pasteur, but in malaria, unlike bacterial diseases, the parasite changes shape, form, and its vulnerabilities multiple times in its life span, making finding a target for the immune system to challenge illusive. Moreover, unlike, for example, yellow fever in which when a person survives an attack, she is then immune for life, malaria is a disease in which people get sick over and over again because the disease does not confer immunity. In fact, whatever immunity seems to occur may actually have been the effect of chronicity. Even in individual cases where immunity has appeared to occur, if the person leaves the endemic area for even just six months, all immunity seems to be lost—an ethical problem well characterized by the early twentieth century. This raises the question about whether it is ethical to give a vaccine unless one is committed—and funded—to keep giving it, since once the immunity wears off, unless it is boosted, the person is once again highly vulnerable, perhaps unsuspectingly so. The husband-and-wife team of researchers, the Wilsons, who studied malaria while stationed in East Africa and who presented to the Royal Society in 1939, noted:

> the main object which I have in mind has been to arouse discussion on what, in my opinion, a question of increasingly pressing importance, namely, the relevance of what has been called "natural immunity" to malaria in deciding on an anti-malaria policy; and secondly to draw attention to some of the lacunae in our knowledge of hyperendemic malaria. Anopheline control under such circumstances in tropical Africa is impossible. . . . During the rains and after every heavy storm innumerable natural hollows fill with rain water or formed swamps; in additions old pig holes, hoof marks and the multitude of man-made extractions which surround every African village and are constantly being renewed—all contributed to the provision of a breeding area so large that the available methods of anopheline control are utterly beyond the resources of such people.[42]

The Wilsons, as I pointed out before, were discouraged about ever ending malaria ("it is impossible"). They raised concerns that even missing a few seasons of malaria could cause a rebound effect and thus worried about activities such as war or even research that took Africans out of their villages and then sent them back, vulnerable and endangered. Starting and then stopping an intervention raises the same ethical issues—in direct correlation with how effective the intervention has been. This raises the problem of durable fidelity—something that is necessary in all interventions. There is something critically unethical about mounting an intervention and then leaving, off to a place of safety. I will return to this problem of fidelity in the conclusion of this book, but note here that it is one of the already existing ethical challenges long prior to gene drives.

It also raises the question of resource allocation. Malaria in the Global North was eradicated because of state-sponsored joint efforts to alter agriculture, water pathways, and the physical environment and to spray chemicals over vast areas of wilderness in the twentieth century. We do not rely on vaccines with only moderate effectiveness, funded enormous project to change the natural world. So, the question arises: Why should African children need to rely on vaccines with a 40% effectiveness? Will vaccines paradoxically allow states to turn from vital functions intended to remediate habitat?

Nevertheless, vaccines were continued and, as I have noted, have finally achieved the first real successes. However, even the 2021 iteration has only achieved 50 percent vaccine efficacy in children aged between six and seventeen months and 34 percent vaccine efficacy in infants—so low a protection that it is not recommended to that group. Ethicists raise the problem that parents may think that their children are completely protected, as they are with other types of childhood vaccines, like polio, and thus not take the precautions needed to protect them with bed nets and other methods. As more trials of other vaccine are proposed, others have raised the problem of equipoise. Is RTS,S a control-arm drug or not? Should it be used for testing other vaccines or not?

Other trials are ongoing and, despite the fact that the "N" (the initial patient sample number) is very small, have shown promise. The most recent vaccine is a variant of RTS,S called R21, which is built on a protein that is excreted by the parasite as it enters the human body at the sporozoite stage. In a trial of 450 children aged between five and seventeen months, the vaccine was up to 77 percent effective at preventing malaria over the course of one year—clearing the 75 percent effectiveness target set by the WHO.[43]

Another enduring ethical question is about success, not failure. We have seen this issue raised again and again and, in some cases, not in an innocent way. In the event that an intervention or set of interventions works, then childhoods in African rural areas would be very different. We have seen how colonialist administrators fretted about this—worrying that a disease-free population would create a social force that might well have destabilized British control over the resources of the colonies. The concern is important, despite the historical complexities of its origin. How should societies plan for success in advance of its onset? For example, by building new schools or social institutions to serve the many children who will survive and not be lost to malaria. Thought needs to be given to these social and economic effects as well, whatever intervention is successful, genetic or not. Of particular importance will be how to enact the critical ethical principles of stewardship of fragile communities and environments, and fidelity to them, not only during research, prevention, and treatment but also after success. Will, for example, the success of a vaccine mean that other critical interventions toward the well-being of communities should be abandoned? In the case of polio, where the disease is spread by the lack of adequate human waste disposal, communities still needed to clean up open sewers, despite a vaccine. In the case of tuberculosis, cities still needed to reduce density and build better housing for the poor, even after effective treatment was employed. The temptation for Koch's magic bullet in the place of public health measures is quite powerful, and as we have seen, it has long history in the story of malaria.

For example. Four days after the WHO approved the vaccine and clearly stated it could not be counted on to end malaria alone, the leadership of the Stockholm, Basel, and Rotterdam Conventions issued a press release called "The End of DDT," in which they suggested the vaccine would lead to an end to the use of pesticides, which they consider harmful, despite the fact that they are still needed, and despite the fact that they regulate them with care.[44]

6.5 Ethical Issues in Existing Research on Malaria

In addition to the considerable existing ethical issues in treatment, long-standing ethical issues arise in the course of research on malaria as well. Like all research on infectious disease, the gold standard for drug or vaccine testing is the clinical trial in which two equally matched populations, one given an intervention and one given a placebo or, in some cases, merely allowed to use an existing treatment strategy, are compared. If the intervention is proven to be effective to anonymized observers, the treatment is a success. But in addition to controlled clinical trials, or when trials are not feasible, it is also ethically permissible to use controlled infection "challenge" studies for testing when the underlying disease actually has a durable treatment strategy. Malaria can be studied in this way and has been for decades. The treatment is in this case is artemisinin. This means that subjects are exposed to malaria and then to new antiparasitic drugs tested against the diseases. Malaria is a terrible disease—it has fevers of up to 106°F, crashing headaches, and bone-wracking pain. So, are these challenge trials—used since Ross infected his servants—really ethical? Ethicists have raised questions about the possibility of consent for a disease of this order, with risk far above minimal. Yet, such challenge trials have been a consistent part of research.

In addition, unlike other diseases in which inoculation with the blood of an infected person is used to create the challenge, malaria studies have a particularly intense mode of infection. Because malaria in the wild is only transmitted from a mosquito bite, accurate challenge tests are usually done by exposure to infected mosquitoes that first "feed" on one live malaria-ridden volunteer and that are then put in little cages and strapped to the naked arm or leg of another volunteer to "feed."

Further, the use of this method extends beyond challenge trials. One of the most important ways that malarial mosquitoes are still caught for study, just as they have been for the last century, is not with traps or by nets swung at clouds of mosquitoes during swarming but by a technique called "human landing catches," in which a section of a volunteer's leg is exposed and is meant to attract female mosquitoes who come to bite and who are far more difficult to catch because they are peripheral to the swarms where males can be caught. Theoretically, the volunteer or a watching inspector is meant to capture the insect before they insert their proboscis, but in some versions, in which the subject is meant to be bitten, as in the protocol for vaccine testing, the subject can be bitten between 50 and 100 times a night. While the bites are painless, the aftermath, if the subject becomes infected, is not. While development on CO_2 releasing machines (used instead of uncovered upper thighs) is proceeding, the machines are tricky to use in resource-poor settings, attract fewer females, need a power source, and are expensive.

Perhaps even more ethically problematic than the human landing catches was the widespread use of human feeding practices in research, where the mosquito was used to get and then give malaria deliberately, transferring the disease between vulnerable patients. Not only was the Statesville prison research performed on a vexed combination of mental patients who had been given malaria to treat their syphilitic disease and prisoners, but in that experiment, as we have seen, the mosquitoes fed on the malarial syphilitics and were then taken to fed on prisoners so that they would become sickened in order that the new drugs for World War II could be tested.[45] Of course, there is no part of this project that, would be approved now, and in today's terms, it is an ethical failure But as described in my previous chapter, nothing about this research concerned the apparently very thoughtful researchers at the time.[46] The use of human landing catches for research is still part of many protocols.

Population research raised questions long before gene drives as well. How are research subjects justly asked for consent for an intervention? How can whole communities provide consent? Prevention strategies, always used across populations and regions, raised other ethical questions. Is it unethical to declare some areas "untreatable" as was done for the entire continent of Africa by the UN planners in the 1955–1956 campaign? What makes an area "too hard" to treat? Many areas and villages strongly resisted being used as test beds for the variety of insecticides used against malarial mosquitoes, as we have seen. The ethical question remains: How far can a state or public health agency go in forcing participation in population-wide studies?

The ethical questions of that 1957 campaign still resonant and are still are part of all malaria prevention research that is population based. The most dramatic example is the use of whole-house spraying of DDT and then more recently developed insecticides. Whole-house spraying meant that everything had to be out of the house before dawn, in the dark, so that the spray would dose the sleeping female mosquitoes resting on vertical surfaces. Then, the insecticide was sprayed on the walls of the home—in most cases, a one- or two-room mud-walled home, so that sleeping and eating areas were all affected—until the walls were wet with the chemical. Then, the family had to stay out of the house, waiting for dawn and then waiting for three hours until it was safe to return. If it rained, then the entire contents of the house may be ruined. This had to be repeated several times over a period of weeks. In some communities, where people bringing in the harvest, largely but not exclusively men, would sleep outside in sheds near the fields, the spraying was useless, for the huts were not sprayed and the harvesters would then bring larvae and resting females back in the folds of their clothing. Home spraying is not a matter of anonymized sweeps of distant planes over neighborhoods, as is done in my city; it is very intimate and very invasive. The insecticide smells, sometimes for days. And it is used both in prevention and in testing strategies.

Despite these ethical issues, prevention and treatment of malaria continued, and the increased efforts have seen significant reductions in malaria incidence (the rate of new cases) and deaths. Between 2000 and 2015, the WHO reported, malaria incidence fell by 37 percent globally, and malaria deaths fell by 60 percent among all age groups and by 65 percent among children younger than five. But by 2015, it was clear that something had changed. The rates were substantially flat. And in 2022, for the first time in decades, the rates of death from malaria climbed to more than 600,000. It was this cessation of progress that changed the ethical calculus—the consideration of worth, risk, and benefit—as new ideas were brought forward, among them, of course, new ideas about gene drives.

All of these earlier ethical questions have been a part of malaria research, treatment, and prevention—moral choices whose parameters have shifted with changes in colonial power relationships, national liberation efforts, and shifting economic realities. These ethical issues did not stop public health officials and researchers from proceeding with the efforts to cope with malaria. And all of these profound ethical issues were part of the research and treatment of malaria for generations of researchers, long before gene drives were considered part of the armamentarium. And yes, they remain as a part of the terrain of the research on which genetic engineering takes place.

6.6 Considering the Ethics of Genetic Engineering Itself

The question I am led to ask is whether gene engineering and gene drives create distinctive ethical issues, in addition to the ethical issues I raised above, which are a part of all malaria research and treatment. Are there ethical issues, that exist only because of the genetic method used to address malaria? What is it about CRISPR-Cas9 that troubles so many? In this part of the chapter, I now turn to consider the ethical issues that arise with any genetic intervention into the existing order—the world we speak of as "the natural." Let me first consider the phenomenology of our discussion because the language is important for our reasoning.

Philosophers, noted Edmund Husserl, have long had a resistance to science as being too literal. The language of science, Husserl argued, did not allow for the kind of nuance and subtlety of the humanities. Without this, modern judgment, including judgment about science, was flawed: "The exclusiveness with which the total worldview of modern man, in the second half of the nineteenth century let itself be determined by the positive sciences and be blinded by the 'prosperity' they produced, meant an indifferent turning away from the questions which are decisive for a genuine humanity. Merely fact minded sciences make merely fact-minded people."[47] But fact-minded science, it turns out, is the basis for much of our lives. And fact-mindedness is important. When we speak, as moral philosophers, my colleagues do not often see the quotidian details of the existing world (human landing catches and all) when we critique science, and yet these details are important to understand, as I have argued here. But do the ethical questions change when science itself changes and when new ways of thinking about biology are brought to the fore? After all, many have argued for the revolutionary nature of this moment, when CRISPR-Cas9 enters, biological orders can be undone, and the genetic code can be unlocked. Google "gene drives" and you will immediately be told by website after website about "the perils and promise" of this moment, or that "we are at a crossroads" because of CRISPR.

Let me divide this next discussion into two parts. The first is to consider the use of the larger project of synthetic biology and genetic engineering to manipulate living organisms. The second is the specific use of gene drives in African countries to eliminate malaria parasites. I argue that a clear focus on the specifics of the case at hand is how we ought to think about the ethics of gene drives. However, first, I want to make some larger points about how genetic manipulation really does affect our view about the future of nature.

This one project, using CRISPR-Cas9 to alter the genes of the mosquito, is part of a larger discipline—a new and more skillful merger of chemistry, engineering, and molecular and computational biology—into a field sometimes called synthetic biology and sometimes called genetic engineering. I mentioned one project—that of making synthetic artemisinin—in the last chapter. I will consider here some of the many ethical issues that are engaged by the emerging field. The field uses the following self-definition: "Synthetic biology is a) the design and construction of new biological parts, devices and systems, and b) the redesign of existing natural biological systems for useful purposes."[48] Another definition is: "Engineering biology (also known as synthetic biology) is the convergence of many disciplines to enable predictive engineering of living systems, the constituent components of living systems, and related biological processes for public benefit, such as curative advanced therapies, advanced material manufacturing, renewable energy sources, more resilient crops, and unprecedented data storage solutions."[49] However, neither of these fully captures the complexity and breadth of the field.

I am not unaware, by the way, that the kind of chemistry that dominated the world when malaria was first treated was synthetic chemistry—it is the basis for all the pesticides and all the chemopraxis to date.

Note that one of the intellectual agendas for synthetic biology/genetic engineering, unlike earlier efforts with the genetic modification of existing organisms, is not only the transformation of existing forms of life, but also the creation of entirely new organisms, processes, capacities, or parts, ones using the basic chemicals or models that exist in nature. Often this is described as a sort of technological improvement over the creatures that have been thrown into existence by naturally occurring evolutionary processes half in jest. And when synthetic biologists described nature as a sort of a parts shop and, in some cases, as a set of plans, rather like the Sears home building blueprints of the 1920s, philosophers reacted just as Husserl predicted, with a sort of visceral horror. The idea that some of the scientists promoted was that to understand the basic, minimal machinery of cells, one had to be able to replicate it—in the way that the fifth-century Greeks sometimes thought of knowledge as practical wisdom: "to make is to know." Some scientists planned to study a bottom-up path, seeing if putting the most primitive forms of RNA together would self-assemble. Others thought that using the processes in nature to recapitulate alternative paths to life would work better, and others imagined that making completely novel organisms, from sequences completely unseen in nature, would be interesting and important. Others saw themselves as "hacking nature," using existing biological processes, like the underlying one in CRISPR-Cas9 or the several naturally occurring gene drives, and repurposing it. In the first years of this new field, there was an explosion of creative possibilities. Synthetic biologists formed a loose, anarchic, interactive community that stressed open discourse, extreme creativity, and transparency in the development of tools. Drew Endy, one of the first practitioners of the field, proposed creating a "BioBrick" library, where parts of DNA sequences could be created, stored, and used by all in a variety of projects that involved "building" new organisms. On the joint website that defined the project, the members of the community added: "We are a group of individuals from various institutions who are committed to engineering biology in an open and ethical manner. We are currently working to help specify and populate a set of standard parts that have well-defined performance characteristics and can be used (and re-used) to build biological systems; to develop and incorporate design methods and tools into an integrated engineering environment; reverse engineer and re-design pre-existing biological parts and devices in order to expand the set of functions that we can access and program; reverse engineer and re-design a "simple" natural bacterium."[50] Such language is rich in its assumptions, and such linguistic claims imply a particular moral framing of the issue—a particular stance toward "naturalness" and indeed to "usefulness" that has not escaped the attention of this author. Neither has the fact that such framing endowed the field with a set of a priori ethical principles. Look again at the self-descriptions I quoted, and note how they both promise a moral end as well as a technical one. Indeed, I spent the first years in the field considering research that scientists believed would support sustainability or crop yields, and it was the ongoing subject of such work that led to my first introduction to the gene drive idea in the first place.[51] I was also interested in the way that ontological norms shifted beneath the feet of this research. I initially considered how one project—the project of the design of an artificial, self-organizing, and self-evolving cellular entity—may cross the border between things that are non-biological and things that are biological—that eat, breathe, grow, and then replicate. I also thought it important to consider how such a self-defined field in biology can undertake the considerable challenge of the establishment of normative rules to govern and manage the uses of such a powerful science and technology. And it did not escape me then that there were also considerable challenges for the emergence of any powerful new field in science that comes of age in a new climate of bio-weaponry, internet access, and globalization—so-called dual-use problems.

Jack Szostak, who would later win the Nobel Prize in Physiology and Medicine in 2009, along with Elizabeth Blackburn and Carol Greider, for discovering how chromosomes are protected by telomeres, had turned his attention to this new field too. His was one of the first projects in genetic engineering that I thought about a great deal. It was the beginning of a different sort of biology, one that was interested in origins, and I was intrigued. That moment where molecules assemble into a life-form, nonbeing into being, seemed to me to be a foundational philosophical problem as well as a scientific one. Here is what I wrote at the time:

"What are we watching?

"After seeing the scientist's PowerPoint demonstration, the moral philosopher walks up to the podium to talk to the molecular biologist and to watch, once more, the little movie he has shown during the talk. It is a short looping clip of small lipid globules that line up, the circles linking into chains, and the chains moving back and forth, back and forth, across the screen. They are moving, it would appear, in response to the magnesium concentration in the solution they are in. In another loop, they cluster, link, and move across temperature gradients. If they were cellular organisms, one would describe this as responsive behavior, and one would watch the linkage of cell to cell to form chains as primitive and evolutionary organization. However, these things/events are not living cells—not quite. They are entirely artificial, made as surely as any machine but of components that, in their entirety, are something entirely new. What they are (beings in the act of being) and what they are doing (ex nihilo generation and supple adaptation)[52] has long been the subject of philosophy. This project—the building of an artificial cell—is a part of a larger goal for both the philosopher and the biologist. As the project of synthetic evolution continues, what are the issues in ethics and philosophy that it evokes? What sort of question is it to ask when one tries to recapitulate life? Is it a matter of ethical permissibility? Transgressive research? Are we "seeing" lifelike patterns because we shape data into familiar stories, "biologizing" physical events? Is life a matter of descriptive criteria or of activities? It is the contention of this essay that asking about life's origins not only uncovers intriguing questions about chance, meaning, and order, but also allows a rather startling discourse about the nature of knowledge in a world with physical realities and enduring cultural narratives.

Szostak had long been interested in how life evolved from the early molecules available in the early Earth environment. What caught his interest at the beginning of his career was a new understanding of the role of RNA. Previously thought to be only capable of transmitting information, discoveries in the early 1980s revealed that RNA was capable of catalyzing enzymes as well, which meant that RNA might have a dual role, not only transmitting information but also doing what protein are exclusively meant to do—catalyzing certain chemical reaction inside cells.[53] Using a few key elements—membrane, "cell" globules, clay, and simple RNA enzymes—he is studying the basic properties of cells. Lately, Szostak has been putting simple RNA enzymes inside little chemical membrane sacks, showing that they can conduct their characteristic activities as if they were in a cell. Thus, some of life's chemistry is compatible with artificial membranes, he says, something that required a careful tweaking of the membrane chemistry. He has also made the sacs grow spontaneously and even divide—with help. "It's a simplified model of the situation we'd really like to have," says Szostak: a growing, dividing, living organism of totally synthetic origins. But even at present, he says, "These simple membrane systems do pretty fascinating things."[54]

Once he made RNAs that could bind to ATP, Szostak was curious about how he could create catalytic RNA—making artificial ribozymes, akin to the actual ribozymes that act as catalytic substrates in a living cell. Not only was he about to generate such molecular structures, but he was about to generate them with far more complexity than is actually found in nature—which led him to speculate if the defining specificity in the actual world was the end of a longer evolutionary process. Molecule by molecule, basic research scientists are discovering the fact-based world, finding increasing clever ways to mimic it, manipulate it, or even, as in Szostak's case, to recapitulate it."

Once again, reader, you might be considering why I would tell this story about basic biological research in a book about gene drives. Here is why. This is a long introduction to the power of the new genetic engineering that is the larger category of which gene drives are a part. We are far beyond the work of altered *E. coli* or Flavr Savr tomatoes here, but I urge you to consider why it is important. This sort of science is epistemology. It changes how we as moderns come to know and then how we speak about what we know and then how we reason about what to do. Why this is critical is that scientists have largely come to agree and accept the basics of classic evolutionary theory of adaptive mutation to ecological niches, which, while a satisfying explanation for the speciation and specification of biological life, still leaves open many questions, not only Szostak's curiosity about how the step from inorganic chemicals in a coincident neighborhood to self-replicating, self-organizing single cells is done, but in other borderline questions about fundamental alterations in the purposes of organisms.[55] This sort of knowledge and this sort of power are familiar to any one of my colleagues in religious studies who do research on the dreams of the alchemists in the late medival and early modern period. This sort of knowledge is what is behind the question of this book: May we make the world? May we know nature in this way, and shape nature in this way? What does it mean for us to have this power?

While speculation about when, how, and what it is that crosses the line from inanimate to animate object, from an event to an entity, is satisfying in a philosophical way, the ethical and ontological issues only emerge when we consider our duties toward the things we create. We are led to ask: what, if any, moral status do the new things we make have? What duties do we have toward a world of genetically made or remade things? If one begins a process and forces evolution, how far may this process be allowed to go? What are the constraints on us as we make or remake the world?

Is Uneasiness a Moral Category?

Yet for many, the ethical issue that was at stake is not the problem of the actual creation of new life-forms and our possible duties toward them, but rather of the disruption in the natural law that this research implies—something that recalls for us the category that Freud named as "uncanny" to name the puzzling sensations evoked by the simulacrums created by inventors of his time. It was precisely the automata of the 1700s, small lifelike dolls with the capacity to move and speak (and that still are maintained in a Swiss village), that led Sigmund Freud to define a category of reaction to all such phenomena—and that serves us well in consideration of why we find so much of genetic engineering so complexly disturbing. Freud called this "the uncanny valley." "The uncanny, the feeling that arises when there is an intellectual uncertainty about the borderline between the lifeless and the living."

If the natural order of the world of things is disturbed, if the basic lines between nonbeing and being, created and made, and begotten and assembled

are blurred, then something about the fixity of our perceived world is awry
First among these objections is the argument that humans possess an essential nature and live within an essential natural order that cannot be altered
without harm. This has been a problem for well over a century. C. S. Lewis,
in an argument very similar to Husserl, expressed this as a concern that the
very acts of rational science—dissection, analysis, and quantification—are a
violation of the sacred integrity that lies behind all of Nature: "Now I take it
that when we understand a thing analytically, and then dominate and use it
for our own convenience, we reduce it to the level of 'nature,' we suspend our
judgments of value about it, ignore its final cause (if any) and treat it in terms
of quantity. This repression of elements in what would otherwise be our total
reaction to it is sometimes very noticeable and even painful: something has
to be overcome before we can cut up a dead man or a live animal in a dissecting room."[56] For Lewis, the understanding of the body as replaceable is disturbing: "The real objection," he says, "is that if man chooses to treat himself
as raw material, raw material he will be, not raw material to be manipulated
by himself as he fondly imagined, but by mere appetite."[57] (Lewis imagines
that new transformative technology will be manipulated by "Controllers"
who will eventually transform Man into mere matter.)

Daniel Callahan echoes his concern, both in the sense that limits need
to be placed on what is decent to do to Nature and in the sense that such
action is a part of a larger danger—that power in the hands of medicine to
heal is really power in the hands of the elite or of the state to manipulate and
control. He argues:

> The word "No" perfectly sums up what I mean by a limit—a boundary point beyond
> which one should no go. . . . There are least two reasons why a science of techno-
> logical limits is needed. First, limits need to be set to the boundless hopes and
> expectations, constantly escalating, which technology has engendered. Advanced
> technology has promised transcendence of the human condition. That is a false
> promise, incapable of fulfillment. . . . Second . . . limits (are) necessary in order that
> the social pathologies resulting from technologies can be controlled . . . while it
> can and does care, save, and free, it can also become the vehicle for the introduc-
> tion of new repressions in society.[58]

The transgressive nature of genetic engineering research is clearly on display
when critics make the claim that such an act is a violation of our human
limits or a recapitulation of creation itself, or when they are concerned that
a second round of creation may well end in a cataclysm. Yet, the judgment

that we can be guided by our moral intuitions has a danger as well. As early as the 1970s, while thinking about early experiments in genetic engineering, ethicist Joseph Fletcher raised a disagreement to that sort of objection: "The belief that God is at work directly or indirectly in all natural phenomena is a form of animism or simple pantheism. If we took it really seriously, all science, including medicine would die away because we would be afraid to 'dissect God' or tamper with His activity. . . . Every widening and deepening of our knowledge of reality and of our control of its forces are the ingredients of both freedom and responsibility."[59]

Returning to the History of Genetic Engineering

Let me return to the story of the first discussions about regulations on genetic interventions that I described in chapter 3. This time, instead of focusing on the regulatory aspects of the work, I will consider two of the larger philosophical issues—ones that the regulators bracketed for "further discussion" but which were always important for bioethics. John Fletcher and Albert Jonson cite the period of the late 1960s as the first mention of modern ethical concerns about genetic engineering. Fletcher notes that Marshall Nirenberg wrote of programming cells with synthetic messages, for example, and of the implications of such an advance in 1967.[60] In 1973, as we saw in chapter 3, Maxine Singer and Dietrich Soll noted such concerns in a letter to the NAS and in 1974, the community of scientists capable of performing this technology, led by the NAS, gathered to create guidelines for their work at Asilomar. The Asilomar guidelines stressed two aspects of regulation. The first aspect was that the concerns about safety should be taken seriously enough to create level 4 biocontainment for the work. The second aspect was that the *E. coli* should be used in the work to replicate the DNA needed to be artificially altered for greater control and, finally, that each and every recombinant DNA experiment should face not only a standard IRB review but also a specialized review by a specialized national committee (the RAC), as I described in Chapter 3. The scientist declared a moratorium on all work until such mechanisms could be established. In 1974, the NIH established the RAC. The RAC held its first public meeting in 1975.[61]

The RAC was created in a more sanguine era. At that time, the full power of genetic engineering was poorly understood. But since 9/11, we can imagine that power being used in disturbing and deadly ways. The discussions, then, about safety changed, for even the complex network of oversight noted above began to seem incomplete when confronted with the actual use of bioterrorism for political ends and the increasing power, scalability, and universalizability of genetic engineering. In 2005–2006, a year-long intensification of this discussion about what is called "the dual use problem" was held, and research was done on how the scientists within the still self-described and self-contained community understood the problem of regulation and the new issues of biosafety and security that lay outside previous RAC discourse. Following the National SynBio 1.0 meeting and an associated NAS meeting, a team of researchers, led by Stephen Maurer of the Goldman School of Public Policy, extensively interviewed the PIs and postdoctoral students of the laboratories at UC Berkeley, MIT, and the University of Texas most centrally involved in the work. They created a draft consensus document aimed at stimulation of robust discussion that could lead to an Asilomar-type agreement. Like that earlier model, the community was, at that time, still small enough to create normative rules. As the techniques and tools are more widely appreciated and the student base grows, more people will need to be accountable to some process of regulation. While, of course, this issue is important for any genetic manipulation, and the role of gain-of-function research and speculation about it certainly became a topic of lay interest during COVID-19, genetic engineering intended for field use and not laboratory use raises even more concerns. I will return to this in the final section of the chapter.

The RAC process was also limited in another way, like much of my field of bioethics. It had no theory of evil, by which I mean that my field has no theory of moral wrongdoing, despite the fact that bioethics was at least partially born of thinking about the cruelty and dehumanization by the Nazi sciences as we shaped the context of research. We often write as if all one needs to do is explain the correct, logical, normative path, and humans will follow it. Our field no longer accepts purely theological concepts such as befallenness or sin, nor do we entirely subscribe to psychological motivations. What have we, as bioethicists, really to say about the gap between the rhetoric of social good and the increasing practice of lucrative spin-off companies or even outright fraud? We can name and describe these lapses, but we know that the problems persist. In fact, many scholars of bioethics think and write largely about the good act and hence theorize nearly exclusively about the good. I have asked it here: what is the good act, and what makes it so?

Many critiques of genetic interventions are concerns that the wealthy will use genetic intervention to "enhance" something or someone, but these critiques do not think this will be done out of evil intent. Scholars largely worry about foolishness, triviality, or the inauthenticity of the rich, who might alter the genetic provenance of their children for competitive advantage or narcissism.[62] However, such critiques so not develop the scenario of using genetic technologies for deliberate harm. (The parents may be misguided but not murderous.) Having no robust theory of evil in bioethics or science allows a certain silence to develop around several core issues in genetic engineering, for all the existing regulations are based on premises of innocent error prevention or overly enthusiastic persuasion by scientists to an unwitting or foolish public as the core problem. The exception to this is a growing attention to the problem of dual use. Yet, even here, the focus is on setting up preventative guide rails rather than on the etiology of the impulse to create weapons from biology.

Further, there is a strong liberty-based rights theory approach within the field, stressing individual autonomy, freedom, and creativity of research as a free-speech act. Hence, while many of the existing regulations are concerned with privacy issues or protection of the patient—or the patent! many others want to allow the free expression of any scientific notion, including ones that seem outlandish but may yield results. It should be noted that all new science is inherently subversive, indicated thinkers from Thomas Jefferson[63] to Thomas Kuhn to Aldous Huxley,[64] in that it exists outside existing structures of knowledge and beneath the text of the known, well characterized or proven. In this sense, the best, most creative, and risky science creates a "knowledge frontier." Like all frontiers or borderland areas, this creates the conditions for powerful trade zones, in which the risk and benefit constraints within existing knowledge terrain are altered. In such a frontier, free exchange (of ideas, goods, services, and knowledge) flourishes under the least restrictive interventions by the state. And like the Ship of Theseus, no matter how secure the science at hand becomes, there will always be the margins where something is known but not enough, so that that ship needs to be built as it is sailing.

The Critical Issue of Biosecurity and Dual Use

In the paper "From Understanding to Action: Community Bases Options for Improving Safety and Security in Synthetic Biology,"[65] Stephen Mauer and his coauthors document extensively how synthetic biologists/genetic engineers understand the potential for the use and abuse of new genetic technology. In particular, any technology that reshapes conditions understood as stable or "natural" creates the intriguing problem of the moral choice faced by the creators—Would the new tool be used for agriculture or other human industry, or would it be used for weaponry? This is as true for genetic engineers as it was for the inventors of metallurgy, wheeled vehicles, gunpowder, forks, or nuclear fission. In many cases (e.g., gunpowder), the technology was tightly controlled by a central authority to prevent dual use by enemies. In others, use was determined by the marketplace from the beginning. However, in all cases, dual use proved to be simply inevitable.

In the most recent period, nuclear arms technology, learned and practiced under clear security guidelines, Western educational systems, and laboratories, was then sold by scientists for personal gain and patriotic passion. Placed against the new sorts of economies and the new sorts of national and religious fervor abroad in the land, the new genetic technologies are a serious cause for alarm. The scale of the experiment, the openness of the field, and the ease of production and their portability present a particular sort of challenge. The same wide-use applicability that makes the science so promising also makes it far more dangerous than conventional weaponry, for a reengineered virus or bacteria could wreck far more havoc than bombs. The norms that would keep such organisms from being deployed or from inadvertent or malicious use are the same for naturally occurring or genetically altered organisms. However, there is no question that they might be used as a weapon against the crops of a nation, or to destroy a critical insect species—honeybees, for example.

Oversight has been inconsistent, and as we have learned during the COVID-19 pandemic, compliance and surveillance is globally inconsistent. In December 2005, in a US government report on the issue of the threat assessment of biological weapons, Milton Leitenberg noted: "The entire area of oversight of problematical 'dual use' research in molecular genetics and its applications in the United States appears to range from inadequate at the local levels to virtually nonexistent at the national level and in terms of BWC treaty compliance."[66] Leitenberg reminds the reader of the pathway of IBC and NIH national oversight and of local IBC rules, but notes: "Failure to adhere to NIH guidelines does not apply except on a voluntary basis to a very large population of institutions that are not recipients of NIH funding, such as US government biodefense laboratories, and US Government contractors as well as hundreds of commercial biotechnology enterprises."[67] He then goes on to note two cases. One involves making a vaccine-resistant strain of anthrax presumably to find ways to combat it ("Project Jefferson"), and one in which a method of countering the action of botulinum toxin is sought, which involves making a biologically stable version of the botulism neurotoxin by using genetic alterations so that it could be studied more easily, but such stabilization would also allow it to be weaponized. (Previously, botulinum toxin was deemed too unstable to have such a dual use.) Neither project has been reviewed by the IBC or the RAC, whose guidelines do not currently include consideration of the security or proliferation implications of dual-use research.[68] In this report, he does note that the NAS has taken this problem on to some extent, recommending that seven categories of "experiments of concern" be added to the NIH oversight process:

> In response to the recommendations of the NAS committee report, the administration announced the establishment of a National Science Advisory Board for BioSecurity (NSABB) on March 4, 2004. Its mandate was to last for 2 years. The NSABB was established by the DHHS and housed within the NIH. The staff of the NSABB was not appointed until 11 months later . . . no membership of the Board was made until its first meeting June 30, 2005. . . . the NSABB will not itself review individual project protocols; it will only respond to requests for guidance. . . . But most importantly, the NSABB is to have *no* (emphasis in original, ed.) oversight over classified BW-relevant research, which is the location in which the most problematical dual-use research is likely to take place.[69]

It is the contention of the still small community of self-identified synthetic biologists that the potential for harm, even for the development of weapons capable of "mass destruction," is not trivial. It is also the opinion of many who I spoke with about the problem that while it is a concern that is always present and even perhaps, some thought, inevitable, actually performing the work could clearly be made more difficult, with far stronger sanctions, earlier warning systems, and plan for incentives for honesty.

It is outside the area of expertise of even an expansive field such as bioethics to assess these concerns. However, it is the contention of this discussion that a clear moral obligation exists in all field of inquiry to protect the society in which it is given the privilege and freedom and funding to exist. This duty is correlative to the right of free inquiry.

At this point, it is important to note that genetic engineering presents a unique risk for bioweaponry, and the reader will remember that small paragraph in the NASEM report that I mentioned in chapter 3. Here, too, NASEM worried that gene drives could conceivably become a weapon.

Meanwhile, we also face more immediate and vivid threats from the unchecked spread by organisms who are "out of place" that are not made in the lab but wreck havoc. Perfectly natural novel organisms can infect humans and sweep across the globe, as we have seen. Ordinary commerce has introduced non-native species that threaten crops and human health. As I write this, the spotted lanternfly (*Lycorma delicatula*), which appeared in the Eastern USA from Asia, threatens the entire Eastern Seaboard and possibly the California wine industry.[70] Lake Michigan, the lake by my city of Chicago, is completely invaded by Asian tiger mussels, which cover the bottom of the lake, and is threatened by Asian carp—large, aggressive fish with the capacity to leap and slap humans in the face—which would eat their way across the entire Great Lakes ecosystem, crashing it with untold effects.

As I finished writing the final version of this book, humanity was coping with the ongoing COVID-19 pandemic in its terrible variant forms; and polio, which had mutated from the attenuated vaccine intended to eradicate it; monkeypox, which was first seen in primate laboratories; a new form of hepatitis; cases of Marburg virus and a multidrug resistant fungus all suddenly emerged as threats. It is sobering to see the way that the microbiological world has such deadly power over our complex modernity, even as we consider altering, making, and changing it, without malice and even without intent to harm.

To Make Is to Know: Notes on an Old Problem about Knowledge

The debates about dual use are not the only set of problems engendered by the technological gesture at the heart of all genetic engineering. At stake as well is the special kind of knowledge that such making implies. For Aristotle, useful knowledge, "practical wisdom," was phronesis. Phronesis implied actually doing an act, making, in order to know—the act of making, not the act of perception or contemplation alone, how wisdom, and indeed rationality and judgment, was achieved. Hence, altering genes, or "making" organisms seems linguistically like a somewhat different moral gesture than earlier forms of medical or scientific interventions, like curing an illness or with drugs

Second, for most of medical history, the sort of technological advance in earlier periods the thing that was changed or enhanced was the sense perceptions of the doctor. Stethoscopes and otoscopes allowed the sounds of the body to be more audible. X-rays, computed tomography scans, and magnetic resonance imaging allow the inner vistas of the body to be revealed. Electroencephalograms and electrocardiograms allow the electrical currents that animate the central and peripheral nervous systems to be charted in quantifiable units. Microscopes allow invasive bacteria to be seen at microscopic and, increasingly, molecular levels. These earlier technologies extended the reach of what Francis Bacon increasingly trusted and what the Greeks did not: the perception and observation of the phenomena of the world and the perception of the outcome of its deliberate perturbation.

> Bacon's method presupposes a double empirical and rational starting point. True knowledge is acquired if we proceed from lower certainty to higher liberty and from lower liberty to higher certainty. The rule of certainty and liberty in Bacon converges . . . For Bacon, making is knowing and knowing is making (cf. Bacon IV [1901], 109–10). Following the maxim "command nature . . . by obeying her" (Sessions, 1999, 136; cf. Gaukroger, 2001, 139 ff.), the exclusion of superstition, imposture, error, and confusion are obligatory. Bacon introduces variations into "the maker's knowledge tradition" when the discovery of the forms of a given nature provide him with the task of developing his method for acquiring factual and proven knowledge.[71]

Thus, the world is known by understanding the parts of the world and, from that, theorizing (knowing) by induction to principles or axioms or laws of nature, physics, and chemistry. In contemporary science, knowing is done largely by "unmaking"—by deconstruction of the component parts in a way that scientists of Bacon's era were unable to imagine, and "making" new organizms. Many of these "making" and "unmaking" techniques, such as the splicing of alternative DNA or the manipulation of cellular structures, allow a sense of inherent interchangeability, as if the real and the person were merely a set of Lego parts, awaiting clever recombination.

New technologies, not anticipated by the first decades of the RAC, changed some of the classic protective paradigms in recombinant DNA and other synthetic research. First, animal models, while required prior to human experimentation, ever since the Nuremberg Trial and the subsequent codes, turned out to be sometimes misleading and may not offer any guidance for the use of technology in humans or with humans or in human environments. Second, the consent of human 'subjects' prior to research is nearly impossible, when the subjects may be the future generations yet to be born. "Future tense consent" may be impossible for very long-term research. Third, new research may use unexpected routes and intellectual disciplines such as nanotechnology, materials engineering, artificial life, computer science, and chemistry that were not anticipated by earlier scholars. Finally, and most importantly, big genetic engineering projects usually do not involve the standard idea of the manipulation of human genes via vectors, patient by patient, but imagine far larger uses—screening of huge populations or environmental alterations in large landscapes. Such a "social scale" may have population implications. The idea that one genetic alteration could affect millions of people allows for serious and just responses to some of humankind's most vexing diseases. Yet, it also suggests a degree of applicability and replicability of some powerful bioagents that is unprecedented in scope and in duration.

What Is a Thing?

Genetic engineering is conceptually important for moral philosophy in another way: for phenomenologists, defining the category of being and hence nonbeing is important. There is a nonbeing in the profound otherness of the established world—living other beings are different from rocks and shoelaces, for example. This otherwise than being is then clearly further queried by things, phenomena, or perhaps actual beings (with some narrative possibility) that have a point of nonexistence and would not exist save for their deliberate creation. As these phenomena change over time, they then share time as well as terrain with us. Creating entities that did not exist is unsettling not only for people with religious objections but also for anyone who suddenly becomes aware of this phenomenon of the new in the quotidian timeline of the present.

In fact, the uneasiness about the real and the natural has been part of several scientific discourses. The idea of simulated life was not limited to the automata machines of the eighteenth century that I mentioned as uncanny. Physical scientists became fascinated with the idea that "life matter" was a series of forces or entities that could be recombined too. Making gold was only one goal of the alchemist. Making life from the manipulation of elements was another: "Not all attempts to replicate artificial life were mechanical, during the Renaissance, a number of astrologers and alchemists developed recipes of more magical creations. Cornelius Agrippa believed, along with his fellow sorcerers, that humans could be grown from mandrake roots. Paraclete published instructions for the manufacture of homunculi . . . Human semen could be put in an airtight jar and buried in horse manure for forty days, . . . magnetized, preserved at the temperature of a mare's womb and fed human blood for forty weeks."[72] The eighteenth-century automata returned to this concept. But in this instance, the signs of the new discipline of science were used to explain the goal: "[The] ambitions of necromancer were revived in the well-respected name of science. Life advances in scientific instrument, and a fondness for magical tricks, mean that automata were thought of as glorious feat of engineering or philosophical toys."[73] As philosopher Umberto Eco noted, it took the emerging power of the Industrial Revolution to use fully the new power of machines that took over the labor and thus "substituted" for the actual person, using mechanics instead of magic and potions. The uncanniness of the assembly line, then, has two sources: first, that human craftsmanship, toolmaking, which is the very sign of humanness, can be entirely recapitulated by a machine; second, that the world of objects and others can be broken down into a series of parts that can be both endlessly recreated, moved about, and used in unforeseen ways and also combined and recombined into a variety of shapes and forms. It remained only for genetics then to appropriate the semiotic principle—parts of a gene are called the "cassette," which can be "swapped out" and changed; "molecular machines" of one organism can be imported into another; a murine model can be "made" and, of course, then sold in catalogs that list their specifications. It is this context in which the projects of all of engineering genetic biology are located.

It is this last consideration that turns our ethical gaze from ontological concerns toward ethical ones: May we make the world? Genetic engineering deals with minimalism as a core concept. Thus, small sections of DNA can be imagined (or replicated from naturally occurring alleles) and synthesized by a laboratory—the instructions arriving via the internet, the product arriving via FedEx. Then, chemical units can be linked to create longer units—perhaps, eventually, whole chromosomes. And this why the destructive dual use issue, or the possibility of a malignant construction, noted above is so disturbing.[74]

The response to the questions I raise in this last section seem to resolve around the level of risk deemed reasonable. The core of the method, after all, is stochastic, exploitative in the evolutionary sense, and thus fully unpredictable in its details. Genetic engineering is a system that is related to, but unlike the first generation of genetic manipulation, and if it is to proceed, it must do so with the ethics of our moral system evolving right along with the science. We cannot yet know the complexity of the issues, and it is a thin response indeed merely to note that science must be "cautious," for what precisely would such an admonition actually mean? This must be considered with care both by people who are enthusiastic about research and by people who are made uneasy about the research. Rather, to be normatively ethical, science must most of all be witnessed, and perhaps this is the way to begin, with publicity. Here, one thinks here of both the public meetings held on Martha's Vineyard to discuss Esvelt's proposals or the Target Malaria village meetings. The public gaze, the academic process, and the commercial users who wait even at the margins of theoretical project are a part of such witness.[75] Honestly, so are the detractors of genetic manipulation and, in fact, so are you, reading this description.

The ethical considerations that attend to all genetic engineering—whether it entails the phenomena that then seem to be a step away from the synthetic, simple organism, or whether it is about the genetic alteration of an existing organism using the tools developed by synthetic biology and genetic engineering—are largely surrounded by the uncertainty of outcome that attends to all basic research. Genetic manipulation for gene drives offers special issues. Can such a process, intended to be based on evolution's principles of mutation, random selection for advantage to niche, and transformation, be said to be regulated at all? What is the meaning of a call to regulate such an experiment? It is the illusive nature of such questions that raises special considerations for ethics. Unlike many questions in bioethics, in which burden, risk, harms, and benefits can be rationally foreseen and considered, the use of evolution's trajectory is entirely speculative. Part of the problem lies in the way that modernity itself is understood, and how our narrative is shaped by the very technology that is the most lifelike and artificial, the creation of the cinematic gaze. For Gaby Wood, who writes about the disruptive effects of the invention of automata in the eighteenth and nineteenth centuries, it was the invention of photography, and of moving photography, that enabled films to create an artificial life, seemingly completely accurate in a way that a painting was not, yet to alter the element of time (that most modern of concepts) by splicing pieces of cuttings of film to create the illusion of a coherent narrative.[76]

Let me develop this concept. Much of the substantive act of genetic modification is based on a similar idea and relies heavily on a similar technological advance in visual narrative, whose typology then both elucidates and distorts the object of the gaze—filmmaking. Like photographic images spliced together, genetic modification takes slices of narrative (in that the genetic code is developed over time and specific context and narrative histories) and "cuts and pastes" it into a new being, hence creating a fictive narrative within the organism, which is then displayed in a PowerPoint movie, which certain features, molecules or cell, labeled (which green fluorescent protein, for example) as if in a specific costume to be seen and understood by the audience in a particular role.

Why this is important, beyond the ironic cultural studies sense, is that it speaks to the concerns often expressed of the disruptive effect of this research (which is understood by the synthetic biology community in the postdoctoral fellow's scientific joke: "44 billion years of evolution—time for a change!"). Genetic engineering extends the disruptive principle (as does all science) that has deconstructed the core narrative of human reproduction, yet extends the project because, unlike descriptive biology or even basic research on how to repair flawed or nonfunctional DNA that causes illness, it rolls the "movie" back to the point of origin, allowing for entirely new plot endings. Understanding this deepens our problem, for short of entirely disallowing the project, at what possible point could society proscribe it? How far should the recapitulation go? It is in the name of these cultural anxieties that normative urges arise.

In these first reflections on genetic manipulation, I asked: Is creation "ours?" It is the question beneath many of the general anti-capitalist sentiments of the NGOs, and it is a fair one to ask beyond the problem of commodification of the organisms that are "made" by genetic manipulation. Do we stand outside it or within it? If the latter, are the acts that scientists struggle to learn and do really just instrumental, technical gestures, simply a part of our inbred genetic character? In other words, is making things in this way simply a more rational approach to technology that humans have long used to transform the natural world into a place more suited for our use? Or is genetic manipulation a substantially new moral gesture, unlike, for example, animal husbandry, at the nanoscale?

In reflecting on this issue, and in moving from descriptive analysis to actual policy, source texts provided the first place to look to think clearly about this question. Genetic engineering, in its replicative and recapitulative modes, draws on classic tropes and established scientific history. But which source texts matter? In whose interests are they interpreted, received, and understood? If we remember that early practitioners of such research in earlier times draw from magical anthologies then cloaked in secrecy, then the forbidden nature of certain sorts of knowledge and the transmission of knowledge is most at stake. If we find the engineering literature persuasive, then we need to focus on the conditions of use for such an experiment, its utility, and whether applications even need be expected for such speculative research—a project closer to cosmology or basic chemistry than to biology. If we conceive of the project within the context of genetic engineering biology, then questions about who should know the data, who should learn, and under what constraints are key. If we imagine this work to be a variant on the first generation of genetic modification, then the questions we would bring to the text are ones of regulation. Who should regulate these sorts of trials, which fall outside traditional categories of genetic manipulation, human or animal subjects, or dangerous materials standards? But if we accept that it is something more, then we understand the questions as deeper ones of epistemic uncertainty. We will return to this in the last chapter.

It is my contention that the tension between and curiosity about the borderline between made and begotten and between artifice and "natural" has been a fascination since antiquity. It reached a turning point in the eighteenth century, when machinery was used in elaborate magical reconstructions of living being, and when "making a copy of the machinery of biology" meant literally understanding the human person as a machine, as an assemblage of mechanical parts.[77] But as a scholar of religion, I can point to passage in the Talmud of the second century where the same concept is debated and the same anxieties raised in considering the limits of alchemy.[78] This idea has been a part of science ever since the metaphors shaped by the most current mechanical device. Hence, in the eighteenth century, the body was "bellow, pumps and pulleys;"[79] in the nineteenth, the work of the body could be replicated and efficiently mass produced; in the early twenty-first, the body is understood as a series of information codes that drive the functions of the molecular machine. This ongoing idea that machines are like people and people are like machines is replicated in several ways in the quest for self-assembling artificial life or real life artificially assembled. First, the impulse for the creation of the machine to understand the processes of the real stands across the liminal space from the deconstruction of the human to machine-like pieces toward the same end. Second, the automatons of the eighteenth and nineteenth centuries were a mix of magical toys, scientific devices, and marketable objects. Philosophers commonly argued that understanding a body of a creature as a thing made it understandable, manageable, and ultimately describable. In making a thing into a life, that process is reversed, and the goal of understanding what is always described as "the mechanism" for biological processes is key. Yet, this creates an immediate category problem. Is the thing a being or a possession? Here again, we can see that philosophers reacted as we do when confronted by the possibility of altering or replicating life.

Commenting on the new artificial automata and indeed any of the new machines of the eighteenth century, Diderot writes of the philosophical problem: "What difference is there between a sensitive and living watch (he means here a human), and a watch made of gold, iron, silver or copper?"[80] Virtanen, writing of the same problem, notes that determining what artificial life actually was remained a difficult task. Describing the problem of watching the automata, he writes: "Would you not believe they had a soul like your own, or at least the soul of an animal."[81]

Such a history raises the question of who actually "owns" the things or lives that are "made." If a thing has "even an animal soul," how do we decide its moral status? Can an unnaturally instigated phenomena which then becomes a part of the natural world, be owned, patented, and sold? How do we imagine the phenomena are controlled? What does the making of an altered life-form say about our desires and propensities? What drove the ethical debate in earlier periods, in which automata excited moral concern? Was the idea that the artifice might be better, more capable, or more real than the actualities of life? This was not only a moral panic in the case of synthetic biology, it is one stated and tantalizing goal—that science could make a "better" or more authentic yeast cell or *E. coli* bacteria, standard, replicable, and engineered for mass production. After all, one such example is artemisinin, manufactured in vats of *E. coli* and so critical to the treatment of malaria, and another is the work by Jack Szostak I described earlier.

At this point in such discussions, bioethicists turn toward concrete normative suggestions (and, surely, all such work is constrained by the obvious and always primary need for safety and containment of any de novo organism). Here, I will suggest that the main goal of ethics is rather a stance of deeply informed and thorough attention, rather than calls for moratoria or cessation of activities. Such attention will require a careful reading of history, some degree of ironic recollection of the history of automata as was briefly related here, and some degree of intellectual courage, for the project may fail (as so many of the projects ultimately did fail), become merely an interesting and clever toy (as many early efforts were), or succeed in ways we have yet to understand fully.

To be sure, there are serious issues raised just in genetic engineering that could apply to a wide range of innovations. Gene drives do not need to carry the burden of the entire field or the anxieties of three decades about recombinant DNA, but every innovation is linked to every other in the public imagination. Creating ethical guidelines will require the virtues of humility and patience. This is a quality of all reflective discourse, perhaps also borrowed from earlier centuries as surely as the science. The ethical quandaries at the borderlands of artifice and inquiry will require, most of all, an ongoing and interactive conversation between philosophers and scientists, both of whom are learning what it is that we see. I will return to these problems in my final chapter, when I consider the problem of uncertainty in emerging science. In this next section, I will consider the moral decisions that are particular to our question: gene drives.

6.7 The Ethical Issues When Genetic Engineering Is Used to Create Gene Drives

Reader, you have patiently allowed me to tell you a great many stories: about the history of malaria, about Africa and its colonial past, about one project of the several that is working on gene drives, and, in this chapter, a summary of some of outstanding issues in both malaria research and treatment and in genetic engineering. I promised that gathering all these issues together would allow you to think more clearly about the ethical issues that surround gene drives, and I have offered my analysis, showing what I consider when I think about the ethics of gene drives. In the final part of this chapter, I will turn from the deep background to the foreground of our concern about gene drives for malaria.

If you read the (many) articles titled "the ethics of gene drives," you will note something peculiar about them. Most of the articles focus on the issue of safety. This is not at all surprising. The 1973 Asilomar conference, as you may remember, was the first time that scientists had met to consider all that was at stake in the use of recombinant DNA technology. All of the concerns were about safety: Would modified *E. coli* spread out of human control? Would modified *E. coli* somehow cause cancer? Would modification of the genome to repair a gene cause a new sort of disease? Many of these issues were addressed by proposing very rigorous safety standards. Initially, all genetic recombination research was done in BSL-4 laboratories, for example. When colleagues raised issues that were largely philosophical—Will we create two classes of humans: enhanced and wild types? Will this change our relationship to the natural world?—or any of the long list of concerns raised by the NGOs detailed in the previous chapters, the conversation would turn back to the more practical, operational issues: safety and containment, consent and monitoring. Moreover, actual gene therapy remained elusive, which meant that discussions about enhancing human traits seemed increasingly like science fiction, neatly accounted for in the film *Gattaca*.

Gene drives, some of which are intended in their final stages to spread as widely as possible, create a special kind of anxiety. Even for drives that are intended to have other end points—temporal disappearance or local spread—the mechanism is intended to spread without human control, out of containment. It is because the very safeguards that allowed the ambitious use of genetic recombination and genetic engineering in biology and medicine cannot be used in the case of gene drives. Thus, the leading ethical question is whether human beings should be able to use genetic technology to intervene in the environment in a way that may or may not be reversible.

This is a different question than the attendant question about whether gene drives can be reversed, which is actually a safety question, or whether they can be designed to be self-limiting, which is also actually a safety or regulatory questions as well. Why it is important to ask the ethical question—whether it is permissible to make that gesture in science—has to be answered first, for if relying technically on such ideas is invalid, relying morally on them is equally invalid. In the first instance, sending a second drive to "reverse" a drive that has gone awry does not really fix the problem, for it means that instead of one drive in the environment, you now have two drives, and if that one goes awry, a third and then ultimately an endless series of interventions will be required in trying to play catch-up. As Burt has clearly said, relying on a second drive is a poor way to cope with unstable technology and avoids having to address the safety issue seriously. This is a convincing argument. There may be other new ways to limit or localize drives, and these too will need to be tested to see how effective they are.

But the larger ethical issue about humans' manipulation of nature is not new, as we have seen. The introduction of a GMO is actually what happens every time a new varietal is introduced. Over the last several years, a vineyard called the Grapery induced "cotton candy grapes," a variety of grapes to which I have become enamored. I am not the only one. There are entire Facebook groups and newsletters devoted to alerting fans when the short season begins. These are a new sort of grape, not bred in the laboratory but altered at the genetic level to be sure, and there is no outcry because the way it was done was conventional. But the object created—a grape that really does taste like cotton candy at a county fair—is the same as if it was done in the laboratory.

Further, the problem of fundamentally changing an environment to eliminate a disease vector is not new either. Consider the spraying of DDT in 1956 or the draining of the swamps in the early part of the twentieth century—radical, regional changes in the environment, impossible to undo fully, even if remediation were possible. To some extent a gene drive, because of gene flow, will not be containable once fully begun. In fact, it is carefully designed to spread as widely as possible for as long as possible. Most *A. gambiae* will be altered—that is the point, and it would eventually occur across Africa. But even ubiquitous *A. gambiae* only have a particular range. Other *Anopheles* species dominate Asia and South America. Yet, here too, since the target is ubiquitous, it would eventually spread to other regions.[82] Human beings have been in the business of changing their environment with whatever tools they have access to since we became human. Our relationship to nature has always been changing, sometimes more slowly, sometimes faster. My grandmother, for example, would grab my hand and tell me to look up every time a plane passed overhead, still dazzled and pleased by the improbability of it.

It is important and it is prudent to consider these problems, and as philosopher Carl Elliott has noted, it has been the great power of the field of bioethics to maintain a critical stance. There are ethical issues that arise in connection with the use of gene drives for malaria in Africa. Many of these have been part of many genetic alteration project, others have been part of many first-in-human trials, and others are the ones—human landing catches, the loss of partial immunity—that have vexed malaria treatment and research since it began. Some have to do with the specific issues in stakeholder engagement or with any interventions in Africa, even with ones devoted to codevelopment as we have seen. This book has been a discussion of these issues, and in taking the stance of the outsider and the critic, I argue that I have upheld my disciplinary responsibility for caution and for aversion to risk in my consideration of this project. I have argued in this book that each of these ethical concerns does have an adequate response and, moreover, that the ethical reality of the current situation—hundreds of thousands of the world's poorest and most vulnerable dying from malaria, one every two minutes—is unethical on the face of it. That this occurs largely in Africa, a continent that has been systematically exploited for generations by the West, whose human power and resources were in fact key to the wealth of the USA, the UK, and Europe, creates a duty of retributive justice in addition to the usual norms of justice and equity that would suggest that the poor have a claim on us based on essential human dignity and human rights. All of this would argue for the research on gene drives to continue and to be supported and for the technology, if possible, to be considered ethically justified.

6.8   The Logic of Bioethics

I have five children, all grown up now with children of their own. None of them ever had malaria or any of the other plagues of childhood—diphtheria, measles, tetanus, and whooping cough for which they got vaccinations, or yellow fever, dysentery, cholera, typhoid fever, or typhus, which ravaged the children in our nation for it first long centuries and which still ravage those in the Global South. When they had fevers, I gave them aspirin and was certain of its provenance. If the fever was too high, I went to the doctor. When one son was hit by a speeding bicyclist, an injury that likely would have resulted in his slow death in an African village, it was a fairly minor affair—an afternoon in the ER, some stitches, and antibiotics. When my children had a mosquito bite, it was a small annoyance, not a forewarning of their death. I am a Californian, and I love nature in the sense that people who love nature speak of it. I love to go hiking in the big mountains and to swim in the dark, inky, indigo of the Pacific, light flashing on the surface, taking the chaos of a wave skidding to shore. "Nature" has never come into my home to sicken and kill my children, and the sea is not despoiled like the water outside of Jamestown. I can walk to large and lovely parks, and I can visit carefully tended and curated places such as Yosemite or the John Muir Woods and think, "Oh, how lovely and free this place is." I understand completely what a privilege that is—this fortuitous accident of my birth in the state of California and of my life in the very clean city of Chicago by its very clear lake and its rule of law. I know how far all of this is from the wooden shack and its picture of pencils and books in the dusty city in Africa, and it is this sobering realization that I argue ought to frame our responses to the concept and enactment of gene drives. Should we use them to make the world? It is the question of this book, but the decision before us is neither ours nor simple.

The ethical issues surely exist beyond the matter of safety or the fascination with regulation. If the calls for a moratorium or appeals to Nature by the critics of gene drives seem so intellectually and morally unsteady, then what are the ethical issues that should be raised? What are the limits on our capacity to change the lives of others? In many articles, the authors in my field worry about the ethical issues and call for a public discussion of them. Yet, they do not define what they are. Arthur Caplan, Brendan Parent, Michael Shen, and Carolyn Plunkett, in an interesting article "No time to waste—the ethical challenges created by CRISPR" say that the technique used to create alterations in organisms will "run roughshod" over existing regulations but don't say how, or why changes in regulations in response to changing technology is an ethical problem.[83] They note the problem that gene drives are intended to eliminate or reduce a species and that this will change an ecosystem, but again, they do not tell us why that is an ethical issue and not a safety issue, or defend the idea that the existing ecosystem of West Africa is the ideal one. Further, the scholar Jeantine Lunshof makes this important point: "Some critics argue that the unpredictable effects that human germline genome editing could have on future generations make it dangerous and ethically unacceptable. Uncertainty, however, is not a useful way to judge ethical acceptability. Others highlight the potential non-therapeutic purposes of germline modification. From the standpoint of ethics, it is not clear why trait modification is by definition a bad thing. Moreover, the criteria for what is therapy and what is 'enhancement' are fluid."[84]

First, let me spend some time reflecting on the nature of contingency—why I am here and my neighbor is in Burkina Faso, for example. My position, and the position of so many of the NGO groups that claim to speak for the people or for Nature, who cannot speak for herself, is one of extraordinary human privilege. The world may be troubling, and it causes legitimate grief and deeply felt outrage, but the injustice does not make me sick, despite the claims about GMOs. The wretched poverty, and the exploitation of the resources that could change that, are not making me sick. We in the West are bystanders, and this contingent luck must humble us and our critiques. Philosophers, such as Peter Singer, use the thought experiment of a child drowning in a nearby pond and consider our absolute duty to save his life. The proper moral agent should not care that she has ruined her fancy new shoes or suit but needs to wade in, and this teaches us that because there are children dying every day in ponds all over the poorest parts of the world, we each should donate, at the very least, the cost of a fancy set of shoes and suit to save them. But really, our position is one step worse: we are not even the guys who wade in to help. We are the ones on the shore who critique the guy wading in to help. Maybe we shout, "You should not wade in because you are wearing a synthetic suit, and it could pollute the pond!" Or we shout, "Don't use that life ring because it was made with the same funds used by the Department of Defense." We are very busy, we bystanders, worrying. It may even be worse. Maybe we are not only bystanders with no stake in the rescue, but also the people who decided that digging a pond near the school, with no guide rails, was fine because we saved money, and who needs guard rails anyway? We liked the pond because it is pretty, and of course, our children all know how to swim. It could get worse if we don't even live anywhere near the pond and the drowning child, but we have read things about it and are against this sort of dangerous rescue operation and think it must be stopped because it is very disruptive of the natural world. This is closer to the problem of bystander critique.

My friend, the smart Stanford professor, when asked about controlling mosquitoes that carry malaria, is worried that that might give scientists too much control over Nature "and it would be like living in Disneyland." Of course, Stanford is already rather like Disneyland for academics, and the professor likes it very much there. But the reason that Americans can live in places that would have been a fantasy land a mere 100 years ago is largely contingent—the lucky accidents of history—and it surely does not grant the bystanders any special knowledge or capacity for judgment. In fact, the position, this orientation, might in fact distort our ordering of the competing moral appeals in the case of gene drives. Yet, many of the moral appeals need a serious response.

Let us consider some core—and competing—moral appeals about which we need to reason.

Appeal 1: Ecology

First, there is the moral appeal of keeping the natural world protected. While I certainly have my concerns about the provenance of the critiques I wrote about in the last chapter, and of course, I have written about my abhorrence at any duplicity when it occurs, I, too, believe that the physical world must be considered when gene drives are proposed. Of course, it is a sober burden that one takes up when one releases a newly "made" organism into the ecology. The deliberate spread of a gene drive means it is designed to go beyond human control, across political and economic borders and deeply embed in the species, which obviously means the food web, water, and soft, warm air of Africa. Up until now, everything in the regulation of genetic engineering was about containment, from the idea of using BSL-4 laboratories proposed at Asilomar to the strict rules about safety recommended by the RAC. Gene drives are not designed to be contained, and while they are (theoretically) limited to one species and, in principle, a genetically unique population within a species in some cases, they are intended to spread beyond human control into the wild world—that is their point.

Since the 1970s, scientists and the general public have been aware that each organism, included humans, lives within a complex ecology, where the many interactions, food webs, predator webs, and shifting climatic conditions all play an intricate role. Further, the stories of the corruption and destruction of these ecologies have been carefully told, and because terrible news is more interesting than ordinary, ordinal news, many people know about the times when human beings tried to alter the physical world, usually for perfectly morally defensible reasons, and it went terribly wrong. Consider the most famous examples—the rats versus mongooses mistake I mentioned earlier. Today, mongooses in the day and rats at night continue to gobble their way through native nestlings and turtle eggs.[85] And then there is kudzu, a vine. Kudzu was introduced from Japan into the USA at the Japanese pavilion in the 1876 Centennial Exposition in Philadelphia. In the 1930s and 1940s, the vine was rebranded as a way for farmers to stop soil erosion. Workers were paid $8 per acre to sow topsoil with the invasive vine. The cultivation ended up creating one million acres of kudzu. It is now common along roadsides and other disturbed areas throughout most of the Southeastern United States as far north as rural areas of Illinois. Worse yet, kudzu produces the chemicals isoprene and nitric oxide, which, when combined with nitrogen in the air, form ozone, an air pollutant and of course a contributor to global warming, as well as a growth inhibitor for many other crop plants. Estimates of its rate of spread differ wildly, from 150,000 acres (610 km^2) annually to "only" 2,500 acres per year according to a US Forest Service estimate in 2015.[86]

Even our forests—theoretically the wilderness itself—is not a naturally occurring place either. The Norway maple was introduced to the Northeastern United States between 1750 and 1760 as an ornamental shade tree, to line the lovely lanes of growing New England towns. About 100 years later, in 1870, settlers to Oregon and Washington brought seedlings along to shade farmhouses with these familiar shade trees. The trees spread into the forests, which were being chopped down to build houses out of redwoods. But Norway maple, valuable for shade because it grows so fast, does so by having shallow roots that spread just under the ground and crowd out native plants. Furthermore, it is likely that the very birds one hears when one is alone in the world are also immigrants. A busy and industrious American Acclimatization Society (AAS) was dedicated to making sure that European plants and animals were brought to North America, in part for economic reasons, in part because people liked familiar creatures around them, and in part because the North American plains and forests looked like they needed "civilization." The chairman of the AAS, Eugene Schieffelin, a Shakespeare enthusiast, decided that Americans needed to have every single bird mentioned by name in the Shakespearean canon flitting about, first in New York's Central Park, which then spread across the country. Similar "Shakespeare Gardens" were planted all over the country; there is one a few blocks from my home, curated to have non-native plants. The European starlings were particularly successful, going from Schieffelin's flock of 100 to millions.

In 1854, the Société zoologique d'acclimatation was founded in Paris by French naturalist, Isidore Geoffroy-Saint-Hilaire whose 1849 treatise *Acclimatation et domestication des animaux utiles* ("Acclimatization and Domestication of Useful Animals") had urged the French government to introduce, and when necessary selectively breed, foreign animals both to provide meat and to control pests. The group inspired the formation of similar groups around the world, particularly in countries that had been colonized by Europeans. Even before the American society's founding, wealthy New York residents and naturalists had deliberately sought to introduce foreign animals. In 1864 the commissioners of Central Park had introduced Java sparrows, house sparrows, chaffinches and blackbirds into the park. The European sparrows were reported to have "multiplied amazingly". They quickly became one of the most common birds in New York, though the others did not seem to do as well. After the society's founding, such efforts were redoubled. The group's annual meeting held at the Great New York Aquarium in 1877 reported that the release of 50 pairs of English skylarks into Central Park had only been a partial success, since most had flown across the East River to take up residence at Newtown and Canarsie in Brooklyn. At the meeting, the recent release of European starlings, Japanese finches and pheasants into the park were noted. The meeting adjourned with the group resolved to introduce more chaffinches, skylarks, European robins and tits, "birds which were useful to the farmer and contributed to the beauty of the groves and fields"—in the city.[87]

In every colony that Europeans founded, non-native species also were part of the enterprise—sometimes because they were thought to be good economically, as we have seen in the case of the mongoose, sometimes because they were fun to hunt. Thomas Austin, a new landowner in Australia, wrote to his nephew in England, to send rabbits to him on the years-long sea voyage, and twenty-four of them survived. Let loose on his property so that he could "devote his weekends to rabbit shooting," the rabbits quickly spread. He is quoted as saying, "The introduction of a few rabbits could do little harm and might provide a touch of home, in addition to a spot of hunting." One hundred and fifty million rabbits later, the rabbits are clearly a disaster.[88] However, in many cases, the new creatures or plants become feral but do not seriously compete with natives—they simply increase the biodiversity of the area. Some species become deeply part of the culture—peaches in the state of Georgia come from China, tomatoes in Italy come from the Americas.

All of these examples have one thing in common, however. They all took place during a particular historical period: the period of colonialization in the nineteenth century. They took place in a time that was innocent of ecological complexities, and they were done by men who either had no idea about the possible consequences or who wanted the consequences to occur—the bringing of wheat, peaches, cows, and starlings, for example. The mid-nineteenth century got a number of things terribly wrong, and the joyful introduction of European species was hardly the worse of them if you consider what else was happening in 1859—slavery at its height in the American South or, in 1890, the forcing of Native Americans into reservations, for example. We tell and retell these stories, and that is a good thing for prudent vigilance, as we know that humans have learned significant lessons in two centuries. Among the moral lessons is that the casual introduction of species into an environment without the most careful controls is staggeringly unwise. This is why African countries require environmental impact statements. This is why the research is done so slowly, in iterative steps, with safety controls. This is why the Bill and Melinda Gates Foundation is funding an elaborate project to map every living species in the food web where A. gambiae are found and to learn about their interactions. In thinking about the appeal to care for the natural world, it is important, as I will note in the next chapter, to give attention to one's own worries about its protection. The attention manifests as a type of what is called in bioethics, pas Aristotle, "prudent vigilance," first suggested by the President's Committee on Bioethics in "New Directions: The Ethics of Synthetic Biology"[89] and later reified by Kaiser and others.[90]

Appeal 2: Extinction Itself

If the first moral appeal raised the principle of non-interference in the natural world, the second appeal is more to the point: no species should be eliminated. Notice how some who oppose gene drives do so on this basis, but don't oppose other methods, which are, after all, intended to be efficacious. Bed nets are fine goes this argument because they allow the mosquito to live unmolested mosquito lives. However, consider the impact on mosquito populations if bed nets were used 100 percent of the time and were 100 percent effective. The intent of a bed net is to eradicate a species, of course, because the inherent goal is to block the mosquito from getting any blood whatsoever, which would mean she could not mature her eggs. If bed nets were 100 percent effective, they too would be eradication devices. Of course, if this were the case, there would be adaptation, and the mosquitoes that happen to prefer biting children sitting down to an early dinner would eventually become dominant, but the point is the same: any effective intervention, whether a gene drive or a blue cotton net soaked with pyrethrin, has the same goal. It is just because bed nets are so difficult to use, in other words imperfect, that they are not effective. For a moral philosopher, however, the logic of the intervention and the intended telos of the intervention are precisely the same. Further, when one considers this, note that this project is intended to eliminate the *Plasmodium* not the mosquito—as I have pointed out, this was done in the industrialized North seventy years ago and surely remains defensible today.

Appeal 3: The Slope Is Slippery

As a moral philosopher, I can argue that slippery-slope arguments are not rational. They are based on a judgment not only that human persons are unrelentingly sinful but also that they are so on a vast and oddly cooperative scale and, finally, that once we begin something, we find it impossible to stop, which is just not the case. While it is often far harder to undo that which is done, the entire premise of bioethics is that we can set limits on human action. What makes this a serious issue, however, is that the case of malaria does suggest the complexity and difficulty of containing (ironically) the use of gene drive technology to one application, malaria control. DDT, once used for malaria control alone, quickly became used ubiquitously. But then again, consider the question carefully. One can clearly imagine using a gene drive for application to disease in which a single vector is responsible, and one can consider the use for entirely other reasons—to eliminate non-native house mice from gobbling up fragile native bird populations on Pacific islands where they had mistakenly been brought in the 1800s, without ceding the entirety of the natural world to gene drive–wielding scientists. Just as in the debate about using genetic interventions for medical therapy but not for enhancement, there will be cases at the borders, but such things can be adjudicated on a case-by-case basis, as I have done with the case of malaria.

But the cases are complex. How are we to think about plans to enact gene drives beyond the use for malaria? Let me give one example about how gene drives might expand quickly, beyond their use for malaria, into a wider gesture of control over the natural world. It turned out, that this very question arose as I prepared this book for publication. I wrote this book over a period of time, from 2018 to 2022, although I was on the Target Malaria Ethics Advisory Board and thus had been thinking about these issues and watching the progress of the project since 2015. Over that period, one of the things that was most striking was the way the project diverged from other similar science projects that I had witnessed firsthand as an ethicist. Of course, the most striking aspect was the long and steady commitment to community engagement and to the African villages in which they worked. But fascinating differences from so many other projects in stem-cell research, synthetic biology, genetic engineering, and nanotechnology were the clarity about the nonprofit aspects of the work and the commitment to making the work transparent, accessible, and low cost, should it ever develop into an effective technology. However, this commitment had to face some vexing challenges.

In 2022, Imperial College London was asked to license the process for targeting the *doublesex* gene for a gene drive to another group, and this group turned out to be a for-profit company, "Biocentis," started by Andrew Hammond and Kyros Kyrou, who left Target Malaria, both of whom, you will remember, had been the young scientists who first published the *doublesex* work, joined initially by Andrea Crisanti, in whose laboratory they had trained (who later left the leadership of Biocentris). The company already mounted an enthusiastic website promising to "empower communities" and create "ground-breaking vector and pest control solutions for a heathier and more sustainable world" that would be "eco-friendly." They promised not to work on malaria, so as not to compete with Target Malaria. They also called their technology "species specific" and a "next-generation self-limiting gene drive technology" that is environmentally friendly and sustainable; reversible and controllable, and effective and affordable, yet applicable to any harmful insect. There are several references to patents: first, that the founders created the intellectual property and hold patents on the CRISPR *doublesex* construct, and second, that Imperial College London has licensed these patents to them, so far exclusively. Readers of the first chapter on the history of malaria will find it interesting that everyone listed on the website as members and leaders of the company, except for Hammond and Kyrou, are Italian, and the company has two offices in Italy, in keeping with the long tradition of Italian interest and expertise in malarial mosquitoes.

Now, in terms of the general landscape of biotechnology, a spin-off company that patents, licenses, and develops its science toward profit is not new, nor is it in itself unethical. I was a professor at Northwestern University, which benefits enormously from profits directly and from large contributions from the smart and generous scientist who developed a drug called Lyrica, which treats a wide range of neuropathic pain in addition to its anti-seizure capacity. Richard Silverman was a basic research scientist, and he too had a company that was able to bring his idea to fruition and sell it to Parke-Davis, which sold it to Pfizer. There are hundreds of such examples, it is, I was told, simply how science drives the market. Or vice versa.

And there is also no question that Hammond and Kyrou as postdocs and graduate students in the Crisanti laboratory did indeed, by 2016, work out the critical method and the critical target for a durable drive. So, why was I concerned? In part, because I had been interested in seeing if Target Malaria could indeed demonstrate how science could be done differently, and the very familiarity of the move away by two of the young and eager researchers indicated how powerful was the pull of the market. Now, to be sure, the Target Malaria team was not involved in the new company, and work on malaria continued without interruption while the Biocentis company headed off in another direction entirely. But the technology—the gene drive—is the same, and the target—*doublesex*—is the same. I have no doubt that their intentions are to alleviate human suffering, as they say, empowering people by allowing them some control over the terrible diseases and harmful crop failures and the death carried into the world by insects. They intend to use gene drives on agriculture, perhaps on vectors other than mosquitoes, and perhaps for other diseases—surely not trivial uses, which indeed would be important and potentially nature altering. But there is no doubt that this is a move toward a far wider application of the concept, and if it is not a slip, it is at least a horizontal step down that slippery slope about which we worry. The ethical analysis of their work, their targets, and their intentions are another matters entirely and are for a different book than this one.

These three appeals are ones that I believe so raise serious questions and doubts about our capacity to regulate gene drives and they will require some serious work by scientists, regulators, and ethicists to think through. On the other hand, however, there are moral appeals that support, and in fact demand, affirmatively, that gene drives be pursued with the utmost rigor, and that stopping this research and implementation would be a moral wrong.

Appeal 4: Civil Society and Economic Life Are Diminished

Malaria is a dreadful disease, both deadly and insidious, constantly eroding childhood and threatening pregnancy. Its course disrupts the civil life held in common and makes serious economic investments far less likely. In addition to the terrible toll of a child dying, sickened children have a hard time reading or concentrating, and sickened adults have a hard time participating in public life and the rates of death have quietly risen over the last three years. Malaria can be eliminated, but only with a determined, fully modern plan, and while vaccines for children are a good start, however imperfect, they will not eliminate malaria by themselves. Meanwhile, as the climate changes, more of the world will be disrupted by disease, and more mosquitoes carrying malaria *Plasmodia* will smarm. Pathogens and people are closer together; temperatures and rainfall, floods, and standing water are all increasing. All of this makes malaria more common—all of this makes the appeal to use every possible tool to combat it stronger. A study in *Nature*, in the summer that I wrote this book, noted that climate change has already aggravated 218 (or 58 percent) of the 375 infectious diseases listed in the Global Infectious Diseases and Epidemiological Network (GIDEON).[91] Because turning away from a carbon-based economy is so very hard for moderns, it will be hard to use moral suasion alone to address the issue and human behavior changes to avoid climate catastrophe. On many issues—surely on the issue of infectious disease—human societies will indeed need a technological response.

Appeal 5: Justice Requires It

In the decades since the introduction of recombinant DNA technologies early in 1970, proposals for the medical exploration of the power of these methods have raised significant concerns and significant optimism, and bioethicists have come to understand making alterations in our DNA code as existential and ontological issues. Experts from many disciplines have debated whether the envisioned scientific advances can perform as expected without spiraling out of control, threatening civil and personal liberties, or whether the balance of benefits and the promises to relieve intractable suffering outweigh potential risks. From the beginning, these discussions have been open to the lay participants, as individuals, as professionals from the media or governments, or as members of NGOs. The debate has, as we have seen, entered the public imagination, standing in for a set of signifying practices. From these discussions has emerged a substantial body of work addressing the ethics of particular genetic technologies, some of which have been successfully introduced and are now simply a part of medical responses such as cancer immunotherapies, and some of which have never been fully realized such as stem-cell tissue replacement. Since the first discussions, the debates have often focused on safety, with an emphasis on potential risks and possible benefits to individuals and their health. However, when we consider, the use of genetic interventions that would affect whole populations or ecologies, we can see how limited a discussion about safety or risk can seem. The questions of what it means to live in a world that is constructed, even more than we know it is presently, and how we can make the world just raise issues far beyond what is achievable and what can be done safely.

The emerging policies that primarily address safety, personal, physical, and environmental risks also need to create a framework for resolving the potential social or moral disputes raised by the success, should it occur, of these new technologies, especially within a multicultural society and against a backdrop of existing inequality in both benefits and burdens of current technologies and economic structures.

Bioethicists have long understood it is possible, should significant scientific constraints be overcome, that new genetic engineering techniques have the potential to create or deepen inequities among people of different races, ethnicities, classes, and physical capacities, especially if the benefits are commercialized as costly luxuries. Genetic interventions that are designed to be permanent would solidify inequity. Concern about these inequities can lead to opposition toward even permitting these technologies to be researched. This distrust is heightened when suggestions that personal genetic benefits are "marketable products" as opposed to health-care services, widely understood as an entitlement benefit. And this anxiety has led to a sense that genetic technologies per se may be unjust.

One of the strongest aspects of gene drive technology in the case of malaria is the radically different approach to distributive justice. By definition, a gene drive offers benefits to everyone in the population, without regard to race, class, or social economic status. Unlike individualized responses to malaria—vaccines, bed nets, or pharmaceuticals, all of which are important, but all of which must be delivered one by one—a solution based on the genetic alteration of the vector makes the intervention fairly accessible to everyone in the region. Of course, should the intervention be proven effective, there will still be issue of justice, for the questions of which regions should benefit first and how to select among regions will need to be addressed as well, at least initially.

Previous ethical assessments have not been able to achieve consensus on theories of justice and have typically been resolved at a lower level of consensus, by applying mid-level ethical principles (e.g., "women and children first") and a general sense of utilitarian necessity. As we have seen, in the earlier chapters, many of the regulatory efforts in gene drive technology by bioethicists have focused on issues of questions of safety or the standard rules for clinical research ethics, while many of the concerns in the NGOs are about the issue of how genetic technology may change our views about illness, mortality, humanity, or nature, however defined. Clearly, much of the attention about the importance of stakeholder engagement is the result of the continuing concerns about justice and the distribution of the social goods of health care. The issue elucidates a core tension relating to distributive justice: How do we foster equitable access to promising new technologies while also accommodating divergent (sometimes not widely shared) viewpoints about what is fair and unfair. In the case of gene drives for malaria, we know that it is largely a disease of the rural poor, children, and pregnant women, whose vulnerability and historical marginalization make a moral claim on us. People who have been the subject of past injustice, in many systems of ethics, are holders of a debt from us, for historically, we in the West have been the beneficiaries of the wealth extracted from their countries, and, in the case of gene drive research, it is currently they who, while standing to gain the most from the elimination of malaria, will of course also be the people on whom the first use of the technology is tested.

However, which theory of justice can operate in this arena? Traditional theories of justice grow out of the organizational principles of classic liberal theory. They largely operate beneath our recognition but yield to rational explanations. Most familiar to Americans is the theory of utilitarianism, mentioned above. In this theory, the goal is to live in a stable, rational society, and these ends justify the means that may involve the taking of individual rights. Utilitarians believe a just system is one that allows the majority to be able to live a flourishing life, free to do what they chose, as long as it does not impinge on the freedoms of others or of the collective. We are familiar with this idea: it allows democratic voting, it allows the taking of private rights of way for public needs, and it undergirds public health policies. However, biotechnologies such as gene drives offer the promise of changing a population's social order, opening up the opportunity for many more capabilities independently of any political or social actions. It is these actions that we generally associate with states and state action, but biotechnologies can increase a person's absolute well-being, as well as suggest the possibility of increasing well-being across society. Other theories of justice, libertarianism for example focus on the maximization of liberty and rely on the market economy to rationalize out workings of justice. We have seen that Target Malaria, as a nonprofit academic consortium, has turned from a marketplace model, but others in the field may well seek to monetize gene drives and would argue that the market is the best way to ensure a fair distribution of goods. Still other theories, as in John Rawl's work, depend on the idea of a social contract, in which a central discourse agreed to by all in advance sets the terms for distribution based on an equality of opportunity.

Gene drives seem to work well, given the assumptions of two other theories of justice: first that of egalitarianism, which divides social good equally to achieve an equality of outcome, and second, the theories of liberation theology, from the Catholic tradition theories which presents a case for a preferential option for the poor, especially for the children of the poor, and argues that both their present suffering and their future diminishment, which compels us to attend to their plight. It is a theological argument, and as a scholar of religion, I am convinced by such arguments and it is also a good point, and one that is a part of Jewish and Islamic texts as well, to remember that the children of the poor are in important ways our future too, for whom we are responsible. But from whatever source or text or tradition, the moral appeal converges in all cases, on the centrality of the appeal for justice asone of the key arguments for the continuation of gene drive research. If we fail to prevent malaria, it will be the poor who are disproportionally burdened, not the wealthy.

Appeal 6: People Who Are Most Directly Affected Should Make the Decisions about Their Lives

Linked to the argument for justice that supports the project is the understanding that even if a gene drive might threaten or worry citizens in the West, if it was a good and ethical moral action in the places most affected by malaria, and if these citizens wanted to proceed, it would be just to do so. This would be so if the harm was ontological—as it is for people who worry that our ideas about "nature" will be distorted by our mastery—or if the harm was in some degree a risk to our physical environment. We can consider our long history with malaria as the proof text for this argument.

When we consider "making" the world, the action of science on the natural world, it is these appeals we will consider. We already "make" the world. We have made it safe for my children and for much of the West, although with climate change, that may no longer be the case. We cannot now abandon the task of making, just when "we" have ordered the forests and wetlands around us to our satisfaction so that they are safe and no longer a deadly threat. You, reader, and I live in a time when it may be possible to actually end a disease, malaria, that has haunted humankind for as long as it is possible to know. It is also true that gene drives may not work, and their failure will be yet another in a long line of failures, as humans confront malaria—the contingency of the effort and the contingency of modernity will both present significant challenges.

These appeals compete. There are three strong arguments against gene drives and three strong ones in its favor. Each is important to consider and evaluate as I have done in this summary. But we are not yet finished thinking! I believe that there is one overriding ethical concern—a fundamental problem of uncertainty that underlies not only this project but also all emerging science. In the final chapter, I will turn to the problem of deep uncertainty in our extraordinarily uncertain time.

Conclusion: Making the Moral World

The World of Uncertainty: A Case Study

Consider J. B. S. Haldane—with his pipe between his teeth, there is a ghost of a smile. He is a modern man, sure of his position, his Oxford firsts in classics and mathematical modeling, and yes, his lectureship in biochemistry at Cambridge. He is the smartest man in a generation, a polymath. He fought in the Great War, emerged as a captain ("the best and dirtiest soldier I have ever known," according to his superiors). Unlike many of his generation, he is an optimist. Haldane knows the danger of guessing at the future ("One can be quite sure that the future will make any detailed prediction look silly"[1]) but is confident that scientists are just better at it ("an actual research worker can perhaps see a little further than the most intelligent onlooker"[2]). He is smart about malaria, and he figures out that sickle cell and thalassemia are genetic mutations caused by pressure from the malaria parasite long before he can prove it. But he cannot know and cannot understand how modern molecular genetics works, for in 1927, all his certainty is speculation—clever and informed, but a fantasy. In his essay, "The Future of Biology," he imagines a world that in many respects anticipates ours. But it does not. He does not know that the twentieth century is rushing toward him in all its chaotic deadliness. He does not see that a second war will be far more catastrophic than the first, or that science will be perverted, his beloved field of genetic research the very locus of the genocidal rationale for the Final Solution. He is the quickest mind of an entire cohort of scientists, which is, he writes, "at present . . . in a stage of measuring and waiting for the idea . . . one man is measuring the length of feelers of 2,000 beetles . . ." and yet he believes that "tomorrow it looks as if we should be overhearing the conversations of bees."[3]

Haldane's great faith in 1927 was in the then-new research in genetics. He anticipated that humans would create embryos, clone them, and alter them, and he thought this would go well. Haldane is so very sure of himself and, in so many cases, wrong. His vision, we can see in hindsight, is framed by his political stance, his social location, and his faith in science itself. Measuring will lead to knowing and knowing to technologies of manipulation and repair. Humans were perfectible, the languages of insects knowable.

In a recent book about the history of science, *The Knowledge Machine: How Irrationality Created Modern Science*,[4] Michael Strevens, a philosopher of science, describes what Haldane considers a central dogma so unshakeable that he can act as its prophet. Strevens describes modern science as beginning after the separation of church and state, and after the "grand gestures," "deep games," and "expansive systems" of earlier systems of natural philosophy, which were abandoned in favor of observational data. The use of experiments to test hypothesis, and the collection of data and the agreement about how to collect such data would prove enough about a system to validate a theory about how something worked and how equations could be produced that predicted this observation, and the question of why it existed would be set aside. Strevens calls this the "Iron Rule" of science.[5] This practice both limited and freed scientists, for the "measurers and the waiting" became critical to the enterprise. However, it is also not the case that a collection of data will necessarily add up to certain knowledge of the thing itself, as we see from Haldane's cheerful claims about immortality or his view that the future might include humans grown in vats.[6]

The Iron Rule prioritizes the collection of data and, inductively, moves from data to rule. Nothing is certain, posits Strevens, unless it is description, enormous data sets, and careful and meticulous description of experiments that can be agreed upon as validating. He argues that the Iron Rule means that the scope of modern science would narrow the gaze to what could be absolutely seen, over and over again from earlier projects of natural philosophy, in which grand theories of everything were proposed. Certainty was waiting. Certainty was replicability. The Iron Rule, however, is destabilized by a closer gaze. We know that data are "cleaned up," that choices are made in what is made notable, that publication limitations themselves shape reportage, that only certain observations are, a priori, established as important, and that phenomenon are complex, occurring in nearly but not perfectly observable patterns. And we are aware that it may well be our capacity for pattern making that is behind even our most objective results. To be a scientific researcher after modernity's many challenges—Freud, Marx, Beauvoir, and DuBois—is to be aware of how little we know not only about the observed phenomena but also about the observer. This deep uncertainty, even about data, creates a world far less iron clad than is supposed. The problem of uncertainty in clinical research is even greater for, of course, human research must be research on, well, fragile, changeable humans with character, agency, and will, but it is a feature of all research, even that where the new precision of CRISPR-Cas9, TALENS, and CAR-T cells holds such power. We are aware at all times, if we are honest readers of science, of the vast chasm of the unknown, and not just peripheral things but things that are central to understanding basic processes and etiologies, the unknown world so much vaster than the known world.[7]

Introduction to the Problem: Uncertainty as Pathlessness

We live in an extraordinarily uncertain time, in a world where, despite increasing evidence of cumulative mastery—cell phones, the internet, microwaves, monoclonal antibodies, and the marvel of CRISPR-enabled gene drives—there is, revealed more sharply since the coming of the pandemic of COVID-19 and the tumultuous events of 2020, an increasing sense of stochastic disorder, a generalized sense of bewilderment in the larger public community, a loss of certainty in norms and truth claims made by experts, and a questioning of scientific testimony.[8] In the USA, of course, the election and the attempt at insurrection were in addition to wildfires, darkened skies, floods, and hurricanes all at record levels, as well as the pandemic. Worldwide, the collapse of economies and the coming of Brexit potentiated the sense of disorder. Running in parallel in academic circles, there is a realization that for all of the refinement in our understanding about how the world works, all the fine-grained control, and the elegance of molecular biology and genomics, and all our theories of human behavior, and all our philosophic arguments, there was far more that is unknown than is known, about COVID-19, or other infectious diseases, and how to control them, or the economy, or politics, and our ordering and our control is very likely to go awry at any time. For scholars of medical research, this can be said to be expected, for science famously is what can be falsified and thus disproven,[9] which means that much of what is believed to be true will be proven incorrect, and this quality of research means that our knowledge base is constantly mutable. By design, premises derived from evidence change as evidence changes, however disconcerting this may be in practice. This is not a new insight. Yet, however rigorous our method, however committed one is to its variables, a life of science still appears to be one of predictability, orderliness, and surety, and it is this very stability that is now at stake. It is difficult enough to find quotidian epistemic ground in ordinary, secure eras, but in the time of pandemics and deep social divisions about values, the work of scientific research—testimony, published text, the workings of the observable biological world, and truth claims—has taken on the quality of an ontological problem. As our control grows, as the theories of genetics unfold into practice, the practices themselves are challenged. Even more, when this takes place within the landscape of social cohesion, it is difficult, but when the landscape is also riven with serious disputes about values and worth, power and purpose, questions of race, gender, and class, the challenges intensify. Even the remarkable achievements—mRNA vaccines made in ten months—take place in a deeply uncertain world.

We all live in an aporetic condition, a landscape without a clear path forward, a complex puzzle, in which we do not agree on the events and lessons of the past, the interpretation of our present moment, or the reliability of the future, all of which were the historical, foundational ground on which our regnant of certainty rested.[10] Yet, the aporesis of science persists. We cannot know the next event, all that is other and yet to be discovered, measured, and theorized. It is this very opening up of oneself to the occurrence of chance that allows, *pas* the French philosopher Jacques Derrida, "an entrance into the future . . . that is the opening into experience."[11] It is, of course, this very quality that undergirds science, the uncharted and unmapped terrain of the real, the researcher, cutting out a slow and iterative trail.

This condition is particularly vivid when considering the field of genetics, the subject of this book, newly endowed with the Nobel Prize–winning technology of CRISPR-Cas9. Genetics dominated the twentieth century narrative of linear certainty, and in the twenty-first century, long after scientists had a more complex idea of genetics and genomics, the public maintained the narrative frame that genetic codes are determinative of our species being, our ipseity. The idea that DNA is utterly determinative is so very common that it has crept into the speech of politics and marketing—"it's in our DNA" is used to describe all manner of characteristics thought to be immutable. Yet, it is there, in our manipulation of the DNA, where our knowledge really is still so primitive, where the linear path is actually not linear at all.

In this final chapter, I will begin by exploring this aporetic concept of uncertainty, which always exists, in addition to the larger framing of social instability that marks our time. I will, reader, return to the specific question of the larger discussion, whether we can "make the world," and whether the world that uses a gene drive spread with the intention of blocking malaria is the sort of world we want. Throughout this book, I have reflected in ways both specific and more general because this is not a book that promises norms or regulations. It is my contention that a broad and open conversation about both the philosophy and the science of gene drives allows us to consider more fully both the limits of our capacity to make the world and the unlimited duty to do so.

Let us begin, as philosophers begin, with definitional taxonomy. Let me argue that there are three sorts of uncertainty that raise ethical issues in scientific research. First, there is the familiar genre of epistemic uncertainty, which is often actually the problem of incomplete knowledge, rectifiable if more research is done or if more perspectives are heard. Here, we can resolve uncertainty: the problem is knowable and logical and can be rationally ordered. This is the uncertainty that is the subject of much of the philosophy of science. It is in part resolved by recourse to Strevens's Iron Rule of evidence, in which plausible theories can be certified by agreed-upon standards of experimentation and rules of observation. Second, there is what we could call technical uncertainty. Here are classic ethical dilemmas: a problem is raised, and there are differing sets of moral appeals that compete for our sense of the rightness of a solution, with no clear agreement on which act is for "the good" or even how to agree on the nature of "goodness" or "rightness." The uncertainty can be methodological or teleological. For example, what ought we to do when there are profound differences in how we regard the moral status of embryos, each argument rooted in foundational and ancient texts? What should we do if our research in genetics suggests that human beings are really very different in small ways that matter greatly, if this will utterly disrupt our systems of justice? We are uncertain about what to do, even knowing all the data, because we do not know how to order them properly or because different actors value outcomes differently or justify them with competing moral appeals. This technical ethical uncertainty can be profound, and bioethics has spent a great deal of time thinking about how to resolve ethical conflict or to assure that there are rules about the minimal agreements (e.g., treating human and animal subjects well, soliciting informed consent for research, crediting authorship correctly) about the values that we do share. Yet, beneath these problems (and the fact that they yield to programmatic, pragmatic, and even political responses gives us a clue that they are not irresolvable) is the deeper problem, the ontological vertigo of an as yet unknown reality, the great, vast darkness of all that is beyond our measure. This is an uncertainty that does not yield to the logic of mandated class on ethics, the comfort of moral calculus, the weighing of risk and benefit, or the precautions of a principle.

How can epigenetics really be understood? What can be done when we know that much of what we perceive as really "real" is a mental deception, given by the structure of our neurons? What can be said about the fact that it may be impossible to ever really measure many phenomena? How can I know if one gesture that I make—say, the placement of a genetic sequence in a particular stretch of DNA in an organism—is the first small step to an inevitably unfolding process of enormous destruction?[12] Why and how, really, did carbon-based life begin on Earth? Why does targeted DNA insert itself in different and unexpected sections of the genome than expected? What is the function of the large sections of DNA that we used to call "junk DNA" (a puzzle that is finally beginning to yield to investigation but was long thought to be unimportant)? Or of dark matter? Of course, a sane and stable investigator does not normally think about such things, well beyond the scope of a particular project, but indeed, these uncertainties surround each ordinal gesture.

However, despite this fraught landscape, moral philosophers, such as myself, teach scientists that decisions can be made and must be made about proper courses of action. This is because we are what philosophers call "plighted."[13] Our plight is this: Human beings are creatures who cannot *not* act—our very inaction or inability to make a choice is, in itself, a moral gesture. Thus, when confronted by a dilemma, defined as a situation in which two courses of action, each with strong but competing moral appeals, are presented, in which both choices have an array of burdens and benefits and various actors who will be affected by our choice, we make a decision, and we proceed on one path or another. This is true, even when we choose not to go forward with a project—we cannot stop, in the sense of returning to a time prior to the discovery, for we are "plighted," and thus we move forward in a world without the scientific concept, proof, or technology, but we move forward into a place in history all the same. Moreover, we create for ourselves a sense that there is one path forward, when in actuality, we confront only an aporetic opening.

Yet Science Proceeds

Philosophers are intrigued with this problem, with the phenomenology of a self, encountering the world as other, with the way that each decision endless opens and simultaneously closes the next set of decisions and reveals and yet conceals different available futures. And while this is interesting, bioethicists and scientists are faced with a practical choice. When confronted with a dilemma in which competing appeals arise to make the case for continuing research, modifying the research to address ethical concerns or, in some case, advocating for stopping it entirely, bioethicists teach how to make an ethical decision and how to use a standard methodology that is used in bioethics. First, we clarify the dilemma, understand all viewpoints, master and agree on the scientific or medical facts, review the history of similar choices, consider the options, identify core values that allow you to rank or weigh them, assess, chose, justify, and proceed. When my bioethicist colleagues Leroy Walters, Jonathan Moreno, Baruch Brody, and I considered this problem as a part of our work in the Howard Hughes Bioethics Advisory Board from 2001 to 2007, our research uncovered a great deal of fragility in ethical decisions in scientific research, in both the clinical and the basic research setting. We came to understand that the actual process of research is framed with uncertainty: What else is unknown to us? What facts are chosen to be credited? Why is it a dilemma *now*? What about possible data error? Is the past always predictive? Can we really accurately weigh risks? What if our values differ? What about competing truth claims? What about competing risk assessments? And while some of these questions were part of standard theories in research ethics, the problem of deep uncertainty was far less understood.

In the case of real-world dilemmas, we also have other complex puzzles with which to contend. Now that we can begin to see more clearly the systematic issues of race and gender, even knowing that we carry biased concepts is not enough: we need to ask how these have shaped our perceptions of both the initial issues and our truth claims. After the scandals in basic stem-cell research—the false claims in the elite Korean laboratory of Professor Hwang Woo Suk that human cloning of stem cells was accomplished in 2006 and the false claims about reprograming of stem cells that were also made in the case of Haruko Obokato, a researcher at Riken Center in Japan in 2014—we are aware of the possibility of deceit, recklessness, and opportunism as human phenomena, and science is no freer of these mendacities than any other human endeavor. In fact, because the stakes are so very high, elite researchers may face even more temptation. In some settings, powerful training hierarchies or fear of professional disgrace or retribution silences junior colleagues, further distorting truthful discourse.

Underlying all research are the essential premises of the scientific tradition. What are these? They can include: that which is now unknown is discoverable; that the known is built on the as yet unknown; that equipoise is needed for a true scientific inquiry; that, in principle, there is always a confirmable hypothesis; that the nature of error is such that it is inevitable but that it can be fortuitous; and finally, that while failure may define all early stages of research, even this failure will be turned to some larger, successful task. These premises, often unarticulated, are widely understood as foundational.

Ethics, too, assumes essential, foundational premises. The first of these is that the future can be known and that one can *rationally* calculate and evaluate moral activity on the basis of a probable world to which one can speak and evaluate. Consequentialist theory is based on this central dogma—for beneficence and nonmaleficence to work as principles requires us to prognosticate, to imagine our choices as if they would come to exist, and then to consider these imaginary effects. Ethical theories rest on the idea that one can shape one's very self by activities that can be known and chosen with reason and a priori judgment. After all, it is reason that is the foundation of philosophical thought, and even if we now understand and can acknowledge the limits of rationality and the way that bias creeps into consciousness, we still believe and act as if the past can generally be counted on as predictive. So, in case A, we think that we know that A → B, and then we weigh good social consequences against harms and burdens or virtuous actions as if they are cumulative. One takes "account" of risk but rarely of our deep inability to actually know the future. After all, our essential premise is unchallenged—that we are capable of "weighing" the future, "balancing" the outcomes, and imagining that we control it, and of course, that is the basis of all risk assessment and our rather touching faith in its protective power but we cannot fully know and thus cannot really set up a plumb line that leads to a certain future.

Some of this has been understood in research ethics in general, however uneasily. There are, we acknowledge, fundamental problems in the central theoretical assumptions behind rational ethical methods. We know that much of the moral calculus is based on a mutable knowledge base. Much of the prognostication is based on partial knowledge because, of course, knowledge is always incomplete and always partial. Most troubling of all, we know that much of what is most important, morally, about the future is unknowable and uncontrollable.

Ethical assessments, moreover, rested on what scientists told moral philosophers about their work. Often, we carefully read final research papers or attended presentations but did not have access to what was left out, innocently, in the first discussions about what is or is not important to consider (something Strevens calls "sterilizing" the work). Often, ethicists, too, think about genetics, for example, as it is portrayed in the popular press—as a sort of cartoon where everything works perfectly—and we accept that simplicity ("CRISPR works like a kind of scissors!"), so we can discuss things like "intent" or "implications," without seeing the instability or uncertainty in the project itself. Now, as Strevens points out, the problems raised by epistemic uncertainty really can be addressed by careful if limited agreements on the sort of experiments that could yield enough data to achieve consensus.[14] But as ethicists, we only know what we are told; we only can start at what we are told is the beginning.[15]

But we do, as ethicists, decide that some experiments are ethical and may proceed as such. In clinical research, the usual way to solve such problems of technical uncertainty is by strengthening rules about informed consent (letting the human subjects in research trials, for example, assess the risk themselves and decide whether to participate in situations of uncertainty where the risk is difficult to assess objectively). The idea is that in most cases, if a human subject agrees to an intervention, it is permissible to proceed. Of course, there will be outlier exceptions, but in general, we think consent is determinative. If one of the first premises in bioethics is that the future can be known and rationally shaped, the process of consent is the second essential premise: that human beings are rational actors, in possession of all the necessary facts to make a decision for themselves as autonomous moral agents, deriving from the principle of autonomy. This principle, too, has problems, which have been widely discussed in the literature of bioethics.[16] Individuals do not adequately calculate risk, thinking that the odds are in their favor when they are not or that the risk is large when it is not. Faced with no viable options, dying patients may have no other choice of action except participation in a trial. In genetic research, as it was presented to me as an ethicist member of the NIH RAC, parents were desperate to find a way to treat their children, and doctors were excited about their findings and wanted to proceed with trials to prove their theory—everything aligned to make consent inevitable. But we found that there were limits to consent, no matter how well a subject is informed. What can we know, and what do we tell? What sort of information is useful and to whom? How well known do the consequences have to be in order to be ethical? How small must the risk be for the experiment to be ethical?

Uncertainties in the process include a socially evolving sense of what is "consent," what is "freedom," and what is "coercive." We came to understand that we could not know what innocent gesture or process in the research might turn out to be a critical ethical mistake when considered across temporal distance (i.e., the concern for special vulnerability was not in the literature prior to the twentieth century—research done on prisoners is a classic example).

We know, even as we teach the doctrine of informed consent, the bioethicist's version of the Iron Rule: that our knowledge could be incomplete in multiple ways. First, we always have incomplete knowledge about the level of risk individuals and communities actually face, and it varied, we found, in different social locations, because risk acceptability is experienced interiorly, to particular communities. In ethical decisions, moreover, there will always be several possible outcomes, and while the probability and value of their occurring can be estimated with a reasonable degree of reliability, and rational individuals could maximize (or satisfy) expected utility, we came to understand that not only subjects but also researchers, and even oversight committees, act rationally at times and, at others, with only partial rationality and much emotionality and yearning.

Second, we came to see that in the cases where there was a need to make decisions under uncertainty, and where there are several possible outcomes, the probability and value of their occurring cannot always be estimated with a reasonable degree of reliability. Rational individuals may adopt different strategies for dealing with this type of uncertainty, unless one strategy dominated because of special factors, sometimes monetary, sometimes the pressures of research competition, sometimes the need to solve a problem and end suffering one felt deeply or urgently. Of course, informed consent norms are not the only recourse to solve this level of uncertainty, but as more research emerged by Richard Thaler and others about irrationality and decision making, this norm seemed even more questionable.[17]

Moreover, we began to understand the profundity of the issue of uncertainty, especially in genetic research, which is always a set of promises about the long-term future, unlike other medical interventions, beyond the lifetime of a particular individual patient. Because the logic of genomic research is linguistically linked to the logic of computer coding, the central dogma seemed to privilege certainty, and while this is no longer the case for scientists, it is still the way the lay public understands genetic intervention. The progression from DNA, RNA, and protein to trait or behavior seems to follow with inevitable logic, and we were initia urged to think of genetic manipulation as a sort of a spell-check. When the genome was "fixed," it would unspool the capacity as promised, as predicted, as the instructions foretold. If molecular genetics is the deconstruction of the real into the smallest possible parts, we expected that putting the parts together would properly allow reconstruction. But it proved far more difficult, far slower, and far more imprecise.[18] Here is where we reach the limits of what the norms provide when making ethical decisions under conditions of deep uncertainty.

We can see how this understanding works in the case of gene drives, where the consent, assent, and approval process of stakeholder engagement is so central. In thinking about the problem of uncertainty in gene drives, where the discordancy between our mechanisms of control and our capacities for stable judgment are most observable when they present as a "limit case" because of the use of de novo genetic interventions, unloosed in the environment, designed to change a species across a wide region, against a disease that potentiates the deep suffering of the world's poorest populations. All these factors came into play as we have seen, all at once.

A Case Study of Uncertainty

We have considered here the case of gene drives for malaria.[19] I tell this story as a case study of uncertainty, for in all stark honesty, we cannot yet know its conclusion—not of the science, or the technology to deploy it, nor of the norms and structures to judge it, nor of the experiments in ethics review, co-development, or stakeholder engagement.[20] Obviously, the elimination of a dreadful disease would be a magnificent human achievement, but it does not take much imagination to pause before the risks of action in the face of the extraordinary uncertainty that surrounds this project. Against the enormity of benefit that eliminating deaths from malaria would bring should this be successful, we considered questions that can be raised about possible harms. Is this enough?

We do not know what the limits of our power should be, or how far we should go in the pursuit of elimination of a species if the species carries a deadly organism. All the way? Part of the way? We do not fully agree on who can make that determination. Westerners tend to think of the dangerousness of proceeding with a new technology, wary of a history of error, but if you live in a malarial region and have lost child after child to wrenching fevers, you might think that blocking new technology is by far the more unethical course of action. If we agreed on the analysis of the past, we might be persuaded that since mosquito populations were suppressed before—in the sixteenth century when the marshlands of the Fens were drained in East Anglia; in the nineteenth century when the crop systems of North America and France were changed, and again in the twentieth century when first Paris Green and then DDT poisoned the habitats of *Anopheles*, and the habitats and the mosquitoes rebounded without their parasites—such an intervention would be acceptable again. But we do not fully agree on the past or how to interpret or evaluate it. If we agreed on the telos, we might argue that a high risk is acceptable, but we do not fully agree on the future either or the worth of various ends. If researchers were more secure in their understanding of the genome and their technical prowess, that would be defensible as a place to begin, but honest researchers are aware of the limits of their capacity.[21] And while epistemic methods and rules of engagement and consent can be established to address many of the ethical challenges of the project, it is without question that the deep uncertainty, the unknowability within the scientific gesture, remains.

Should research be stopped because this deep uncertainty is fully revealed? Should it be halted while, meanwhile, actual specific vulnerable children die who might well be saved by fully funding the research and allowing it to proceed in the face of uncertainty? Are the ethical guardrails of our standard practices of research ethics enough, even if they do not really address the fundamental uncertainty? We will return to this central ethical problem.

Can Ethical Research Be Done under Conditions of Uncertainty?

Researchers turn to ethicists because decisions about the validity and worth of their work must be made. Yet, the argument of this book describes the nearly impossible problems associated with making decisions under uncertainty, and once the reality and scope of the aporesis is understood, one surely is drawn to ask: It is ethical to proceed with research at all, especially projects in genetic research such as gene drives, which, if used, would affect not only a handful of children with a dreadful illness but also whole populations, regional species, and local ecologies? Indeed, some, including many in the European Parliament and many scholars in Europe, have codified the answer to this: no. And this is because, in foundational EU documents, what is called the "precautionary principle" is a statutory part of regulations.

I discussed the history and use of this principle extensively in chapter 3 of this book, so I will not rehearse these arguments here because[22] while the precautionary principle has been both attacked and defended, that is not my primary focus. I raise it to explain why it has proven to be inadequate by sketching some objections here. Does it help us move ahead in conditions of uncertainty? I would argue that it does not, in large part because it avoids the profundity of the problem, for what we actually need to assess as we consider genetic research is not only one proposed intervention, it is our condition itself. We will move ahead into the temporal future, for there is no escaping chronicity, and there is no escaping our "plightedness." Our present, even standing still, is as racked with uncertain outcomes as the future suggested by any intervention. Any new "technology, process, or product" might threaten us, but it also might stop it. Further, choosing the particular moment in time in which we reside means choosing what we now know and have, and validates it as inviolable: not only the environment, but also the burdens it bears, the power relationships, the implicit bias, and the pleasures of privilege that shape our assessments as well as other measures. Nonaction is not safer, it simply makes the moral claim that our present situation is fine, safe enough, whereas it is actually morally unacceptable.

Return with me to the problem of gene drives and the uncertainty about the future they might bring, and one can see that concern about possible outcomes avoids attention to the desperate injustice of the present, the unfair lethality of the burden of disease on the poorest humans, not to mention the species-killing technologies now used, the insecticides, and destruction of wetlands. We are "plighted" in this a second way as well, in that we live in a world that is full of human suffering, brokenness, and hunger, not just a place of serene order whose beauty and grace is threatened by technology. Decisions are linked to other decisions, happening and unfolding all at once, horizontally, simultaneously, and not only in a lineal fashion. Maintaining the status quo is not actually "better safe" because there is not really a safe to stand on, at least not for far too many. And with only safety and certainty to guide us on the one true road, "too little in this world would change. We would live in a world closed down to the novelty of an event—a rupture always necessarily outside the limits of knowledge and current logic."[23]

The Risks of Knowledge

There are serious risks, however, to the approach I have described thus far, of seeing an aporetic uncertainty and knowing that reality is held together by the illusion of order, with constant doubt and with constant awareness of the void that surrounds any act, as any scientist getting this far in this book can forcefully explain. I too know that risk. Following the line of this argument might lead one to assume that knowledge was simply a matter of standpoint epistemology,[24] which might be well enough for academics in the humanities disciplines, where the stakes are the judgment of literature, or the worth of an argument about hypotheticals, not so very high, surely not life and death, but are utterly inadequate when it comes to scientific research. The idea that uncertainty should be understood as fundamental, the feature not a bug, can be understood by scientists to be a sort of nihilism, promoted by philosophers unwilling to turn from speculation to the serious tasks of science. There is a *real*, my colleagues in science remind me, there is a real world. This is correct.

It is important to understand that my claim about deep aporetic doubt is not merely deconstruction but rather a call to the most liberatory aspects of scientific knowledge. Understanding that the future is open does not mean that truth is entirely undermined. Clarifying the reality that objectivity is difficult to achieve, that the Heisenberg effect is profound, or that attending to the complexities of epistemic doubt does not mean that nothing can ever be known, measured, or observed, for that would be taking the concept of aporesis into absurdity. But suggesting that science lives and acts in a time of great uncertainty and yet must proceed creates important and sobering moral choices. In fact, noting it and making this legible allows the scientist to remain open to possibility, discovery, and failure, a core feature of the enterprise of experiment. As the philosopher Michael Anker notes, understanding that you are faced with uncertainty is not an excuse to defer or to hesitate prior to action. It means that each decision is both a response to the urgency to act and a recognition that each decision opens a new terrain of unknowability, a new pathlessness, and a new need for a decision. "Every decision reorganizes the fabric of life, but each move in itself does not lead to a conclusive point of certainty; it leads to a new, uncertain, undecidable, and aporetic space from which once again we must decide and act."[25]

At the beginning of this book and throughout, I described the four considerations that an early discussion among genetic scientists, ethicists, lawyers, and theologians put forward to think about heritable genetic modifications in human beings:

(1) Are there reasons in *principle* why using this technology should be impermissible?

(2) What contextual factors should be taken into account, and do any of these prevent development and use of the technology?

(3) What purposes, techniques or applications would be permissible and under what circumstances?

(4) What procedures, structures, involving what policies, should be used to decide on appropriate techniques and uses?[26]

So let me return to "the real world." , that world imagined in point number four.

I noted at the time that while these four questions have stood us in good stead as a field in the consideration of medical genetic interventions at the individual level, they would be inadequate to address fully the problem of region-wide, heritable, genetic modification. Nevertheless, let me briefly summarize what this book can claim about each one. I have returned to these questions throughout this book.

First, I have argued that there is no principled reason that humans should not attempt to eliminate mosquitoes from the environment because it has been done over and over again. There is no principle that argues that species cannot be altered to make a better world for humans. There is no principle that argues that breeding is permissible for such alteration but genetic manipulation is not. May we make the world? Clearly, it is what human beings have done, over and over again. We will fail and we will err, but it will not be because there is a principle of noninvolvement that is violated.

Second, the contextual factors that need to be taken into account all argue for its permissibility, not its danger. Gene drives will not make an unjust world more unjust. They will not create two classes of humans. They will not create wealth for the wealthy. In fact, they will do just the opposite. If malaria is eliminated with gene drives alone or in combination with other modalities, a great and oppressive burden would be lifted from the backs of the poorest in our world. The context of the research is one in which these disease burdens are so rarely addressed that a project directed at them creates a particular duty to enact them if we can. Should other uses for gene drives be proposed, that would be another story. There is nothing inevitable about a wider use of the technology. To block the development of gene drives for malaria because perhaps, at some later point, they could be used as weapons or to benefit the privileged unjustly is not only absurd but also unethical.

Third, this last point leads us to the third consideration. DDT, if it had only been used, and used swiftly and completely, with adequate funding and support, all over the globe, on malarial mosquitoes, might have eliminated malaria. But because it was used for agriculture, for all manner of insect control, and for use in everyone's private little gardens, it was ubiquitous, and that led not only to Carson's issue about the food chain and songbirds and pelicans, but also to the development of resistance to DDT in *Anopheles* mosquitoes. And while researchers are doing many things to try to lessen the rapidity and possibility of resistance leading to the failure of a gene drive, such as putting two targets in at once, we will still need to restrict the technology carefully to avoid a repeat of the problem. Gene drives will not be appropriate for every vector, every plant disease, or every invasive species. Each case will need to be considered separately. In many, many cases, I would argue that they will be a better option than widespread spraying of pesticides, which surely do make the world—and make it far more toxic and far more carcinogenetic. But the discussion will still need to proceed. Clearly, the moral panic that attended an RNA vaccine's first-in-human use reminds us how deeply the fears about anything "genetic" run in the public imagination.[27] The problem of the fears of the demos, noted in the fourth century BCE in Athens, is an old one.

Thus, a final note about the relationship between democracy, witnesses, and truth telling can be made with a brief consideration of parrhesia. Parrhesia derives from the Greek term for the practice of truth telling in the public square, the agora, and the Senate. Sometimes, parrhesia means that experts must speak against the majority if the majority go astray. But to tell the truth was only one obligation of the citizen. It was equally important to hear the truth. Parrhesia is a relationship, requiring tellers and listeners to have the courage to say and to receive difficult truths. The dissolution of this relationship—and its replacement by false flattery or abstract rhetoric—was the single worst outcome for the Greek imagination. In our reflections about gene drives, it is important to remember that citizens have virtues as well. Sometimes, the public debates create confusion—a din that threatens to drown the slower, difficult work of real science, the lessons learned from failure, and repeated failure, the courage it takes to listen to an account of failure and to stay within the relationship, willing to allow the science to continue. It is important to remember how very early in the process of creating gene drives we are, even after more than a decade of research and stakeholder engagement. It may be far too early to evaluate the project, and perhaps even too early for a book such as this one. There will be other projects besides Target Malaria. There has been incremental and very slow but steady progress in the realm of basic science, watching the colonies in their cages and seeing the stakeholders at work. all of this is very beautiful, and there is really no other word. But there will be nothing close to clinical success for many years. In part, this is why it is so important to allow the research to unfold.

The fourth consideration raised in the AAAS report is normative. How do you set up regulatory bodies and rules for gene drives? I want to make a few points. First, African regulators, using the stakeholder process so much a part of this first gene drive project, should be trusted. It should not need to be said, but it does need to be said, that thoughtful, careful regulators, academic researchers, philosophers, and theologians in Africa have the first and more direct stake in this process and do not really need external critics who have little knowledge of the African context. As we have seen in this book, the history and the context of the African malaria disease dynamic is complex and particular to that history.

Ethicists make both descriptive and normative claims. This book is in large part descriptive, elucidating some epistemic and ontological challenges. Yet, I am also making some normative claims. It is the contention of this chapter that if the way to think about the ethical challenges of uncertainty emerges from within the scientific disciplines alone and is focused on epistemic uncertainty, this solution will necessarily be limited and ultimately unstable. And if the deep uncertainty is ignored, and we hustle instead to create ethical codes and rules that do not take it as central, addressing only the technical aspects of uncertainty with consent, then the rules will be insufficient little wooden bridges over the void. This is because addressing science is mutable, the world probable, the real uncertainty vast.

Yet, there is a way for science to proceed ethically, and there is, I believe, a way that scientists and their publics, philosophers, and critics do make the world ethically. What must remain stable are the ethical commitments that call for a worthy life within conditions of immutable uncertainty, for these ever have been the subject of moral philosophy since its beginnings in the memory of cultures as diverse as scriptural discourses, Greek narratives, Confucian philosophy, Arabian poetry, and Socratic debates.[28]

A wide range of moral philosophers understood the limits of knowledge. It is not new to know that the world is more dark than light, more unknown than known. They understood what it was to live in a time of chaos, and yet they engaged in the robust inquiry of ethics, asking: What is the good act, and what makes it so? What is the worthy life, and how might it be achieved? How is the good society structured? It is here, in the reflection on these questions, that we can consider norms for decisions and rules for how to move ahead in science in times that seem as terrifying and capricious as the premodern world, a world of volcanic eruption, constant war, epidemic disease, and yet a world where philosophers first thought: What do we mean by justice? and How can one know truth? And within this discipline, many turned to the question of virtue and how it could be named, maintained, and taught.

Decision making under conditions of uncertainty is difficult to structure rationally in the experimental context, perhaps especially when genetic research now promises so much and perfect control seems so nearly possible. At the most technical and straightforward, it seems to require, at a minimum, adequate updated information, a process in which core values are surfaced and clarified and protection against exploitation of vulnerability potentiated by uncertainty. All of this becomes critically important in times of crisis and ever more important when a deadly pandemic occurs and when truth itself becomes a matter of opinions and politics. To return again to gene drives, much can be done to make science more ethically trustworthy. For example, the many proposals named by the many commissions and committees that have drawn up careful technical rules for safety, containment, iterative projects, environmental impact reports, stopping rules, publishing and licensing norms, and the structures of community engagement so important to the success of the project are useful and should be heeded. But the deep, aporetic uncertainty about the long outcomes and implications of the work will be complex, will be unknown, and will always remain so. To promise otherwise is the wrong sort of promise.

In other words, not only is it possible to consider scientific research ethically justifiable to continue under conditions of uncertainty, but I also consider the recognition that uncertainty is a profound feature of science and, moreover, constitutive of human freedom is itself central to the work. As Michael Anker concludes, freedom, in the absolute sense, is the phenomenon of living in a world without absolute measure. "We stand thus in the opening of freedom, in the aporia of anxious indeterminacy. What we do here, or what we do in relation to the aporia of freedom, makes all the difference in regard to how the world unfolds."[29]

If we can make truly free (and I would add "truly ethical") decisions, "a decision worthy of being called a decision," we must understand that our decisions create new worlds. "Aporias thus draw us toward the possibility of ethical becoming, the possibility of living an 'ethical life' in a world without absolute measure."[30] It is to this "ethical life" to which I now turn to conclude.

Conclusion: The Possibility of an Ethical Life

Should gene drives be created under these conditions? Beyond our commitment to the rules of science and the technical utilitarianism that these rules provide, beyond even the core ethical understanding of the absolute primacy of the theo-philosophical recognition that the Other must be regarded as one's kin, both of which are imperative, let me suggest that we will need to commit to four other things if gene drives can be regarded as ethical when so much is at stake. These are the virtues of veracity, courage, humility, and fidelity—the stable core of Aristotelian moral order. If scientific knowledge is the sort of knowledge that is constantly mutable, perhaps these more enduring attributes may provide some guideposts. In a pathless sea, we turn to the character of the crew.

First, investigators must always tell the truth without exception. This requires clarity and sincerity for everyone involved: investigator, subject, and polity. We must be honest about risk, honest about the unknowable nature of the future, truthful about failure in research, and truthful about mortality, morbidity, and fragility in the clinical research context, especially when we consider the power of genetic research, for the genome is now regarded with the same degree of moral seriousness as medieval scholars considered the soul—definitional, inviolable, special. This degree of truthfulness requires humility, and it is difficult in a time of contention, but it is critical. The duty to repair that is so deeply a part of making the world comes from the facticity of the broken world. Understanding that one cannot fix with science the aching loss at the core of human life—our contingency, our fragility—allows humility to enter the practice of science.

Second, investigators and their institutions must be courageous, risking complete failure, risking political pressure, and risking upending previous normative structures of power. It takes great courage to challenge the hierarchies of the laboratory, for example, or to admit to the funders that a long path of research will not yield results after so promising—and promised—a start. It takes courage to defend your work in a time when there is such anger at elite knowledge and disdain for intricacy, nuance, and complexity. It requires courage, not timidity and not rashness, for what good is aporetic freedom if one is afraid to act?

Third, honesty about uncertainty ought to lead to a sense of humility. Science holds power—predictive power, explanatory power—and where religion alone promised salvation, medical science now does so. But scientific expertise is not necessarily generalized to expertise in all epistemologies, and researchers need to have a sense of humility as well as courage, for a boastful or arrogant claim has no place in the laboratory. It is the wrong sort of promise to promise revolution or redemption. Surely, the continual surprises that have unfolded in the COVID-19 pandemic alone should render the ethical scientist humble.

Finally, if there are the wrong sort of promises, then there are the "right sort of promises" that can be made in science, and the promise of faithfulness, of fidelity, is that sort. The ends of research may not meet the telos of the concept, harm may come, and it should never be borne alone. Investigators cannot know, really, fully, or completely, what their research will accomplish, for the space that is opened by research science is always an open space. Every decision leads to a new place where a new decision is called for, and "the incessant change and flux of all phenomena (whether it be named subject, object, or thing) disallows any true stability or absolute form of certitude."[31] A decision is made to proceed, the world shifts, and new decisions unfold within the first. For postmodern philosophers, it is this place of indeterminacy that allows creativity. The openness to possibility is the openness to the Other who might come next, the very ipseity of the future, bearing the name of the future.

But if knowing the profundity of uncertainty does not allow us to know all the implications and consequences of our work, then what makes the work ethical and responsible must be something else—and it is the promise of fidelity: that the researcher will stand by, being witness to the consequences of her acts and taking responsibility to repair any harm they may bring. Subjects, environments, and societies are not objects that can ever be abandoned, profit taken, and damages forgotten. This is the realpolitik of that lovely philosophy of openness of inquiry as freedom of speech. Its correlate is the openness and utterness and incessant responsibility for the Others who bear the weight of your work. This is the duty that is correlative to the freedom of creativity. This promise—this "I will stand by you"—needs to be inscribed in all of the technical norms that we write, but its seriousness must first be deeply understood. If science were not uncertain, if it were a small human activity, one could make a firm little ethics rule about how it ought to be played. But it is not. Scientific research is one of the great human moral gestures, one of the great works that is possible to us, and it is an uncontainable, unruly, and yet powerful response to human suffering, and that is why it is so.

This observation and this ordering, this counting and this experiment, in all its grandeur, anxiety, and risk, once fully understood, endures. It must also be responsible at this scale, across continents and lifetimes. This is not to abdicate the necessity to follow the regulations that we ethicists are so intent on erecting, for they are necessary, the boundaries and ligations upon which the process rests, but it is to ask for far more.

Think of the enormity—the audacity of the attempt to eliminate malaria! How to respond to the uncertainties that surround us, to the shaken world, the wary publics, the terror of the pandemic, the life and death stakes of malaria in Africa? It is not only by the work of research; it is by the construction of the self of the researcher, the moral agency of the investigator, who is shaped by the inquiry and who understands its gravity.

But it is not only the scientist, of course, who is the world maker. It is the citizen, the reader, the one who would judge the act as well. We participate in the project, even as we critique, and in my case, even as I critique the critique of science. In my writing, arguments about the nature, goal, and meaning of the moral gesture of science, the worth of it, and the question of whether science makes the world a more moral and ethical place are key. The problem of how to help the suffering of the Other is foundational to texts that are at the core of the conversation that is the point of a field of ethics.

But it is not so easy living in the long wait of a world in need of redemption, not in our secular time when modernity has deconstructed the messianic and we worry that the future will never open before us at all. It has long been the contention of the field of ethics that we stand as outsiders to the moral work of science, raising the questions of the stranger to the practitioners of the research. If this is the case, and I believe that it is, then ethics raises ever more *strange* questions, impertinent questions of meaning and human purpose, difficult and dangerous questions of "why" and difficult and risky discussions that recall things that all citizens know—the stakes of the questions, the people who will bear the real cost of research and treatment, and the tragic loss at the heart of medicine. This is not a new attachment. The academy, from the Greeks of the fifth century BCE through the 1600s and Bacon, Kant, and the entire eighteenth century, assumed that ethical questions—questions about wholeness and causality—had a central place in human knowledge. However, since the rise of the German and post-Civil War American university systems, the very hallmark of the university is skepticism, the method of knowledge is to understand increasing smaller parts of wholes and to ask questions about how and what not "why" about the natural world. In ethics, one learns quickly that skepticism, irony, and critique is simply how one approaches a problem. Bioethics is a field that, quite literally, has lost its faith—not only in God or the clergy but, it would seem, in the very capacity for scientists to be honest, for doctors to be selfless, for exchange to be anything but coercive. We are a long way from the Scottish enlightenment idea of the elegance and veracities of social relationships, further still from the demands of scripture. In other work, I have argued that religious and philosophical texts and traditions call forth a necessity: to attend to the sacrifice that is imperative for a just and decent society, to call us to remember that the most wretched and lost and desperate is our sibling, who belongs in our house, who is entitled to our hospitality, and who is the subject of our care. That argument is not only made in theological traditions.

Thus, the question about the permissibility of gene drives is also this: Do gene drives create a better moral life? And for this, there are no quantitative measures, there is only the discursive debate that is found in text and traditions about the worth and meaning of a good life. However, here, one can surely say that living in a world in which we could do better to end malaria and yet ignoring the problem or turning away because of our own fears and interests does create a tragic world. We make choices to do actions. Actions are the objects of our choices, and acts are choices largely for their ends, about which we can deliberate. But the act and the end are only a part of the moral activity, which also includes reasons for acting, then norms that motivate us, and, for many, these norms are understood as divinely important, good, and inevitable.

It is this that renders our lives worthy of value, and makes the activities, the science, the ethics, the world in which we live, decent, meaning having the quality of this illusive partnership that is the basis of the repair of the world. Our actions, then, are not only self-determinative but also world determinative. If we see the moral imperatives that motivate this, we see that the sort of world we will create is the real question lying behind all of emerging science. It must be the core question for ethics as well. This is why we are troubled by the problems we create when we use the language of owning, buying, and payment in science, by the way, for it blinds us to sacrifice and suffering, the debt and forgiveness at the heart of the work.

I have said that while our capacity must be limited, our duties are limitless.

Not only is the virtue of fidelity one that we as citizens need to ask of scientists, but it is one that we must enact as well. It recognizes that it is an accident of history that we in the West, with the technology, are here, while others are elsewhere; this context creates duties to those others. We must proceed with some constraints because of the principle of fidelity—fidelity to the neighbors with whom we share the world. Fidelity also demands a commitment to the entire range and scope of the project at hand. This is true, by the way, for both action and inaction—the body that regulates and decides and who profits from a policy decision is accountable to repair any harms that occur. Unlike precaution, which takes no responsibility for the negative consequences of inaction, a principle of fidelity means that ill effects must be addressed and paid for, and this payment is part of the price of the decision. Unlike risk analysis, which assumes that failure was a risk "paid for" in advance, as it were, by the acceptance of benefits, a principle of fidelity would take into account the responsibility for repair in response to any harm, beyond even the compensatory benefits that the technology might have already created. In a world in which every exchange takes place on a global scale, in which our actions may affect vulnerable others in continents and times we cannot know, only the principle of fidelity reminds us we are responsible for the enormity of now and the infinity of the world to come. It is unknowable what will occur—hence we commit only to what has occurred—our relationship to the other who is our neighbor. In other work, I have called this a theory of hospitality because the demands of justice are inadequate to describe the sacrifice implied by such a theory, one that will need faith beyond all the power of the marketplace and its seductions and exchanges.

Ethical questions such as this, virtues such as the ones I have named, and duties such as the ones I suggest only have real power if citizens and scholars raise them honestly. It is the public arguments of ethics that remind us that the made world is not ours alone, nor are scientists and the watchers of scientists without an audience. It is the poor of the world; it is they for whom the work is done and the books about the work are written. Only we must recognize and enact our duty to see them. Only when the poor become visible can we perceive that we are surrounded by moral limits. It is the limit on our taking that is set by what is owed to the others at the margins, and thus the fragility that edges the very breath of our being reminds us to see the contingency at the edge of the project's science. As reader, as citizen, and as participant, it is up to each of us to raise the moral question and to be this witness. But it is also to remember the moral task as well. The ethics of gene drives in an uncertain, limitless, vertiginous time begins in the inevitability and certainty of these duties and the limitless, endless creation of that virtuous life. We must make the world; we must make it good.

Notes

Introduction

1. Carol Magee, *Africa in the American Imagination: Popular Culture, Radicalized Identities, and African Visual Culture* (Jackson: University Press of Mississippi, 2012).

2. David Peterson Del Mar, "Africa in the American Imagination," The Organization of American Historians, August 3, 2017, http://www.processhistory.org/del-mar-africa-us-imagination/; Manny Otiko, "Africans Push Back Against Western Media's Images of Suffering Continent," Atlanta Black Star, July 9, 2015, https://atlantablackstar.com/2015/07/09/africans-create-twitter-hashtag-showcase-positive-images-continent/; Grant Schreiber, "Changing the Way Americans See Africa," RealLeaders, February 6, 2019, https://real-leaders.com/changing-the-way-americans-see-africa/; Julius A. Amin, "America's Legendary Ignorance about Africa Persists," The Conversation, September 19, 2016, https://theconversation.com/americas-legendary-ignorance-about-africa-persists-65353; Jonathan Zimmerman, "Americans Think Africa Is One Big Wild Animal Reserve," The New Republic, July 9, 2014, https://newrepublic.com/article/118600/america-must-stop-stereotyping-africa-continent-animals; Charles A. Ray, "Does Africa Matter to the United States?" Foreign Policy Research Institute, January 11, 2021, https://www.fpri.org/article/2021/01/does-africa-matter-to-the-united-states/. To be fair, this might be a view held by Africans about America, where I live—that it is disease-ridden and dangerous and violent, full of people resisting the most basic public health rules, and on the brink of civil war.

3. Burt, Austin, Koufopanou, Vassiliki, "Homing endonuclease genes: the rise and fall and rise again of a selfish element," Currrent Opinions in Genetic Development, 2004, December 14 (6): 609–615.

4. I found later that Burt and many others had been working on the genetic control of vector-borne diseases for decades, but in bioethical circles, we were largely fixated on far more esoteric topics, such as cloning or organ transplants or stem-cell research, none of which were directed toward the diseases of the poor.

5. Austin Burt and Robert Trivers, *Genes in Conflict: The Biology of Selfish Genetic Elements* (Cambridge, MA: Harvard University Press, 2006), 1.

6. Burt and Trivers, *Genes in Conflict*, 3.

7. "AAAS Principles for Heritable Genetic Intervention," in *Designing Our Descendants: The Promises and Perils of Genetic Modifications* (Washington, DC: AAAS Press, 1999), frontispiece.

8. I have been a member of my institution's IRB, several NIH DSMBs, and the RAC.

9. Randall M. Packard, *The Making of a Tropical Disease: A Short History of Malaria*, ed. Audrey R. Chapman and Mark S. Frankel (Baltimore: Johns Hopkins Press, 2007).

10. World Health Organization, "World Malaria Day," https://www.who.int/teams/global-malaria-programme/reports/world-malaria-report-2012.

11. World Health Organization, "World Malaria Day," https://www.who.int/teams/global-malaria-programme/reports/world-malaria-report-2012.

12. National Institute for Communicable Diseases, The National Health Laboratory Services, May 10, 2023, http:// www.nicd.ac.za.malaria

13. UN Intergovernmental Panel on Climate Change, "UNIPCC 2018 Report on Effects of 1.5 degrees C," http://report.ipcc.ch/sr15/pdf/sr15_chapter3.pdf.

14. UNIPCC 2018 Report.

15. UNIPCC 2018 Report.

16. Laurie Zoloth, "Heroic Measures: Just Bioethics in an Unjust World," *The Hastings Center Report* 31, no. 6 (2003): 33–40.

Chapter 1

1. Sonia Shah, *The Fever: How Malaria Has Ruled Humankind for 500,000 Years* (New York: Picador Press, 2010), 14.

2. Randall Packard, *The Making of a Tropical Disease* (Baltimore: Johns Hopkins Press, 2007), 19.

3. Centers for Disease Control and Prevention, "Malaria Parasites," CDC, July 16, 2020, https://www.cdc.gov/malaria/about/biology/parasites.html.

4. Shah, *Fever*, 15.

5. Harrison, Gordon, *Mosquitoes, Malaria, and Man: A History of the Hostilities since 1880* (New York: E. P. Dutton, 1978).

6. Bill Gates, "The Deadliest Animal in the World," Gates Notes (blog), *Mosquito Week*, April 25, 2014, https://www.gatesnotes.com/Health/Most-Lethal-Animal-Mosquito-Week.

7. Gates, "Deadliest Animal," 14.

8. Shah, Sonia, https://scroll.in/article/872185/why-has-malaria-plagued-humans-for-500000-years-a-ruthless-protozoan-creature-has-the-answer

9. Shah, *Fever*, 25.

10. Shah, *Fever*, 26.

11. Shah, Fever, p 27.

12. James L. A. Webb Jr., *The Long Struggle Against Malaria in Tropical Africa* (New York: Cambridge University Press, 2015), 12.

13. Karen M. Masterson, *Malaria Project* (New York: Penguin Random House, 2015), 16.

14. Shah, *Fever*, 32.

15. These earlier historians assumed that evolution tended toward accommodation. However, as we have seen with COVID-19, this may not always be the case. All the parasite needs for successful reproduction is for enough bitten carrier human victims to live long enough to be bitten again. So, their death may or may not affect that in area of dense infection. Clearly, the move from *P. vivax* to *P. falciparum* was an instance of a pathogen becoming more rather than less deadly.

16. Masterson, *Malaria Project*, 15.

17. Harrison, *Mosquitoes, Malaria, and Man*.

18. Shah, *Fever*.

19. Shah, *Fever*; P. W. Hedrick, "Population Genetics of Malaria Resistance in Humans," *Heredity* 107, no. 4 (2011): 283–304.

20. Dominic P. Kwiatkowski, "How Malaria Has Affected the Human Genome and What Human Genetics Can Teach Us about Malaria," *American Journal of Human Genetics* 77, no. 2 (2005): 171–192.

21. Masterson, *Malaria Project*, 12.

22. Harrison, *Mosquitoes, Malaria, and Man*, 120.

23. Shah, 30.

24. Harrison, *Mosquitoes, Malaria, and Man*, 37.

25. Webb, *Long Struggle Against Malaria*, 12.

26. Alexandra's Orewa, "Influences On and Reasons Why William Shakespeare Wrote *The Tempest*," Word Press, August 7, 2015, https://alexandrasorewa.wordpress.com/2015/08/07/influences-on-and-reasons-why-william-shakespeare-wrote-the-tempest/.

27. Shah, *Fever*, 45, 48.

28. Shah, *Fever*, 49.

29. Centers for Disease Control and Prevention, "Laveran and the Discovery of the Malaria Parasite," CDC, September 23, 2015, https://www.cdc.gov/malaria/about/history/laveran.html.

30. Shah, Fever, 142.

31. Shah, *Fever*, 143.

32. Shah, *Fever*, 144.

33. Shah, *Fever*, 147.

34. Shah, *Fever*, 149.

35. Shah, *Fever*, 149.

36. Harrison, *Mosquitoes, Malaria, and Man*, 2.

37. In 2018, filled to the brim with antimalarial medicine and wearing insecticide-soaked clothes, a bed net, a little hat with a net for my face, and insect repellent, I visited remote areas in Sri Lanka and Myanmar, and saw that there was no university, dorm, school for children, or clinic that had screens. Moreover, thousands of people, including children and pregnant women, in Rangoon, Columbo, Bagan, and the rural countryside, worshipped large Buddhas at nighttime, dusk, and dawn, calmly meditating amid black swarms of mosquitos. My worry and elaborate precautions were seen as a little silly—something that foreigners did. The Myanmar monks, who of course wear nothing but dark maroon or orange robes, so that their arms and legs are exposed (women wear a pink color, and cover their arms and legs), had had "malaria many times." Shah makes the comment that while Westerners see malaria as a deadly and terrible disease, many in countries where it is endemic see it as akin to a common cold or influenza.

38. Harrison, *Mosquitoes, Malaria, and Man*, 3.

39. Harrison, Mosquitoes, Malaria, and Man, 4.

40. Harrison, *Mosquitoes, Malaria, and Man*, 147.

41. Harrison, *Mosquitoes, Malaria, and Man*, 156.

42. Harrison, *Mosquitoes, Malaria, and Man*, 151.

43. Webb, *Long Struggle Against Malaria*,. Introduction.

44. Webb, The Long Struggle Against Malaria, 50.

45. Webb, *Long Struggle Against Malaria*, 54.

46. Eliana Ferroni, Tom Jefferson, and Gabriel Gachelin, "Angelo Celli and Research on the Prevention of Malaria in Italy a Century Ago," *Journal of the Royal Society of Medicine* 105, no. 1 (2012): 35–40.

47. BlueNile, "Lessons from Successful National Malaria Campaign of Italy 1900–1962," Malaria World, March 16, 2015, https://malariaworld.org/blogs/lessons-successful-national-malaria-campaign-italy-1900-1962.

48. Harrison, *Mosquitoes, Malaria, and Man*, 4.

49. William C. Gorgas, *Sanitation in Panama* (New York: D. Appleton & Co., 1915).

50. William Gorgas, "Yellow Fever Meets Its Nemesis," *Epidemiology* 22, no. 6 (2011): 872.

51. I am aware of the irony here.

52. Matti Friedman, "The Man Who Battled Israel's Most Formidable Enemy—The Mosquito," *The Times of Israel*, April 25, 2012, https://www.timesofisrael.com/remembering-the-man-who-battled-israels-most-formidable

53. Matti Friedman, "The Man Who Battled Israel's Most Formidable Enemy—The Mosquito," *The Times of Israel*, April 25, 2012, https://www.timesofisrael.com/remembering-the-man-who-battled-israels-most-formidable-enemy-the-mosquito/.

54. Friedman, "Man Who Battled Israel's Most Formidable Enemy."

55. Friedman, "Man Who Battled Israel's Most Formidable Enemy."

56. Friedman, "Man Who Battled Israel's Most Formidable Enemy."

57. Palestine Department of Health, *A Review of the Control of Malaria in Palestine (1918–1941)* (Jerusalem: Department of Health, 1941).

58. Muhammad Umair Mushtaq, "Public Health in British India: A Brief Account of the History of Medical Services and Disease Prevention in Colonial India," *Indian Journal of Community Medicine* 34, no. 1 (2009): 6–14.

59. Harrison, *Mosquitoes, Malaria, and Man*, 106.

60. Packard, The Making of Tropical Disease, 110.

61. Packard, *Making of Tropical Disease*, 117.

62. Gabriel Gachelin and Annick Opinel, "Malaria Epidemics in Europe after the First World War: The Early Stages of an International Approach to the Control of the Disease," *Historia, Ciencias, Saude—Manguinhos* 18, no. 2 (2011): 431–469.

63. Gachelin and Opinel, "Malaria Epidemics in Europe."

64. Émile Marchoux, UN Commission Report on Malaria 1924–1931.

65. Marchoux, UN Commission Report.

66. Packard, *Making of Tropical Disease*, 171.

67. Packard, *Making of Tropical Disease*, 112.

68. Packard, *Making of Tropical Disease*, 113.

69. Shah, *Fever*, 99.

70. Masterson, *Malaria Project*, 200.

71. Masterson, *Malaria Project*, 211.

72. Masterson, *Malaria Project*, 249.

73. Of course, this drug became famous when it was promoted as a drug to treat COVID-19. It did not work. The second malaria drug, ivermectin, also promoted as a cure for COVID-19, will be encountered later in this narrative. But it is, of course, interesting that malaria became in this way part of the story of COVID-19 in 2020.

74. Harrison, *Mosquitoes, Malaria, and Man*, 217.

75. Harrison, *Mosquitoes, Malaria, and Man*, 286.

76. Harrison, *Mosquitoes, Malaria, and Man*, 239.

77. Usually, challenge trials are avoided as unethical unless there is treatment that works reasonably well. Drugs are tested either on people who already are sick with the disease in question or on healthy volunteers for safety first and then on people with the disease.

78. Harrison, *Mosquitoes, Malaria, and Man*, 289.

79. Harrison, *Mosquitoes, Malaria, and Man*, 289.

80. Jonathan Moreno, ASBH panel on Nuremberg, 2017.

81. Shah, *Fever*, 198.

82. Shah, *Fever*, 195.

83. Shah, *Fever*, 195.

84. Bagster D. Wilson, "Implications of Malarial Endemicity in East Africa," *Transactions of the Royal Society of Tropical Medicine and Hygiene* 32, no. 4 (1939): 435–465.

85. Wilson, "Implications of Malarial Endemicity."

86. From Miller, as cited in Shah: Since a fully immune adult shows no signs of illness attributable to malaria, he should not be given treatment for the few parasites he may carry, and babies should only be given enough to remove danger to life; the object in both cases being to interfere as little as possible with the state of full immunity. Ibid.

87. Ibid.

88. Ibid.

89. Shah, *Fever*, 95.

90. Webb, *Long Struggle Against Malaria*, 24.

91. Shah, *Fever*, 207.

92. Patrick T. O'Shaughnessy, "Parachuting Cats and Crushed Eggs the Controversy over the Use of DDT to Control Malaria," *American Journal of Public Health* 98, no. 11 (2008): 1940–1948. See also Shah, *Fever*, 209.

93. Shah, *Fever*, 211.

94. Harrison, *Mosquitoes, Malaria, and Man*, 251.

95. Harrison, *Mosquitoes, Malaria, and Man*, 247.

96. Packard, *Making of Tropical Disease*, 206.

97. Masterson, *Malaria Project*, 322.

98. Shah, *Fever*, 213.

99. Packard, *Making of Tropical Disease*, 207.

100. Packed, *Making of Tropical Disease*, 297.

101. Shah, *Fever*, 217.

102. Webb, *Long Struggle Against Malaria*, 90.

103. Webb, *Long Struggle Against Malaria*, 92.

104. Webb, *Long Struggle Against Malaria*, 74.

105. Webb, *Long Struggle Against Malaria*, 74.

106. Harrison, *Mosquitoes, Malaria, and Man*, 3.

107. Packard, *Making of Tropical Disease*, 217.

108. Webb, *Long Struggle Against Malaria*, 94.

109. Shah, *Fever*, 219.

110. David Hipgrave, "Communicable Disease Control in China: From Mao to Now," *Journal of Global Health* 1, no. 2 (2011): 224–238.

111. Shah, *Fever*, 112.

112. Robert S. Desowitz, *The Malaria Capers: Tales of Parasites and People* (New York: W. W. Norton and Company, 1991), 15.

113. Shah, *Fever*, 113.

114. Shah, *Fever*, 113.

115. Shah, *Fever*, 103.

116. Shah, *Fever*, 90.

117. Packard, *Making of Tropical Disease*, 195.

118. Shah, *Fever*, 221.

119. Shah, *Fever*, 223.

120. Webb, *Long Struggle Against Malaria*, 134.

121. Packard, *Making of Tropical Disease*, 113.

122. Packard, *Making of Tropical Disease*, 115.

123. Shah, *Fever*, 227, 239.

124. Packard, *Making of Tropical Disease*, 247.

125. Packard, *Making of Tropical Disease*, 249.

126. Packard, 249.

127. Packard, *Making of Tropical Disease*, 190.

128. Amy Maxmen, "The Enemy in Waiting," *Nature* 559 (July 2018): 458–465; aksi this article, "How to Diffuse Malaria's Ticking Time Bomb, Nature.

129. Maxmen, "Enemy in Waiting." 455.

130. Ed Yong, "We're Already Barreling Toward the Next Pandemic," *The Atlantic*, September 29, 2021, https://www.theatlantic.com/health/archive/2021/09/america-prepared-next-pandemic/620238/?utm_source=newsletter&utm_medium=email&utm_campaign=atlantic-daily-newsletter&utm_content=20210929&silverid=%25%25RECIPIENT_ID%25%25&utm_term=The%20Atlantic%20Daily.

131. Yong, "We're Already Barreling."

132. WHO, "Global Technical Strategy for Malaria 2016–2030," May 1, 2015, https://www.who.int/publications/i/item/9789241564991.

133. WHO, "Global Technical Strategy."

134. WHO, "Global Technical Strategy."

135. WHO, "World Malaria Report 2018," November 19, 2018, https://www.who.int/publications/i/item/9789241565653.

136. WHO, "World Malaria Report 2018."

137. WHO, "World Malaria Report 2018."

138. WHO, World Malaria Report, 2018.

139. Priya Pal, Brian P. Daniels, Anna Oskman, Michael S. Diamond, Robyn S. Klein, and Daniel E. Goldberg, "*Plasmodium falciparum* Histidine-Rich Protein II

Compromises Brain Endothelial Barriers and May Promote Cerebral Malaria Pathogenesis," *mBio* 7, no. 7 (2016): e00617-16.

140. WHO, "World Malaria Report 2018."

141. Our World in Data, "Malaria," https://ourworldindata.org.

142. Gretchen Vogel, "In Landmark Decision, WHO Greenlights Rollout in Africa of the First Malaria Vaccine," *Science*, October 6, 2021, https://www.science.org/content /article/landmark-decision-who-greenlights-rollout-africa-first-malaria-vaccine?utm _source=Nature+Briefing&utm_campaign=caf0465157-briefing-dy-20211007&utm _medium=email&utm_term=0_c9dfd39373-caf0465157-43632917&.

143. Target Malaria press release on vaccine, October 10, 2021.

144. Gretchen Vogel and Leslie Roberts, "Vaccine Trial Meets Modest Expectations, Buoys Hopes," *Science* 334, no. 6054 (2011): 298–299.

145. Michael Cotton, "The Mosquirix (RTS.S) Malaria Vaccine," *Tropical Doctor* 50, no. 2 (2020): 107.

146. P. Doshi, "WHO's Malaria Vaccine Study Is a 'Serious Breach of International Ethical Standards,'" *BMJ* 368 (2020): m734.

147. Doshi, "WHO's Malaria Vaccine Study," m734.

148. Doshi, "WHO's Malaria Vaccine Study," m734.

149. Doshi, "WHO's Malaria Vaccine Study," m734.

150. Helen Branswell, "In Major Decision, WHO Recommends Broad Rollout of World's First Malaria Vaccine," *STAT*, October 6, 2021, https://www.statnews.com /2021/10/06/in-major-decision-who-recommends-broad-rollout-of-worlds-first -malaria-vaccine/?utm_source=STAT+Newsletters&utm_campaign=9dba8a4fba-MR _COPY_01&utm_medium=email&utm_term=0_8cab1d7961-9dba8a4fba-150696433.

151. Yasemin Saplakoglu, "World's First Malaria Vaccine Approved in Major Breakthrough Against Deadly Infection," *ScienceAlert*, October 6, 2021, https://www .sciencealert.com/who-recommends-worlds-first-vaccine-for-parasites-in-war-on -malaria.

152. Apoorva Mandavilli, "A 'Historic Event': First Malaria Vaccine Approved by W.H.O.," *The New York Times*, October 6, 2021, https://www.nytimes.com/2021/10 /06/health/malaria-vaccine-who.html.

Chapter 2

1. National Academies Report, National Academies of Sciences, Engineering, and Medicine, "Gene Drives on the Horizon: Advancing the Science, Navigating Uncertainty, and Aligning Research with Public Values," National Academies Report, Committee

on Gene Drive Research in Non-Human Organism: Recommendations for Responsible Conduct, Board of Life Sciences, Division on Earth and Life Studies, The National Academy of Sciences, Engineering, and Medicine, The National Academies Press, Washington, DC, 2017. In the first version of this manuscript, the reviewers described my singling out Burt for attention as excessive, however, this was done in the NASEM report which that I am describing. The committee here, too, was careful to attend to the importance of his role.

2. "West Nile Solution: Kill Them All," interview with Austin Burt, *The Globe and Mail*, May 17, 2003.

3. Austin Burt and Graham Bell, "Red Queen versus Tangled Bank Models," *Nature* 330 (1987): 118.

4. Charles Darwin, *On the Origin of Species* (1889). http://darwin-online.org.uk /Variorum/1872/1872-429-c-1869.html.

5. Darwin, *Origin of Species*.

6. Austin Burt, "The Evolution of Fitness," *Evolution: An International Journal of Organic Evolution* 49, no. 1 (1995): 1–4.

7. Darwin, Origin of Species.

8. Wikipedia, "The Red Queen Hypothesis," https://en.wikipedia.org/wiki/Red _Queen_hypothesis.

9. Lewis Carroll, *Alice in Wonderland*.

10. Austin Burt and Robert Trivers, *Genes in Conflict: The Biology of Selfish Genetic Elements* (Cambridge, MA: Harvard University Press, 2006), 1.

11. Austin Burt, "Site-Specific Selfish Genes as Tools for the Control and Genetic Engineering of Natural Populations," *Proceedings of the Royal Society Journal* 270, no. 1518 (2003): 921–928. If such genes can be engineered to target new host sequences, then they can be used to manipulate natural populations, even if the number of individuals released is a small fraction of the entire population. For example, a genetic load sufficient to eradicate a population can be imposed in fewer than twenty generations if the target is an essential host gene, the knockout is recessive, and the selfish gene has an appropriate promoter. There will be selection for resistance, but several strategies are available for reducing the likelihood of it evolving. These genes may also be used to engineer natural populations genetically by means of population-wide gene knockouts, gene replacements, and genetic transformations. By targeting sex-linked loci just prior to meiosis, one may skew the population sex ratio, and by changing the promoter, one may limit the spread of the gene to neighboring populations. The proposed constructs are evolutionarily stable in the face of the mutations most likely to arise during their spread, and strategies are also available for reversing the manipulations.

12. Burt, "Site-Specific Selfish Genes," 2.

13. Burt, "Site-Specific Selfish Genes," 3.

14. Burt, "Site-Specific Selfish Genes," 5.

15. Burt, "Site-Specific Selfish Genes," 13–14.

16. A. S. Serebrovsky, "On the Possibility of a New Method for the Control of Insect Pests," *Zoologicheskii Zhurnal* 19 (1940): 618–630.

17. NASEM, "Gene Drives on the Horizon," 12.

18. C. F. Curtis, "Possible Use of Translocations to Fix Desirable Genes in Insect Pest Populations," *Nature* 218, no. 5139 (1968): 368–369.

19. NASEM, "Gene Drives on the Horizon," 12.

20. Andrew F.G. Bourke, "Hamilton's Rule and the Causes of Social Evolution, Philos-Trans Royal Society, London Biological Science 2014, May 19 369 (1642) : 29130362.

21. Burt and Trivers, *Genes in Conflict*, 18.

22. In theory, killer X chromosomes could work in the same way, but it is not known whether killer X chromosomes can cause species extinction because there is no evidence of their existence.

23. Burt and Trivers, *Genes in Conflict*, 76.

24. Burt and Trivers, *Genes in Conflict*, 185.

25. Burt and Trivers, *Genes in Conflict*, 186.

26. https://academic.oup.com/g3journal/article/12/6/jkac081/6565321

27. Burt and Trivers, *Genes in Conflict*, 202.

28. Burt and Trivers, *Genes in Conflict*, 467.

29. Burt and Trivers, *Genes in Conflict*, 217.

30. Burt and Trivers, *Genes in Conflict*, 225.

31. Burt and Trivers Genes in Conflict, 226

32. Burt and Trivers, Genes in Conflict, 227.

33. Burt and Trivers, Genes in Conflict, 228

34. Burt, "Site-Specific Selfish Genes."

35. NASEM, "Gene Drives on the Horizon," 3.

36. NASEM, "Gene Drives on the Horizon," 13.

37. V.M. Gantz et al., " Highly efficient Cas9 mediated gene drive for population modification of the malaria vector mosquito Amopheles stephensi, Proceedings of the National Academy of Science USA, 2015 December 8, 112 (59) E6736–43. doi 10, 1073/pnas. 1521077112.

38. A. Burt, Site-specific selfish genes as tools for the control and genetic engineering of natural populations, *Proc Biol Sci*, 2003, 270, 1518: 921928, and cited in https:// academic.oup.com/g3journal/article/12/6/jkac081/6565321. 1518.

39. Ethan Bier, "Gene Drives gaining speed", Nature. https://www.google.com /search?q=htthttps%3A%2F%2Facademic.oup.com%2Fg3journ.

40. Burt, NAS talk, op cite.

41. Bier, op cite.

42. Burt, NAS talk, at 14:49 "driving Y'.

43. L. Casey Chosewood and Deborah E. Wilson, eds., *Biosafety in Microbiological and Biomedical Laboratories*, 5th ed. (Atlanta, GA: Centers for Disease Control and Prevention, 2009).

44. EU Protocols on Biosafety Containment Levels. Directive 2000/54/EC of the European Parliament and of the Council of 18 September 2000 on the protection of workers from risks related to exposure to biological agents at work (seventh individual directive within the meaning of Article 16(1) of Directive 89/391/EEC).

45. Directive 2000/54/EC of the European Parliament and of the Council of 18 September 2000 on the protection of workers from risks related to exposure to biological agents at work (seventh individual directive within the meaning of Article 16(1) of Directive 89/391/EEC).

46. Wikipedia, "Biosafety," https://ehs.unc.edu/manuals/biological.

47. Wikipedia, "List of Biosafety Level 4 Organisms," https://en.wikipedia.org/wiki /List_of_biosafety_level_4_organisms.

48. Target Malaria, "Who we are," http://targetmalaria.org.

49. Target Malaria, "Together, We Can End Malaria," https://targetmalaria.org/.

50. Target Malaria, "Together, We Can End Malaria."

51. Ibid.

52. Target Malaria, "Together, We Can End Malaria."

53. Target Malaria, https://targetmalaria.org/what-we-do/our-development-pathway /genetically-modified-sterile-male/

54. https://targetmalaria.org/what-we-do/our-development-pathway/genetically -modified-male-bias/

55. Ibid.

56. ISSA.org, "Policy Briefs: Environmental, Socio-economic and Health Inpact Asssesment (ESHIA) for gene drive organisms.

57. Philanthrophy News Digest.org. October 27, 2016.

58. Valentino M. Gantz et al., "Highly Efficient Cas9-Mediated Gene Drive for Population Modification of the Malaria Vector Mosquito *Anopheles stephensi*," *Proceedings of the National Academy of Sciences of the United States of America* 112, no. 49 (2015): E6736–6743.

59. Interview with Ethan Beir, UCSD, in October 2019 by Laurie Zoloth.

60. Sitara Roy et al., "Cas9/Nickase-Induced Allelic Conversion by Homologous Chromosome-Templated Repair in *Drosophila* Somatic Cells," *Science Advances* 8, no. 26 (2022): eabo0721.

61. Kyros Kyrou et al., "A CRISPR-Cas9 Gene Drive Targeting *Doublesex* Causes Complete Population Suppression in Caged *Anopheles Gambiae* Mosquitoes," *Nature Biotechnology* 36, no. 11 (2018): 1062–1066.

62. Kyrou et al., "A CRISPR-Cas9 Gene Drive."

63. Ibid.

64. Andrew Hammond et al., "Gene-Drive Suppression of Mosquito Populations in Large Cages as a Bridge Between Lab and Field," *Nature Communications* 12, no. 1 (2021): 4589.

65. Hammond, et al., p. 4589

66. This turns out to be hard—for genetic changes in insects can change the phenotype, and if a male has an altered phenotype, he may not be seen as a fit mate. Typically, genetically altered organisms can be less fit than wild types as well. Conversations with. Burt in 2018.

67. Ibid.

68. Hammond et al., "Gene-Drive Suppression of Mosquito Populations."

69. Ewen Callaway, "Gene Drives Thwarted by Emergence of Resistant Organisms," *Nature* 542, no. 7639 (2017): 15.

70. Kyruou et al., "A CRISPR-Cas9 Gene Drive."

71. Although, while the gene is conserved in all insects, the target site is different on different insect species.

72. Virginie Courtier-Orgogozo et al., "Evaluating the Probability of CRISPR-based Gene Drive Contaminating Another Species," *Evol Appl* 13, no. 8 (2020): 1888–1905.

73. (Benedict et al. 2008; Esvelt et al. 2014; Webber et al. 2015; National Academies of Sciences and Medicine 2016; Rode et al. 2019).

74. Which they do not describe in detail.

75. I want to note here that the TM reviewers of my book were very skeptical about this paper, writing "What are the mechanisms? It is not just the target site that needs to be conserved. E.g. how does the DNA get into the germline of the other species (I presume via mating, virus??) would the whole transgene be transferred (which is several kilobases long—this might limit uptake from potential viruses) would the regulating elements such as the prooster work in those species? (in the dsx paper by Kyrou 2018 Cas9 is expressed by an *A. gambiae* germline specific promoter? I think all of these are good questions.

76. Nicole Lou, "High Hopes for New Monoclonal Antibody for Malaria," *MedPage Today*, August 3, 2022, https://www.medpagetoday.com/infectiousdisease/generalinfec-tiousdisease/100049?xid=nl_mpt_morningbreak2022-08-04&eun=g1989701d0r&utm _source=Sailthru&utm_medium=email&utm_campaign=MorningBreak_080422&utm _term=NL_Gen_Int_Daily_News_Update_active.

Chapter 3

1. The reviewers wanted me to add George Church's lab, which indeed is true, but Church and Esvelt could hardly be called people who worked in "relative obscurity."

2. National Museum of American History, "Recombinant DNA in the Lab," https:// americanhistory.si.edu/collections/object-groups/birth-of-biotech/recombinant-dna -in-the-lab.

3. Maxine Singer and Soll Dietrich, "Letter from Maxine Singer and Dieter Soll to Philip Handler," National Library of Medicine Digital Collections, https://collections .nlm.nih.gov/catalog/nlm:nlmuid-101584580X26-doc.

4. https://www.hhs.gov/ohrp/regulations-and-policy/belmont-report/index.html

5. https://repository.library.georgetown.edu/handle/10822/548744

6. The term is itself contested. Some, such as Mildred Cho, contend that "no ther-apy has ever resulted."

7. The Ethics of Human Gene Therapy, by LeRoy Walters and Julie Gage Palmer. New York: Oxford University Press, 1997. 209 pp. Also: Rewriting the "Points to Consider": The Ethical Impact of Guidance Document Language Article, Feb 1999, also https://pubmed.ncbi.nlm.nih.gov/3457268/

For the most complete account of both the complex history and the resulting complex scaffold of committees, see LeRoy Walters and Julie Gage Palmer, *The Ethics of Human Gene Therapy* (New York: Oxford University Press, 1997).

8. LeRoy Walters, Senate testimony, February 2, 2000, as cited in King, Rewriting Points, op. cit., 382.

9. https://en.wikipedia.org/wiki/Mary-Dell_Chilton

10. https://www.ncbi.nlm.nih.gov/books/NBK195894/

11. King, Rewriting Ibid., 385.

12. King, Rewriting Ibid., 386.

13. Walters and Palmer, *Ethics of Human Gene Therapy*.

14. Alta Charo, address to the American Society for Bioethics and Humanities, Boston. October, 2002.

15. King, op. cit., 385.

16. Meir Rinde, "The Death of Jesse Gelsinger, 20 Years Later," *Science History Institute*, June 4, 2019, https://www.sciencehistory.org/distillations/the-death-of-jesse-gelsinger-20-years-later.

17. Rinde.

18. Rinde.

19. Rinde, "Death of Jesse Gelsinger."

20. "AAAS Principles for Heritable Genetic Intervention," in *Designing Our Descendants: The Promises and Perils of Genetic Modifications* (Washington, DC: AAAS Press, 1999), frontispiece.

21. Lee Ann Patterson and Tim Josling, "Regulating Biotechnology: Comparing EU and US Approaches," European Policy Papers #8, Archive of European Integration, 2003, http://aei.pitt.edu/28/.

22. Alta Charo, "Governance of Dual Use Research in the Life Sciences: Advancing Global Consensus on Research Oversight," in *Proceedings of a Workshop, Chapter 2, Governance in Theory and Practice* (Washington, DC: National Academies Press, 2018).

23. Laurie Zoloth, "Introduction," in *Second Texts, Second Opinions: Essays toward a Jewish Bioethics* (Oxford: Oxford University Press, 2022).

24. Charo, "Governance," 12.

25. Helen Longino, *Science as Social Knowledge: Values and Objectivity in Scientific Inquiry* (Princeton, NJ: Princeton University Press, 1990).

26. Longino, Helen, Science as Social Knowledge: Values and Objectivity in Scientif Research, https://www.jstor.org/stable/j.ctvx5wbfz.

27. My reviewers pointed out that there are other differences—EU regulations are based on processes, and USA ones on products, but the point of this section is not

to articular all the many differences, of which there are many, but to highlight the principle of precaution in the debates about genetic engineering.

28. Directorate General for Environment (European Commission), University of the West of England (UWE), Science Communication Unit, *The Precautionary Principle: Decision-Making under Uncertainty* (Luxembourg: Publications Office of the European Union, 2017).

29. Directorate General for Environment (European Commission), *Precautionary Principle*, 3.

30. Ibid.

31. Ibid.

32. Wikipedia, "The Precautionary Principle," https://en.wikipedia.org/wiki/Precautionary_principle.

33. Wikipedia, "Precautionary Principle."

34. EUR-Lex, "Convention on Biological Diversity—Cartagena Protocol on Biosafety," November 17, 2020, https://eur-lex.europa.eu/EN/legal-content/summary/convention-on-biological-diversity-cartagena-protocol-on-biosafety.html#:~:text=The%20Cartagena%20protocol%20to%20the,%2F2003%20%E2%80%94%20see%20summary.

35. Ecologic Institute, "The Precautionary Principle in the European Environment, Health and Food Safety Policy," March 2004, https://www.ecologic.eu/1126.

36. Frank B. Cross, "Paradoxical Perils of the Precautionary Principle," *Washington and Lee Law Review* 53, no. 3 (1996): 851–925.

37. Cross, "Paradoxical Perils."

38. Loretta M. Kopelman, David B. Resnick, and Douglas L. Weed, "What Is the Role of the Precautionary Principle in the Philosophy of Medicine and Bioethics?" *Journal of Medicine and Philosophy A forum for Bioethics and Philosophy* 29, no. 3 (2004): 255–258.

39. Kopelman, Resnick, and Weed, "What Is the Role of the Precautionary Principle."

40. The House of Lords, Science and Technology Select Committee, "Genetically Modified Insects," December 17, 2015, https://publications.parliament.uk/pa/ld201516/ldselect/ldsctech/68/68.pdf.

41. Jonathan Weiner, "Precaution in a Multi-Risk World," in *Human and Ecological Risk Management: Theory and Practice*, edited by Dennis J. Paustenbach (New York: John Wiley, 2002), 1509–1532.

42. Ibid.

43. Weiner, "Precaution in Multi-Risk World," 14.

44. Aristotle, https://www.goodreads.com/quotes/689892-nature-does-nothing-in-vain-therefore-it-is-imperative-for#:~:text=Therefore%2C%20it%20is%20imperative%20for,to%20be%20content%20and%20complete.%E2%80%9D

45. Naing, Aung Htay, and Kim, Chang, Kil, "A brief review of applications of anti-freeze proteins in cryopreservation and metabolic genetic engineering., 3 Biotech, 2019, Sept 9. (9) 329. Doi: 10.1007/s13205-019-1861-y

46. Keith R. Hayes et al., "Risk Assessment for Controlling Mosquito Vectors with Engineered Nucleases: Controlled Field Release for Sterile Male Construct and Risk Assessment Report," CSIRO Health and Biosecurity, May 2, 2018, https://publications.csiro.au/rpr/pub?pid=csiro:EP178126&sb=RECENT&expert=false.

47. Who. 1991. Report of the meeting: Prospects for Malaria Control by Genetic Manipulation of its Vectors, Tucson, Arizona, 27–31 January 1991, TDR/BCV.Mal-ENT/91.WHO, Geneva Switzerland; WHO (2010) Progress and Prospects for the Use of Genetically Modified Mosquitoes to Inhibit Disease Transmission. Report on planning meeting, 1:Technical consultation of current status and planning for future development of genetically modified mosquitoes for malaria and dengue control. Geneva, Switzerland, 4–6 May 2009.

48. Ibid.

49. Stephanie James et al., "Pathway to Deployment of Gene Drive Mosquitoes as a Potential Biocontrol Tool for Elimination of Malaria in sub-Saharan Africa: Recommendations of a Scientific Working Group," *American Journal of Tropical Medicine and Hygiene* 98, no. 6 Suppl. (2018): 1–49, 7.

50. Ibid.

51. Of course, what appropriately means is left undefined.

52. James et al., "Pathway to Deployment," 8.

53. James et al., "Pathway to Deployment," 10.

54. The House of Lords, Science and Technology Select Committee, "First Report of Session 2015–16: Genetically Modified Insects," December 17, 2015, https://publications.parliament.uk/pa/ld201516/ldselect/ldsctech/68/68.pdf, 2.

55. The House of Lords, "First Report of Session 2015–16," 2.

56. The House of Lords, "First Report of Session 2015–16," 3.

57. https://www.pirbright.ac.uk/publications?keywords=gene+drive+regulations&contributors=&year=&pdf=All

58. www. Probright.

59. And perhaps they meant that in the event of a complete species collapse, laboratory stocks could potentially restart a wild colony, should that be necessary (and of

course, if there were no human cases of malaria, then the mosquitoes would not have parasites to carry).

60. The House of Lords, First Report of Session 2015–16, 39.

61. The House of Lords, "First Report of Session 2015–16," 39.

62. https://www.who.int/news-room/fact-sheets/detail/dengue-and-severe-dengue#:~:text=About%20half%20of%20the%20world's,million%20infections%20occurring%20each%20year.

63. https://nas-sites.org/gene-drives/2015/10/03/second-public-meeting/.

64. NASEM, "Gene Drives on the Horizon: Advancing Science, Navigating Uncertainty, and Aligning Research with Public Values," National Academies Press, Washington, DC, 2016.

65. NASEM, "Gene Drives on the Horizon," 3.

66. NASEM, "Gene Drives on the Horizon," 67–68.

67. NASEM, "Gene Drives on the Horizon," 75.

68. NASEM, "Gene Drives on the Horizon," 79.

69. NASEM, "Gene Drives on the Horizon," 79–80.

70. NASEM, "Gene Drives on the Horizon," 79.

71. NASEM, "Gene Drives on the Horizon," 112.

72. NASEM, "Gene Drives on the Horizon," 116.

73. NASEM, "Gene Drives on the Horizon," 128.

74. NASEM, "Gene Drives on the Horizon," 132.

75. NASEM, "Gene Drives on the Horizon," 143.

76. Not a strong point in malaria research, as Grassi might add.

77. NASEM, ibid. 159.

78. NASEM, "Gene Drives on the Horizon," 160.

79. NASEM, "Gene Drives on the Horizon," 161.

80. NASEM, "Gene Drives on the Horizon," 161.

81. Gene Drives on the Horizen.

82. Gene Drives on the Horizon, Ibid., 164.

83. Gene Drives on the Horizon, 166.

84. African Union and New Partnership for Africa's Development, "Gene Drives for Malaria Control and Elimination in Africa," 2017, https://www.nepad.org/publication/gene-drives-malaria-control-and-elimination-africa.

85. Claudia Emerson et al., "Principles for Gene Drive Research," *Science* 358, no. 6367 (2017): 1135–1136.

86. Gregory E. Kaebnick et al., "Precaution and Governance of Emerging Technologies," *Science* 354, no. 6313 (2016): 710–711.

87. Kaebnick et al., "Precaution and Governance of Emerging Technologies," 2.

88. John Min et al., "Harnessing Gene Drive," *Journal of Responsible Innovation* 5 (2018): S40–S65.

89. Min et al., "Harnessing Gene Drive," 560.

90. Austin Burt et al., "Gene Drive to Reduce Malaria Transmission in Sub-Saharan Africa," *Journal of Responsible Innovation* 5 (2018): S66–S80.

91. Burt et al., "Gene Drive," 575.

92. Burt et al., "Gene Drive," 577.

93. Paul Mitchell, Zachery Brown, and Neil McRoberts, "Economic Issues to Consider for Gene Drives," *Journal of Responsible Innovation* 5 (2018): S180–S222.

94. Mitchell, Brown, and McRoberts, "Economic Issues," 120.

95. Mitchell, Brown, and McRoberts, "Economic Issues," 118.

96. https://en.wikipedia.org/wiki/Easterlin_paradox

97. Mitchell, Brown, and McRoberts, "Economic Issues," 187–188.

98. J. Kuzma et al., "A Roadmap for Gene Drives: Using Institutional Analysis and Development to Frame Research Needs and Governance in a Systems Context," *Journal of Responsible Innovation* 5 (2018): S13–S39.

99. Thompson, Paul, "The role of ethics in gene drive research and governance," Journal of Responsible Innovation, https://research.ncsu.edu/ges/files/2017/11/jri-si-thompson-roles-ethics-gene-drive-research-governance-2018.pdf

100. Thompson, "The role of ethics".

101. Thompson, The role of ethics.

102. Keith R. Hayes et al., "Identifying and Detecting Potentially Adverse Ecological Outcomes Associated with the Release of Gene-Drive Modified Organisms," *Journal of Responsible Innovation* 5 (2018): S139–S158.

103. Weiss Evans, Samuel and Palmer, Megan J, , "Anomaly Handling and the Politics of Gene Drives," *Journal of Responsible Innovation* 5 (2018): S223–S242.

104. Sam Weiss Evans and Megan J. Palmer, "Anomaly Handling and the Politics of Gene Drives," *Journal of Responsible Innovation* 5 (2018): S223–S242.

105. Evans and Palmer, "Anomaly".

106. George Annas et al., "A Code of Ethics of Gene Drive Research," *The CRISPR Journal* 4, no. 1 (2021): 19–14.

107. African Union Report on Gene Drive Technology. https://au.int/sites/default /files/documents/33126-doc-06_the_vision.pdf

108. Annas et al., "Code of Ethics," 5.

109. Annas et al., "Code of Ethics," 6.

110. Annas et al., "Code of Ethics," 23.

111. Kanya C. Long et al., "Core Commitments for Field Trials of Gene Drive Organisms." *Science* 370, no. 6523 (2020): 1417–1419.

112. Kent Redford and William Adams, *Strange Natures: Conservation in the Era of Synthetic Biology* (New Haven, CT: Yale University Press, 2021).

113. A reviewer wished me to add something about DDT here, but I will address the issue of DDT in a later chapter. The point I am making here is about the neglect of the issue of this tropical disease from the center of debates in bioethics. Another reviewer questioned this comment because he thought that bioethicists had played a role in the DDT debates. However, most of that controversy occurred outside and before the regent of bioethics as a field. Bioethics journals have focused far more on cloning than malaria, by literature count.

Chapter 4

1. Anthony Stavrianakis, Gaymon Bennett, and Lyle Fearnley, *Science, Reason, Modernity: Readings for an Anthropology of the Contemporary* (New York: Fordham University Press, 2015), 2.

2. One reviewer noted that China and Russia were also playing roles in the countries we are discussing, but it is in their capacities as "the West" structurally, as opposed to their geographic positionality.

3. Stavrianakis, Bennett, and Fearnley, *Science, Reason, Modernity*, 3.

4. Stavrianakis, Bennett, and Fearnley, *Science, Reason, Modernity*, 3.

5. Louis Menand, *The Metaphysical Club: A Story of Ideas in America* (New York: Farrar, Straus, and Giroux, 2001).

6. Stavrianakis, Bennett, and Fearnley, *Science, Reason, Modernity*, 10.

7. Stavrianakis, Bennett, and Fearnley, *Science, Reason, Modernity*, 21.

8. Farmer died during the writing of this book. Yet, his work and extraordinary dedication to the health of the rural poor was something that I thought about frequently as a model for ethical discourse.

9. Paul Farmer, *Fevers, Feuds, and Diamonds: Ebola and the Ravages of History* (New York: Farrar, Straus, and Giroux, 2020), 240.

10. Farmer, *Fevers, Feuds, and Diamonds*, 240.

11. Farmer, *Fevers, Feuds, and Diamonds*, 240.

12. Farmer, *Fevers, Feuds, and Diamonds*, 270–273.

13. Farmer, *Fevers, Feuds, and Diamonds*, 499.

14. Farmer, *Fevers, Feuds, and Diamonds*, 501.

15. Farmer, *Fevers, Feuds, and Diamonds*, 506.

16. Megan Vaughan, *Curing Their Ills: Colonial Power and African Illness* (Palo Alto, CA: Stanford University Press, 1991).

17. Vaughan, *Curing Their Ills*, 35.

18. David Arnold, *Colonizing the Body: State Medicine and Epidemic Disease in Nineteenth Century India* (Berkeley: University of California Press, 1993), 29.

19. Arnold, *Colonizing the Body*, 38.

20. Arnold, *Colonizing the Body*, 38.

21. Arnold, *Colonizing the Body*, 201.

22. Helen Tilley, *Africa as a Living Laboratory: Empire Development, and the Problem of Scientific Knowledge, 1870–1950* (Chicago: University of Chicago Press, 2011), 1–2.

23. Tilley, *Africa as Living Laboratory*, 4.

24. Tilley, *Africa as Living Laboratory*, 5.

25. Tilley, *Africa as Living Laboratory*, 5.

26. Tilley, 5.

27. Tilley, *Africa as Living Laboratory*, 5.

28. Tilley, *Africa as a Living Laboraroty*, 5

29. Tilley, *Africa as Living Laboratory*, 5.

30. Tilley, *Africa as Living Laboratory*, 11.

31. Tilley, *Africa as Living Laboratory*, 17.

Notes to Pages 171–180

32. Tilley, *Africa as Living Laboratory*, 170.

33. Tilley, *Africa as Living Laboratory*, 171.

34. Tilley, *Africa as Living Laboratory*, 190.

35. Tilley, *Africa as Living Laboratory*, 181.

36. Tilley, *Africa as Living Laboratory*, 185.

37. Tilley, 189.

38. Tilley, *Africa as Living Laboratory*, 210.

39. Tilley, Africa as a Living Laboratory, 210

40. Tilley, *Africa as Living Laboratory*, 211.

41. Tilley, *Africa as Living Laboratory*, 218.

42. Tilley, *Africa as Living Laboratory*, 171.

43. Tilley, *Africa as Living Laboratory*, 325.

44. Ernest Harsh, *Burkina Faso: A History of Power, Protest, and Revolution* (London: Zed Books, 2017).

45. Harsh, *Burkina Faso*, 235.

46. Harsh, *Burkina Faso*, 232.

47. Harsh, *Burkina Faso*, 234.

48. Paulina Tindan, Aminu Yakubu, and Jantina De Vries, "Genomics Research in Africa: Taking Stakeholder Engagement Seriously," *BMC* Series blog, October 18, 2019, https://blogs.biomedcentral.com/bmcseriesblog/2019/10/18/genomics-research-in -africa-taking-stakeholder-engagement-seriously/.

49. Davy, Humphry, as cited in Holmes, Richard, The Age of Wonder: The Discovery of the Beauty and Terror of Science Vintage, London, March 2, 2010.

50. Holmes, Richard, The Age of wonder.

51. Holmes, Richard, The Age of Wonder.

52. Holmes, Richard, The Age of Wonder.

53. Holmes, Richard, The Age of Wonder.

54. Delphine Thizy et al., "Proceedings of an Expert Workshop on Community Agreement for Gene Drive Research in Africa-Co-Organized by KEMRI, PAMCA, and Target Malaria," *Gates Open Research* 5 (2021): 19.

55. Although, as I noted, it is imagined to happen after the fact not before the science.

56. James et al., "National Academy of Sciences, Engineering and Medicine Report," 2016.

57. https://prjournal.instituteforpr.org/wp-content/uploads/2015v09n01NiWangD elaFlorPenaflor.pdf

58. Although the team is aware of the issue.

59. Delphine Thizy, talk to the Ethics Board of Target Malaria.

60. John L. Teem, Aggrey Ambali, Barbara Glover, Jeremy Ouedraogo, Diran Makinde, and Andrew Roberts.

61. John L. Teem et al., "Problem Formulation for Gene Drive Mosquitoes Designed to Reduce Malaria Transmission in Africa: Results from Four Regional Consultations 2016–2018," *Malaria Journal* 18, no. 1 (2019): 347.

62. Elinor Chemonges Wanyama et al., "Co-developing a Common Glossary with Stakeholders for Engagement on New Genetic Approaches for Malaria Control in a Local African Setting," *Malaria Journal* 20, no. 1 (2021): 53.

63. Wanyama et al., "Co-developing Common Glossary."

64. Thizy et al., "Proceedings of an Expert Workshop."

65. Thizy et al., "Proceedings of an Expert Workshop."

66. A. J. Roberts and D. Thizy, "Articulating Ethical Principles Guiding Target Malaria's Engagement Strategy," *Malar Journal* 21, no. 35 (2022).

67. WHO, *Guidance Framework for Testing Genetically Modified Mosquitoes*, 2nd ed. (Geneva: World Health Organization, 2021).

68. This sentence was adding by Thizy during the review process to clarify things for the reader.

69. Target Malaria website, https://targetmalaria.org.

70. Target Malaria website.

71. South Cook County Mosquito Abatement District, "Mosquito Control: Our Integrated Approach," https://www.sccmad.org/programs. We are reassured they know what they are doing. . . .

72. Elinor Ostrom, *Governing the Commons: The Evolution of Institutions for Collective Action* (Cambridge: Cambridge University Press, 1990).

73. Ostrom, *Governing the Commons*, 2.

74. Garrett Hardin, "The Tragedy of the Commons. The Population Problem Has No Technical Solution; It Requires a Fundamental Extension in Morality," *Science* 162, no. 3829 (1968): 1244.

75. And this is true for community consent as it is for individual consent by persons in any research.

76. These are not their real names. In order to protect confidentiality, I have used fictional names for the real people in this project.

77. Golden Rice.

78. Daniel Kevles, "The Historical Contingency of Bioethics," *Princeton Journal of Bioethics* 3, no. 1 (Spring 2000): 51–58.

79. While was not a planned part of their work.

Chapter 5

1. Nagel, Thomas, The View from Nowhere, Oxford University Press, 1986. Also see MacIntyre, Alasdair, After Virture, Notre Dame Press, 1981 for an extensive critique of this problem..

2. And the team at Target Malaria has been very responsive to my critiques to boot. At one point, I described a video of David Beckham that they had on their site as moderately racist, and the next day, they took it down. (Beckham!)

3. Who so kindly met with me.

4. In researching this book, I contacted several of the groups whose work is described below, and asked to interview them, so as to better understand their arguments. All that I wrote to refused. However, they each publish extensively; they have held several online conferences (only some of which are open to the public.)

5. ETC Group, "A Brief History," https://www.etcgroup.org/content/etc-group-brief-history.

6. ETC Group, "A Brief History."

7. Acres, USA magazine. Acres, USA's website tells us that it is The Voice of eco-agriculture. This interview, done in 2019, is no longer available on their website.

8. Trudi Zundel, "Reckless Driving: Gene Drives and the End of Nature," September 1, 2016, https://www.etcgroup.org/content/reckless-driving-gene-drives-and-end-nature.

9. Zundel, "Reckless Driving."

10. Zundel, "Reckless Driving."

11. ETC Group, "Driven to Extinction, " October 14, 2020, https://www.etcgroup.org/content/driven-extinction.

12. Shiva herself is the subject of enormous controversy. She has claimed a doctorate in physics and a background as "one of India's leading physicists," yet this is not the case. Her claims about farmer suicide have been carefully investigated and rejected as

false. Her speaking fee—$40,000 per lecture—has been criticized. This controversy can be explored fully in the New Yorker article, "Seeds of Doubt," Dr. Shiva's reply, and the New Yorker's answer, all of which are publicly available on the internet but which are not the subject of this chapter, which is to explore the content of the objects, not the character, however dubious, of the objectors.

13. Vandana Shiva, "Biodiversity, GMOs, Gene Drives and the Militarised Mind," IPS News Agency, January 14, 2023, http://www.ipsnews.net/2016/07/biodiversity -gmos-gene-drives-and-the-militarised-mind/.

14. Shiva, Biodiversity, citing her twitter account @drvandanashiva.com.

15. Shiva, Biodiversity.

16. Shiva, "Biodiversity."

17. Shiva, blog posting.

18. Shiva, Biodiversity.

19. Shiva, "Biodiversity."

20. Shiva, "Biodiversity."

21. Jihad, which is a term for "struggle" in the Arabic, refers to the usually internal religious struggle of a devout Muslim, and which was also used by militant Islamist groups to refer to a military fight against the West. Shiva is herself, a Hindu.

22. Annam: Food and Health, Navdanya website.

23. https://www.navdanya.org/bija-refelections/2020/03/18/ecological-reflections -on-the-corona-virus/.

24. Biosafety Information Centre, "Call for a Global Moratorium on Gene Drive Releases," November 13, 2018, https://biosafety-info.net/articles/biosafety-science /emerging-trends-techniques/call-for-a-global-moratorium-on-gene-drive-releases/.

25. Biosafety Information Centre.

26. https://ifg.org/2014/09/08/save-the-date-techno-utopianism-and-the-fate-of-the -earth-conference-october-25-26/.

27. Johannes Fabian, *Time and the Other: How Anthropology Constructs its Subject* (New York: Columbia University Press, 1983), 18.

28. Kathryn Schulz, "The Pitfalls of Contemporary Nature Writing," *The New Yorker*, July 16 and 19, 2021, 74–80.

29. Schulz, "Pitfalls of Contemporary Nature Writing," 7, p. 9.

30. Encyclopedia.com, "Cassava," May 29, 2018, https://www.encyclopedia.com /plants-and-animals/plants/plants/cassava.

31. BioCassava project on Gates Foundation website, 2005.

32. Encyclopedia.com, "Cassava."

33. Richard Norgaard, "The Biological Control of Cassava Mealybug in Africa," *American Journal of Agricultural Economics* 70, no. 2 (1988): 366–371.

34. USDA National Agricultural Library, "The New World Screwworm," https://www.nal.usda.gov/exhibits/speccoll/exhibits/show/stop-screwworms--selections-fr/introduction.

35. James E. Novy, "Screwworm Control and Eradication in the Southern United States of America," Food and Agriculture Organization of the United Nations, http://www.fao.org/3/u4220t/u4220T0a.htm.

36. Novy, "Screwworm Control and Eradication."

37. Novy, "Screwworm Control and Eradication."

38. Novy, "Screwworm Control and Eradication."

39. Jason Bittel, "Why the Government Breeds and Releases Billions of Flies a Year," *National Geographic*, December 11, 2019, https://www.nationalgeographic.com/animals/2019/12/north-american-screwworm-barrier/#:~:text=A%20program%20in%20Panama%20breeds,livestock%20from%20flesh%2Deating%20larvae.

40. Sarah Zhang, "America's Never-Ending Battle Against Flesh-Eating Worms," *The Atlantic*, May 26, 2020, https://www.theatlantic.com/science/archive/2020/05/flesh-eating-worms-disease-containment-america-panama/611026/.

41. Teach- in TechnopUtopianism and the Fate of the Earth, The Great Hall at The Cooper Union, New York, sponsored by the International Forum on Globolization. http://ifg.org/techno-utopia.

42. Ibid. International Forum on Globalization.

43. Leon Kass, "Ageless Bodies, Happy Souls: Biotechnology and the Pursuit of Perfection," *The New Atlantis*, Spring 2003, https://www.thenewatlantis.com/publications/ageless-bodies-happy-souls.

44. Susan Rubin and Laurie Zoloth, eds., *Margin of Error: Mistakes in Bioethics and Medicine* (University Press, 1998).

45. https://www.frontiersin.org/articles/10.3389/fmicb.2019.01404/full

46. UC Berkeley news release, April 2006. See also *Nature Biotechnology*, July 2006; abstract of article, Keasling et al.: "Malaria is a global health problem that threatens 300–500 million people and kills more than one million people annually[1]. Disease control is hampered by the occurrence of multi-drug-resistant strains of the malaria parasite *Plasmodium falciparum*[2,3]. Synthetic antimalarial drugs and malarial vaccines are currently being developed, but their efficacy against malaria awaits rigorous clinical

testing[4, 5]. Artemisinin, a sesquiterpene lactone endoperoxide extracted from *Artemisia annua* L (family *Asteraceae*; commonly known as sweet wormwood), is highly effective against multi-drug-resistant *Plasmodium* spp., but is in short supply and unaffordable to most malaria sufferers[6]. Although total synthesis of artemisinin is difficult and costly[7], the semi-synthesis of artemisinin or any derivative from microbially sourced artemisinic acid, its immediate precursor, could be a cost-effective, environmentally friendly, high-quality and reliable source of artemisinin[8, 9]. Here we report the engineering of *Saccharomyces cerevisiae* to produce high titres (up to 100 mg l⁻¹) of artemisinic acid using an engineered mevalonate pathway, amorphadiene synthase, and a novel cytochrome P450 monooxygenase (*CYP71AV1*) from *A. annua* that performs a three-step oxidation of amorpha-4,11-diene to artemisinic acid. The synthesized artemisinic acid is transported out and retained on the outside of the engineered yeast, meaning that a simple and inexpensive purification process can be used to obtain the desired product. Although the engineered yeast is already capable of producing artemisinic acid at a significantly higher specific productivity than *A. annua*, yield optimization and industrial scale-up will be required to raise artemisinic acid production to a level high enough to reduce artemisinin combination therapies to significantly below their current price."

47. C. J. Padden and Jay D. Keasling, "Semi-Synthetic Artemisinin: A Model for the Use of Synthetic Biology in Pharmaceutical Development," *Nature Reviews Microbiology* 12, no. 5 (2014): 355–367.

48. Mark Peplow, "Synthetic Biology's First Malaria Drug Meets Market Resistance," *Nature* 530, no. 7591 (2016): 389–390.

49. The snake is just a snake, nature morally neutral, people intended to create by picking up the shattered pieces, the jigsaw puzzle of the fallen sky, trying to figure it out. From a Christian perspective, as Elshtein reminds us, the tree at the center of the moral universe is the Cross, but for the Jewish philosopher, it is the Torah, Law, justice, the pact of solidarity, and witness that is Etz Chaim, the tree of life at the center of the lost world.

50. Levinas, Emmanuel, Existence and Existents, https://mercaba.org/SANLUIS /Filosofia/autores/Contempor%C3%A1nea/L%C3%A9vinas/Existence%20and%20 existents.pdf

51. Or, in some cases, by the most privileged members of countries, South African cities.

52. A reviewed noted that the terms genetic technology, genetic engineering, and gene transfer are used interchangeably. This is because the terms all refer to different ways or describing research at the genetic level, or levels of specificity in the science of molecular biology, However, in other disciplines, and in the literature I am describing here, they are indeed used interchangeably. There is not even certainty on whether the field is called synthenic biology or molecular engineering or engineering biology.

53. WHO, "Vitamin A Deficiency," https://www.who.int/data/nutrition/nlis/info/vitamin-a-deficiency.

54. Ed Regis, *Golden Rice: The Imperiled Birth of a GMO Superfood* (Baltimore: Johns Hopkins University Press, 2019), 2.

55. Regis, *Golden Rice*, 15.

56. Jorgo Riss, Jagona Munic, and Benedikt Härlin, "Please Support a Global Moratorium on the Environment Release of Gene Drive Organisms," Greenpeace, June 30, 2020, https://www.greenpeace.org/static/planet4-eu-unit-stateless/2020/07/30062020-NGO-gene-drive-letter.pdf.

57. Greenpeace, "Golden Rice," Greenpeace Southeast Asia, March 1, 2013, https://www.greenpeace.org/southeastasia/publication/1073/golden-rice/.

58. "AAAS Principles for Heritable Genetic Intervention," in *Designing Our Descendants: The Promises and Perils of Genetic Modifications* (Washington, DC: AAAS Press, 1999), frontispiece.

Chapter 6

1. *New York Times*, September 22, 2021.

2. Euzebiusz Jamrozik et al., "Ethical Aspects of Malaria Control and Research," *Malaria Journal* 14 (2015): 518.

3. In fact, the subject of hastily called and seemingly urgent discussions the week I edited the final draft of this paper, at the NIH.

4. WHO, "Annual Malaria Report 2017," November 19, 2017, https://www.who.int/publications/i/item/9789241565523. Note that the US billion is not money from the USA, just the number in US dollars. The USA actually gives far less than this.

5. Jamrozik et al., "Ethical Aspects of Malaria."

6. Ruud Der Muer.

7. Jamrozik et al., "Ethical Aspects of Malaria."

8. Randall M. Packard, *A History of Global Health: Interventions into the Lives of Other Peoples* (Baltimore: Johns Hopkins University Press, 2016), 96.

9. Packard, *History of Global Health*.

10. Packard, *History of Global Health*.

11. Packard, *History of Global Health*, 105.

12. Packard, *History of Global Health*, 72.

13. Packard, *History of Global Health*, 89.

14. Packard, *History of Global Health*, 109.

15. Packard, *History of Global Health*, 156–157.

16. Packard, *History of Global Health*, 159.

17. https://www.who.int/teams/social-determinants-of-health/declaration-of-alma-ata#:~:text=The%20Alma%2DAta%20Declaration%20of,goal%20of%20Health%20for%20All.

18. Http://www.who.int.governance, Constititution of the World Health Organization

19. Packard, *History of Global Health*, 228.

20. Packard, *History of Global Health*, 229.

21. Packard, *History of Global Health*, 254.

22. Packard, *History of Global Health*, 250.

23. Jamrozik et al., "Ethical Aspects of Malaria".

24. V. A. Rauh et al., "Impact of Prenatal Chlorpyrifos Exposure on Neurodevelopment in the First 3 Years of Life among Inner-City Children," *Pediatrics* 118, no. 6 (2006): e1845–e1859.

25. WE-Empower, Inc., "Synthetic Pesticides in Africa: The Good, the Bad, and the Ugly," *AgriLINKS*, February 28, 2019, https://agrilinks.org/post/synthetic-pesticides-africa-good-bad-and-ugly.

26. Gibreel A. A. Nesser et al., "Levels of Pesticides Residues in the White Nile Water in the Sudan," *Environmental Monitoring and Assessment* 188 (2016): 374; E. M. Osoro et al., "Organochlorine Pesticides Residues in Water and Sediment from Rusinga Island, Lake Victoria, Kenya," *IOSR Journal of Applied Chemistry* 9, no. 9 (2016): 56–63; Edwin Dobb, "Why Poison Is a Growing Threat to Africa's Wildlife," *National Geographic*, August 2018, https://www.nationalgeographic.com/magazine/2018/08/poisoning-africa-kenya-maasai-pesticides-lions-poachers-conservationists/; and WE-Empower, Inc., "Synthetic Pesticides in Africa."

27. US Environmental Protection Agency, "DDT—A Brief History and Status," April 21, 2022, https://www.epa.gov/ingredients-used-pesticide-products/ddt-brief-history-and-status.

28. https://www.brsmeas.org/Implementation/.

29. P. Ndebele and R. Musesengwa, "Viewpoint: Ethical Dilemmas in Malaria Vector Research in Africa: Making the Difficult Choice Between Mosquito, Science, and Humans," *Malawi Medical Journal* 24, no. 3 (September 2021): 65–68.

30. Newstory about suppository.

31. Jamrozik et al., "Ethical Aspects of Malaria."

32. Sonia Shah, *The Fever: How Malaria Has Ruled Humankind for 500,000 Years* (New York: Picador Press, 2010), 14.

33. Laurie Zoloth, "At the Last Well on Earth: Climate Change as a Feminist Issue," *Journal of Feminist Studies in Religion* 33, no. 2 (2017): 139–151.

34. Denise L. Doolan, Carlota Dobaño, and J. Kevin Baird, "Acquired Immunity to Malaria," *Clinical Microbiology Reviews* 22, no. 1 (2009): 13–36.

35. Ingrid Chen, "'Asymptomatic' Malaria: A Chronic and Debilitating Infection That Should Be Treated," *PLoS Medicine, Policy Forum* 13, no. 1 (2016): e1001942.

36. Chen, "'Asymptomatic' Malaria."

37. Amy Maxmen, "The Enemy in Waiting," *Nature* 559 (July 2018): 458–465.

38. Maxmen, "The Enemy."

39. Jamrozik et al., "Ethical Aspects of Malaria."

40. Jamrozik et al., "Ethical Aspects of Malaria."

41. Menna Smit, "Safety and Mosquitocidal Efficacy of High-Dose Ivermectin When Co-Administrated with Dihydroartemisisin-Piperaquine in Kenyan Adults with Uncomplicated Malaria (IVERMAL): A Randomized, Double-Blind, Placebo-Controlled Trial," *Lancet Infectious Diseases* 18, no. 6 (2018): 615–626.

42. D. Bagster Wilson, "Implications of Malarial Endemicity in East Africa," *Transactions of the Royal Society of Tropical Medicine and Hygiene* 32, no. 4 (1939): 435–465.

43. Heidi Leford, "Malaria Vaccine Shows Promise—Now Come Tougher Trials," *Nature* 593, no. 7857 (2021): 17.

44. http://www.brsmeas.org/Implementation/MediaResources/PressReleases/TheendofDDT/tabid/8971/language/en-US/Default.aspx.

45. Franklin G. Miller, "The Stateville Penitentiary Malaria Experiments: A Case Study in Retrospective Ethical Assessment," *Perspectives in Biology and Medicine* 56, no. 4 (Autumn 2013): 548–567.

46. However, it did interest the defense lawyers in the Nuremberg trial, who used it to prove how widespread the practice of using prisoners in research was.

47. Bennett et al., op. cit.

48. Engineering Biology Research Consortium, "What Is Synthetic/Engineering Biology?" https://ebrc.org/what-is-synbio/.

49. National Institute of Standards and Technology, "Engineering Biology," March 10, 2020, https://www.nist.gov/mml/bbd/primary-focus-areas/engineering-biology#:~:text =Engineering%20biology%20(also%20known%20as,advanced%20therapies%2C%20 advanced%20material%20manufacturing%2C.

50. Website for project: http://syntheticbiology.org/Who_we_are.html.

51. These issues are obvious to any bioethicist, humanities scholar, or historical or social theorist who reads that preceding definition, and they include: a sense that nature is a commodity whose existence can be improved for human use; a sense that the biological world can be understood as a sort of machine, with parts that bear scant relationship to a particular whole; that the givenness of order as we find it is mutable and temporal; and a sense that our intervention is sanguine, for such a world can be taken apart and reconstructed much like any machined element of society. Reflected as well is a positive and pragmatic idea that the power of basic research can be harnessed. This footnote is not intended as a critique of these ideas but rather as a note that the author and the reader understand that such are the ideas behind the declarative sentences. The ontological and epistemic phenomenon of this work is not the subject of this limited white paper.

52. Mark Bedau, "The Nature of Life," in *The Philosophy of Artificial Life*, ed. Margaret Boden (Oxford: Oxford University Press, 1996).

53. Howard Hughes Medical Institute, "Jack W. Szostak, PhD," 2006, http://www .hhmi.org/research/investigators/szostak_bio.html.

54. New Scientist, "Is this life?"

55. Could one set in place the core chemical requirements for biological life by assembling the elements presumed to be available in primordial Earth, and, by creating conditions for evolutionary processes, set them in motion, create a model system, and watch it evolve? What would be the implications of such a project: an RNA world set in motion by single-stranded RNA? Szostak is not alone in this intellectual project, the creation of an "RNA World," although he did indeed win the Nobel Prize for his research in finding ways to locate genes in mammals and develop the critical tools for manipulating them. Below are some other examples.

David W. Deamer, professor emeritus of chemistry and biochemistry at the University of California, Santa Cruz, and a cadre of pioneers expanded their quest to understand life three decades ago, launching an attempt to build a "protocell." According to Deamer, such an entity must meet ten requirements for life, including (1) having membrane enclosures that (2) can capture energy, (3) maintain ion gradients, (4) encapsulate macromolecules, and (5) divide. Macromolecules must be able (6) to grow by polymerization, (7) to evolve in a way that speeds growth, and (8) to store information. Add to that (9) information store the ability to mutate and (10) to direct growth of catalytic polymers.

Albert J. Libchaber of Rockefeller University engineered a DNA plasmid to express proteins and put them into membranous sacs. They could produce proteins for a few hours but would eventually peter out when the raw materials ran low inside the compartment. They needed to keep the supply coming. So, he and Vincent Noireaux, now an assistant professor at the University of Minnesota, designed them to produce a channel-forming protein, alpha hemolysin. Suddenly, finished proteins tagged with green fluorescent protein inserted themselves into the artificial membrane allowing nucleotides and other molecules to enter. These "cells" survive for up to four days, but it's only a small victory. In the quest to build life, defining success is hard, Libchaber says. Is it success simply to create a cell that functions? Or must it also reproduce? "I think in our case at least, the first step has been achieved." Next, he wants to make them divide—something that's only been done thus far through physical manipulation.

The idea of developing a synthetic biological organism that can divide into copies of itself is more than a goal of purely investigative research: one clear plan for the work is in its application and use. For engineers, such restructuring is a part of how their field is intended: using biological parts is merely a difference in kind and not intent. In their manifestation, naturally occurring solutions to problems may be discarded in favor of one with a better (more intelligent) design. It was a new way of thinking about genetic alteration.

56. C. S. Lewis, "The Abolition of Man," in *On Moral Medicine*, ed. Stephen E. Lammers and Allen Vehey, 274.

57. Lewis, "Abolition of Man."

58. Daniel Callahan, "Science, Limits and Prohibitions," *Hastings Center Report* 3, no. 5 (November 1973): 5–7.

59. Joseph Fletcher, "Technological Devices in Medical Care," in *Who Shall Lie*, ed. Kenneth Vaux (Fortress Press, 1970).

60. John Fletcher, *Human Gene Therapy* (Georgetown, 1990), 57.

61. Nancy King, "RAC Oversight of Gene Transfer Research: A Model worth Extending?" *Journal of Law, Medicine and Ethics* 30, no. 3 (2002): 381–389.

62. There is extensive literature on this topic that makes this argument: Eric Parens, beginning with a Hastings Center project, extending to a report in the *Hastings Center Report*, and following with a book on the issue, makes the claim cogently, and Leon Kass and Francis Fukayama, in both individually authored books and in the President's Council Report, make the claim as well.

63. Letter to José Francesco Corrê a Da Serra—Monticello, April 11, 1820.

64. Quote Fancy, "Aldous Huxley Quotes," https://quotefancy.com/aldous-huxley-quotes.

65. Stephen Maurer, Keith Lucas, and Starr Terrell, "From Understanding to Action: Community-Based Options for Improving Safety and Security in Synthetic Biology," Goldman School of Public Policy, University of California at Berkeley, funded by the MacArthur foundation, 2006, for presentation at SynBio 2.0 Berkeley, California, May 2006.

66. Milton Leitenberg, *Assessing the Biological Weapons and Bioterrorism Threat* (US Government, 2005), Washington DC, 82–115.

67. Leitenberg, Assessing, p. 99

68. Leitenberg, *Assessing the Biological Weapons*, 82.

69. Leitenberg, *Assessing the Biological Weapons*, 83.

70. Ginia Bellafante, "Die, Beautiful Spotted Lanternfly, Die," *New York Times*, September 16, 2021, https://www.nytimes.com/2021/09/16/nyregion/spotted-lanternfly -nyc.html.

71. Stanford Encyclopedia of Philosophy, "Francis Bacon," December 29, 2003, revised December 7, 2012, http://plato.stanford.edu/entries/francis-bacon/#5.

72. Op. cit., Edison, 16.

73. Edison 16.

74. Stephen Mauer et al., *Carnegie Project on Self Governance in Synthetic Biology* (project report, 2006).

75. Here, we can add that several in the field—Esvelt, Burt, and others—have long promoted this.

76. Op. cit., Edison, Chapter 3.

77. Wood, Gaby, *The Quest for Artificial Life* (2006).

78. Laurie Zoloth, "Rabbinic Magic," *Journal of Medicine and Philosophy*.

79. Wood, Gaby.

80. Wood, Gaby.

81. Edisonpage 16.

82. When modified to those species.

83. Arthur L. Caplan, "No Time to Waste—The Ethical Challenges Created by CRISPR: CRISPR/Cas, Being an Efficient, Simple, and Cheap Technology to Edit the Genomes of Any Organism, Raises Many Ethical and Regulatory Issues Beyond the Use to Manipulate Human Germ Line Cell," *EMBO Reports* 16, no. 11 (2015): 1421–1426.

84. Jeantine Lunshof, "Regulate Gene Editing in Wild Animals," *Nature* 525, no. 9551 (2015): 127.

85. https://www.google.com/search?q=mongoose+in+hawaii&rlz=1C5CHFA _enUS626US626&oq=mongoose+in+hawaii&aqs=chrome..69i57j0l5.6657j1j8&sour ceid=chrome&ie=UTF-8.

86. Wikipedia, "Kudzu," https://en.wikipedia.org/wiki/Kudzu.

87. Lunshof, "Regulate Gene Editing in Wild Animals."

88. https://www.google.com/search?q=how+many+rabbits+are+there+in+australi a&rlz=1C5CHFA_enUS626US626&oq=how+many+rabbits+are+there+in+aus&aqs =chrome.0.0i512j69i57j0i22i30l3j0i390.8770j0j15&sourceid=chrome&ie=UTF-8.

89. Presidential Commission for the Study of Bioethical Issues, *New Directions: The Ethics of Synthetic Biology and Emerging Technologies* (Washington, DC: Author, 2010).

90. M. Kaiser, "Precaution or Prudent Vigilance as Guiding the Path to Global Food Security?" in *The Ethics of Consumption*, ed. H. Röcklinsberg and P. Sandin (Wageningen: Wageningen Academic Publishers), 71–76.

91. C. Mora et al., "Global Risk of Deadly Heat," *Nature Climate Change* 7 (2017): 501–506.

Conclusion

1. J. B. S. Haldane, "The Future of Biology," in *On Being the Right Size and Other Essays*, ed. J. M. Smith (Oxford: Oxford University Press, 1985), 15.

2. Haldane, "Future of Biology," 13.

3. Haldane, "Future of Biology," 14.

4. Michael Strevens, *The Knowledge Machine: How Irrationality Created Modern Science* (New York: Liveright Publishing Corporation, 2020).

5. Joshua Rothman, "The Rules of the Game: How Does Science Really Work?" *The New Yorker*, September 28, 2020, 67–71.

6. Haldane, "Future of Biology," 24.

7. I must point how here that one of my science colleagues, on his review of this manuscript, was appalled that I said this. How can you honestly know, he asked, how can you even say that? Well, I thought as I read his comment, it seems to me to be obvious. Consider only the solar system, how little we know, then consider even one of the many puzzles in genetics, how epigenetics works across generation. Even in bioethics, we are constantly learning and reevaluating, and our discipline, moral philosophy, has been at it far longer that scientists. I might also add that it is a truism in many religious traditions, and especially in Jewish thought, and even ritualized in two places in the practice, once, when the larger half of the Afikomen is hidden at

the Passover Seder, and once in the way the Sukkat is built, when the booth is made covered with branches so there is more shade than sun.

8. Cary Funk, Brian Kennedy, and Courtney Johnson, "Trust in Medical Scientists Has Grown in U.S., but Mainly Among Democrats," Pew Research Center, May 21, 2020, https://www.pewresearch.org/science/2020/05/21/trust-in-medical-scientists-has -grown-in-u-s-but-mainly-among-democrats. While there has been some literature to suggest that the pandemic has made scientific testimony more credible, this has only been the case among Democrats. World-wide, this has translated to opposition to mask, lock-downs, and vaccine resistance.

9. Karl R. Popper, *The Logic of Scientific Discovery* (XXX: Routledge, New York, 1959); Richard Rudin, "The Scientist Qua Scientist Makes Value Judgments," *Philosophy of Science* 20, no. 1 (1953): 1–6.

10. Rudin, "Scientist Qua Scientist."

11. Jacques Derrida and Maurizio Ferraris, *A Taste for the Secret*, trans. G. Donis (Malden, MA: Blackwell Press); Michael Anker, *The Ethics of Uncertainty* (XXX: Atropos Press, New York, 2009).

12. One of the scientific reviewers suggested "just do a risk assessment" but that of course, misses the point that one cannot by definition know what perfectly innocuous gesture may, in a decade be the one unforeseen thing that was crucial a larger historical sequence. In fact, entire internet discussion turn on this fact. ("what small thing changed history the most?" gets thousands of responses.)

13. Christine Korsgaard, *The Sources of Normativity*, ed. Onora O'Neill (Cambridge: Cambridge University Press, 1996).

14. Strevens, *Knowledge Machine*.

15. In classic Jewish theology, one is not to inquire what came before Bereshit or the first word in the Hebrew Bible. The first letter of the first word faces only in one direction—forward—and from that, the rabbinic commentators take the normative advice of not inquiring behind the start of the story. It is a little like this.

16. Ruth R. Faden and Tom L. Beauchamp, *A History and Theory of Informed Consent* (Oxford: Oxford University Press, 1986).

17. Richard H. Thaler and Cass R. Sunstein, *Nudge: Improving Decisions About Health, Wealth, and Happiness* (New Haven, CT: Yale University Press, 2008).

18. Drew Endy, in talk at the SynBio 3.0 conference in London.

19. Austin Burt et al., "Gene Drive to Reduce Malaria Transmission in Sub-Saharan Africa," *Journal of Responsible Innovation* 5 (2018): S66–S80; Austin Burt and Andrea Crisanti, "Gene Drive: Evolved and Synthetic," *ACS Chemical Biology* 13 (2018): 343–346.

20. C. M. Collins et al., "Effects of the Removal or Reduction in Density of the Malaria Mosquito, *Anopheles gambiae* s.l., on Interacting Predators and Competitors in Local Ecosystems," *Medical and Veterinary Entomology* 33, no. 1 (2019): 1–15.

21. And honest researchers can articulate what is plausible and what is implausible which can take a great deal of courage.

22. Collins et al., "Effects of the Removal or Reduction in Density of the Malaria Mosquito," 4.

23. Anker, *The Ethics of Uncertainty*, 61.

24. Alasdair MacIntyre, *After Virtue* (Notre Dame, IN: University of Notre Dame Press, 1981).

25. Anker, *The Ethics of Uncertainty*, 61.

26. "AAAS Principles for Heritable Genetic Intervention," in *Designing Our Descendants: The Promises and Perils of Genetic Modifications* (Washington, DC: AAAS Press, 1999), frontispiece.

27. I served as a reviewer for vaccine exception requestions for a large American health care system and this fear was raised consistently. My UK reviewers said, however that they did not think it was an issue in the UK, but it was in the USA.

28. Strevens, *Knowledge Machine*.

29. Anker, *The Ethics of Uncertainty*, 81.

30. Anker, *The Ethics of Uncertainty*, 83.

31. Anker, *The Ethics of Uncertainty*, 103.

Index

Accommodation in evolution, 7–8, 325n15
Accra, Ghana, 194
Acquired immunity, 46, 47–48, 253
  and chronic low-level malaria, 46, 47, 48, 253–254
  and inattention to Africa in WHO campaign, 52
  loss of, 9, 46, 47, 54, 70–71, 72, 172
  natural, 47, 257
  in vaccine response, 71, 74, 256–257
Acres, USA, 201–204
ACT (artemisinin-based combination therapies), 59, 62, 63, 67, 140, 251
Adams, Jane, 165
Adams, William, 161
Adaptation, 24, 79, 267
  in mosquito biting time, 24, 60, 291
Adenovirus in *OTC* gene therapy, 121, 122
Aedes, 101, 141
Aedes aegypti, 11, 83, 146
Africa, 57–62. *See also specific countries and regions*
  agriculture in, 6, 7, 8, 57, 175
  Anopheles gambiae in, 46, 157, 159–160
  bed nets in, 59–60, 68, 159
  bioethics in context of, 197–198
  cassava in, 213–216

colonialism in, xxvi, xxxiv, 12, 16–18, 157, 163, 166–173, 197–198, 240
community engagement in, 158, 180, 183, 292
control over care in, 167
COVID-19 vaccines in, 238
endemic malaria in, 46–47, 52, 71
epidemic malaria in, 57, 58
gross domestic product in, 158, 174
health-care system in, 52–53, 57, 58
history of malaria in, 5–7, 166–175
HIV infection and AIDS in, 57, 58, 166, 167
inattention to, in anti-malaria efforts, 57
incidence of malaria in, 60, 62, 67–68, 173, 253
insecticide use in, 69, 248–249
as living laboratory, 169–171
malaria vaccine trials in, 71–75
migration in, 53
military impact of malaria in, 39
pilot anti-malaria programs in, 48, 52, 54
Plasmodium falciparum in, 46, 62
scramble for, xxvi, 16, 170
sickle cell disease in, 8–9
slaves taken from, 12, 13, 166, 169, 215, 240
stakeholder engagement in, xxxiv, 160, 163–198, 234, 315

Africa (cont.)
　Target Malaria in, 97, 163, 166, 173,
　　180–189
　traditional and indigenous
　　knowledge in, 171–172
　view in US on, xix, 323n2
　WHO anti-malaria campaign in,
　　46–47, 48, 52, 53–54, 62
African chrysanthemums, 39, 60
African Malaria Conference (1950), 52
African Medicines Regulatory
　Harmonization, 158
African Network on Biosafety Expertise,
　158, 205
African Research Survey, 170
African Union, 113, 147, 157–160
　community engagement process in,
　　183
　Gates Foundation funding in, 205
　gene drives in, 101, 157–160, 183,
　　205
　and New Partnership for Africa's
　　Development (NEPAD), 157, 205
Agency for International Development
　(US), 246–247
Agragene, 102
Agriculture
　in Africa, 6, 7, 8, 57, 175
　climate change affecting, 175, 251,
　　252
　DDT use in, 50, 222, 248, 249
　gene drives in, 202, 208
　golden rice in, 192, 205, 231–232,
　　233–234
　Green Revolution in, 206, 207, 210
　in India, 32–33
　in Italy, xvi, 27
　and malnutrition in crop failure, 33
　regulation of GMOs in, 119, 125, 131,
　　134, 137
　screwworms as pest in, 216–219
　Shiva on, 206–207
　in United States, 25, 119, 125

Agrippa, Cornelius, 276
AIDS, 57, 58, 59, 166, 167
Algeria, Laveran in, 16–18
Alice in Wonderland (Carroll), 78, 79–80
Allele frequency, gene drives affecting,
　78, 81–82
Allenby, Edmund, 30
Alma-Ata, Declaration of, 245–247
Alving, Alf, 43, 44
American Acclimatization Society, 289
American Association for the
　Advancement of Science (AAAS),
　xxiii, 123–124, 147
　on four questions in ethical
　　assessment, xxiii, 124, 234–235,
　　313–315
American colonies, malaria in, 12,
　13–15
American Society of Tropical Medicine,
　37
American South, xxvi, 25, 36–37
American way in malaria control, 24–26
Amyris Biotechnology, 224
Anemia
　in pregnancy, 255
　sickle cell, 8–9, 125
Angola, 158
Anker, Michael, 312, 317
Annas, George, 156
Anopheles, 4, 11, 20, 21
　in American South, 37
　gene drives in, 89, 90
Anopheles arabiensis, 6, 97
Anopheles coluzzii, 97, 103, 136
Anopheles culicifacies, 32
Anopheles funestus, 6, 97
Anopheles gambiae, xvi, xxi, 6
　in Africa, 46, 157, 159–160
　African Union on gene drive for, 157,
　　159–160
　and Allied forces in WWII, 39–40
　community questions on, 183
　in ecological risk assessment, 195, 290

in Kyrou and Hammond research, 105

male-biased, 188

NASEM report on gene drives for, 146

as super-transmitters, 6–7

in Target Malaria, 97, 99, 136, 183, 188, 195

as target of gene drives, 284

Anopheles Mascariensisi, 7

Anopheles melas, 7

Anopheles moucheti, 7

Anopheles nili, 7

Anopheles Paludi, 7

Anopheles stephensi, 89, 101

Anthrax, 273

Anthropocene, xvii

Aporetic uncertainty, 302, 303, 316
  ethical research in, 310
  freedom in, 317
  and risks of knowledge, 312–313
  in science, 302

Appendix M on recombinant DNA technology, 117, 118

Aquinas, Thomas, 132

Arabs in Palestine, in anti-malaria interventions, 31, 32

Arctic Circle, malaria in, 15, 34

Arendt, Hannah, xviii, 42, 193

Aristotle, 132, 274, 290

Arnold, David, 168

Artemether, 67

Artemisia annua, 56, 349n46

Artemisinin
  in Africa, 59
  in challenge trials, 259
  in China, 56–57
  in combination therapies (ACT), 59, 62, 63, 67, 140, 251
  price of, 57, 59, 349n46
  resistance to, 24, 59, 62, 67, 251
  synthetic biology project on, 223–224, 263, 281, 349n46
  in Thailand, 63

Artesunate, 67

Asexual reproduction, 2, 79

Asilomar State Park meeting, 117, 126, 137, 139, 270
  bioethics as concern in, xxiii, 115–116
  on need for safety and oversight, 118, 134, 144, 269, 282, 288

Asymptomatic malaria, 48, 253–254

Atabrine (Quinacrine), 38, 39, 40, 41

Austin, Thomas, 290

Australia, 214, 223, 290

Automata, 276–277, 278, 280, 281

Autonomy principle, 124, 307

Aykroyd, Wallace, 243

Bacillus malariae, 18

Bacon, Francis, 275

Bacterial diseases, 17–18, 33
  syphilis in, 42–44, 65, 116, 155, 260

Bacterial DNA, 88–89, 114

Bad air as source of malaria, 17

Balkans, malaria in, 15

Baltimore, malaria in, 12

Bana village, sterile male mosquitoes released in, 135, 136, 186–187

Banks, Joseph, 178

Bantu people, 6, 7, 9

Barber, M. A., 37

Barefoot doctors in China, 55

Basel, Rotterdam, and Stockholm Conventions, 249, 259

Bataan, military impact of malaria in, 38, 39

Bed nets, 21, 24, 59–60, 68
  access to, 241
  adaptation of mosquitoes to, 24, 60, 291
  children sleeping under, 60, 72, 75, 159, 248
  climate change affecting use of, 251
  in combination with other control strategies, 140
  distribution of, 72

Bed nets (cont.)
  effectiveness of, 234, 291
  eradication as goal of, 291
  as fish nets, 60, 195, 248
  insecticide treated, xxvii, xxxi, 59, 60, 69, 248
  World Bank sale of, 58, 60
Bedouins, 31, 32
Being and nonbeing categories, 276
Bell, Graham, 78
Belmont Report, 117, 118
Benedict, Mark, 109
Benefits and harms compared, 278, 309–310
  in House of Lords report, 142
  in NASEM report, 144–145
  uncertainties in, 309–310
Bengal famine (1943), 243
Bennett, Gaymon, 164
Berg, Paul, 114
Berger, Peter, 228
Berlin Conference of International African Association (1884), 169
Bermudas, 14
Beta carotene in golden rice, 231–232, 233–234
Biased gene conversion, 85
Bias in sex ratio, male, 87, 94, 100, 103, 188, 192
Bicycles, for travel to health care clinic, 250
Bier, Ethan, 89, 101–102, 103
Bignami, Amico, 19, 20
Bill & Melinda Gates Foundation, 59, 98, 150, 224
  opposition to, 202, 204–205, 206, 210, 223
  species mapping project of, 290
BioCassava Plus, 214
Biocentis, 292, 293
Biodiversity, 205–206, 232
  African Union report on, 159–160
  community concerns about, 183

NASEM report on, 148–149
UN Convention on, 149, 203, 204, 205
"Biodiversity, GMOs, Gene Drives, and the Militarised Mind" (Shiva), 205–206
Bioethics, xxii–xxiv, 115–116, 342n113
  in African context, 197–198
  Asilomar meeting on, xxiii, 115–116
  foundational narratives of, xxii–xxiii
  in gene drives, xxiii–xxiv, 197
  logic of, 285–298
  in public health, xxiv–xxv
  theory of evil lacking in, 270, 271
Biofuelwatch, 205
Biological control of cassava mealybug, 96, 213–216
Biological weapons, 270, 272. See also Dual use problem
Biosafety, 94–96, 270, 271–274. See also Safety issues
Birds
  DDT affecting, 50–51
  GBIRd group concern for, 110, 161, 232
  introduction and spread of, 223, 289
  mice as threat to, 110, 146, 161, 232, 292
  Ross research using, 21
Bites of female mosquitoes, xxi, 3–5, 6
  adaptability in timing of, 24, 60, 291
  bed nets in prevention of (see Bed nets)
  Celli interventions for prevention of, 26–27
  in climate change, 251
  doublesex gene affecting, 105
  incubation period between bite and illness, 11
  Plasmodium transmission in, 2, 3–5
  preference for human blood in, 4, 5–6, 91
  in research trials, 260

Blackburn, Elizabeth, 265
Blackwater fever, 24
Blindness in vitamin A deficiency, 231
Blood meal of female mosquitoes, xxi,
    2, 3, 19, 91
  preference for human blood in, 4,
    5–6, 91
Blood tests, 49, 63, 254
Blumenberg, Hans, 164
BMJ, 72
Bonifacio Integral, 27–28
Boston, malaria in, 12
Botswana, 158
Botulinum toxin, 273
Boyer, Herbert, 114
Brandeis, Louis, 30
Brandt, Allan, 65
Brazil, cinchona tree in, 12–13
Breeding
  DNA alteration in, 220–221
  of rice, 231–232
Bright lines in gene therapy, 123,
    124
British Association for Science, 169
British Medical Association, 21
British Royal Society, xx
Brody, Baruch, 305
Brown, Zachery, 154
Brucellosis, 55
Bubonic plague, 64
Burden of proof in precautionary
    approach, 130, 132
Burkina Faso, 105, 173–175, 176, 189
  Bana village in, 135, 136, 186–187
  colonial history of, 240
  community engagement in, 103, 188,
    191
  as initial site for Target Malaria, 163,
    173
  insectary in, 103, 135–136
  malaria vaccine in, 74
  mark-release-recapture technique in,
    187

National Biosafety Committee of,
    103, 187
  selection as site for mosquito release,
    96–97, 103
Burt, Austin, xx, xxi, xxii, xxvi–xxvii,
    77–82, 84–96
  on biosafety, 94–96
  on cassava mealybug control, 96,
    213–214, 216
  on DNA repair mechanisms, 85
  on fifth force, 80–81, 90
  on gene drives, xx, 77–78, 85, 90–96,
    153–154, 193, 283
  on homing endonuclease genes,
    85–87
  House of Lords testimony of, 141
  at Imperial College London, xx, xxx,
    79
  Journal of Responsible Innovation
    article, 152–154
  NASEM presentations of, 143
  NAS presentations of, 77–78, 90–94,
    213–214
  Red Queen theory, 78, 79–80
  on selfish genetic elements, 80–82,
    90, 332n11
  STS Association presentation, 151
  on suppression and modification
    strategies, 90–93
  on Target Malaria, 96, 98–101, 103
  on uncertainties, 91–93
Burt laboratory at Imperial College
    London, xxx, xxxiv, 84, 88, 113, 141
Byron, Lord, death from malaria, 15
Bystander critique of interventions,
    ethical issues in, 234, 286–287, 298

Caged mosquitoes, xvi, 95, 99, 105–106
Callahan, Daniel, 268
Cambodia, 62
Canada, mosquito population in, 78
Cane toads, 223
Caplan, Arthur, 286

CAR (chimeric antigen receptor) T cells, 88, 125, 301
Carbon dioxide, mosquito detection of, 2, 260
Caribbean Islands, WHO anti-malaria campaign in, 49
Carotene in golden rice, 231–232, 233–234
Carroll, Lewis, 78
Carson, Rachel, 50–51, 248, 314
Cartagena Protocol on Biosafety, 129, 134–135
Carter, Jimmy, 117
Cascata delle Marmore (Marmore Falls), xv–xvii
Cas proteins, 89
  and CRISPR-Cas9 technique (see CRISPR-Cas9 technique)
Cassava, 96, 213–216
Casuistry, 118, 120
Cats, DDT affecting, 49
Cattle, screwworms as pest of, 216–219
Cattle Growers' Association, 217
Celli, Angelo, 26–27, 65, 111, 239
Centers for Disease Control and Prevention, 119
Central Park (NYC), birds introduced into, 223, 289
Cerebral malaria, 17, 56, 60, 69
  malaria vaccine increasing risk for, 72, 73
Challenge trials, 43–44, 259, 328n77
Charo, Alta, 120, 126
Charpentier, Emmanuelle, 88–89
Chikungunaya, 146
Children
  adverse effects of malaria in, 232, 294
  artemisinin-based combination therapy in, 59
  asymptomatic malaria in, 254
  bed nets for, 60, 72, 75, 159, 248
  incidence of malaria in, 174
  intermittent therapy in, 67

malaria reinfection in, 70–71, 72
malaria vaccine in, 71–75, 257–258, 294
mortality rate from malaria, 60
suppository drug therapy in, 250
vitamin A deficiency in, 231
Children's Bureau, 242
Chile, WHO anti-malaria campaign in, 49
Chimeric antigen receptors (CARs), 88, 125, 301
China
  CRISPR-Cas9 technique in, 123–124
  Cultural Revolution in, xxvi, 55
  Four Pests campaign in, 55
  history of malaria in, 6, 10, 54–57
  Manson research in, 19
  public health initiatives in, 37, 54–55
Chinese Communist Party, 54–55
Chinese wormwood, 56, 223–224.
  See also Artemisinin
Chloroquine, 45
  price of, 57
  resistance to, 51, 56, 67, 252
  in WHO anti-malaria campaign, 50
Cholera, 64, 65
Christianity, 10
Christophers, Samuel Rickard, 33, 251
Chronic low-level malaria, 46, 47, 48, 253–254
Church, George, 89, 151, 336n1
Cinchona trees, 12–13, 38
Cleaning the tropics, Gorgas approach to, 28–29
Climate change, xxviii, 248, 251–252
  agriculture in, 175, 251, 252
  ethical issues in, 251–252, 294
  incidence of malaria in, xxviii–xxix, 248, 251–252, 294
Clinical Gene Transfer Research (CGTR) committee, 119, 120
Clinical trials
  adverse reactions in, 121–122
  challenge trials in, 43–44, 259, 328n77

ethical issues in, 259–261
human landing catches of
mosquitoes in, 259–260
on hydroxychloroquine (sontochin),
42, 43–44
on leukemia therapy, 125
on malaria vaccine, 71–75, 260
regulation of, 137
on syphilis, 43–44, 116, 155, 260
Cloning research, 113
Clothing in mosquito bite prevention,
26, 27
Coal mine accidents, 177–180
Co-development approach in Target
Malaria, 173, 176, 184, 186,
191
Coggeshall, Lowell, 43
Cohen, Jonathan, 229
Cohen, Stanley, 114
Colonialism, 34
in Africa, xxvi, xxxiv, 12, 16–18,
157, 163, 166–173, 197–198,
240
control over care in, 167
economic impact of, 240, 243
in India, 32–33, 169, 243, 251
and military role in malaria control,
63
native population growth as concern
in, 222
non-native species introduced in,
289–290
in North America, 12, 13–15
and public health efforts, 243
in South America, 13
in WHO anti-malaria campaign, 53
Commons, 189–190
Commonwealth Scientific and
Industrial Research Organization
(CSIRO), 135–136
Community engagement, xxx, xxxiii
in Africa, 158, 180, 183, 292
NASEM report on, 145–147

in primary health care, 247
Scientist Working Group report on,
140
in Target Malaria, 98, 100, 135, 180,
292
Compaoré, Blaise, 174
Compaoré, François, 174
Confidentiality issues, 253
Conflict of interests, 122, 186
Congo, Democratic Republic of, 173
Consent issues, xxv, 190–191, 260,
346n75
Belmont Report on, 117
in community prior to field studies,
185–186
ethics in, 260, 307–308
of future generations in long-term
research, 275
in genetic engineering, 124
in golden rice research, 233–234
in malaria vaccine trials, 72–73
in opposition to gene drives, 202
in OTC gene therapy, 121, 122
in Target Malaria, 98, 176, 187,
188
in uncertainty, 307–308
in WHO anti-malaria campaign,
49, 53
Consequentialist theory, 306
Containment protocols, 94–95, 284,
288
biosafety levels in, 95
in recombinant DNA research, 116
reversal drives in, 152
in Target Malaria, 99–100
Contextual factors, in four questions of
ethical assessment, xxiii, 124, 235,
313–314
Convention on Biological Diversity
(UN), 149, 203, 204, 205
Corruption in Burkina Faso, 174, 175
Courage, commitment to, 317, 318
Courtier-Orgogozo, Virginie, 109

COVID-19 pandemic, xix, xxv, xxix, 274
   COVID-19 vaccines in, 75, 238
   ethical issues in, 133, 227, 238, 241, 256, 318
   and gain-of-function research, 270
   incidence of malaria in, xxvii–xxviii, 60, 70
   malaria vaccines in, 71, 73, 75
   oversight and regulations in, 272
   pathogen transmission in, 8, 325n15
   research challenges in, 105, 136, 149
   Shiva on, 207
   and Target Malaria, 136, 189
   uncertainties in, 301, 318
Craig, George B., 83
Crisanti, Andrea, 84, 88, 141, 156, 292
Crisanti laboratory at Imperial College London, xxxiv, 84, 94, 113
CRISPR-Cas9 technique, 89–94, 108, 123
   in Bier research, 101, 103
   in China, 123–124
   ethical issues in, 262–264, 286
   in Kyrou and Hammond research, 104
   in leukemia, 125
   NASEM report on, 143–144
   opposition to, 204, 207
   risks in, 155
   uncertainty in, 301
CRISPR-nickase, 103
Cross, Frank, 129–130
Cuba, 28
Culex, 20
Cultural Revolution in China, xxvi, 55
Cummings, Claire Hope, 205
Curtis, Chris F., 84

Darien colony in Panama, 14–15, 217
Darwin, Charles, 78–79
Data collection, and Iron Rule of science, 300
Data Safety Monitoring Boards, xxiv, 125

Davy, Humphrey, xxxiv, 177–180, 188
Davy lamp, 178, 180
DDT, 24, 41–42, 45–47, 310, 342n113
   in agriculture, 50, 222, 248, 249
   in China, 55
   environmental impact of, 49, 50–51, 248–249
   ethical issues in use of, 248–249, 261
   home use of, 245, 261
   in Integrated Vector Management, 249
   and malaria vaccine, 259
   regulation of, 239, 249
   resistance to, 49–50, 51, 108, 314
   in WHO anti-malaria campaign, 46, 49–51
   widespread use of, 222, 248, 314
Deamer, David W., 353n55
Death rate in malaria. *See* Mortality rate in malaria
Decision making in uncertainty, 308–313, 316
   in dilemmas, 304, 305
   for nonaction, 311
Declaration of Alma-Ata, 245–247
Declaration of Helsinki, 238
Defense Advanced Research Projects Agency (DARPA), 204, 206–207
Deforestation in Burkina Faso, 175
Del Chilton, Mary, 119
Dementia in syphilis, 42–43
Dengue fever, 42, 101, 143, 144, 146, 201, 251
Dentatus, Manius Curius, xvi
Derrida, Jacques, 302
Dewey, John, 165
Diabaté, Abdoulaye, 187
Diagnosis of malaria
   in asymptomatic infection, 253–254
   blood tests in, 49, 63, 254
   PCR technique in, 254
Dichlorodiphenyltrichloroethane. *See* DDT

Dickens, Charles, 15
Dictionary project in Target Malaria,
    183–184, 192
Diderot, Denis, 281
Dilemmas, 304, 305
Directed targeting, 87
Distributive justice, 296
DNA
    bacterial, 88–89, 114
    and H3Africa data, 176
    historical alteration in breeding
        practices, 220–221
    and homing endonuclease genes,
        85–86
    as identity, 220, 302
    as immutable characteristic, 302
    knocking in or knocking out
        process, 88
    mitochondrial, transfer of, 124
    opposition to alteration of, 220
    PCR analysis of, 84, 254
    recombinant (see Recombinant DNA)
    repair system in damage of, 85–86,
        88–89, 93
Dobzhansky, Theodosius, 83
Doctors' Trial at Nuremberg, xxii–xxiii,
    xxiv, 44, 116, 147, 237–238, 240
Doctors Without Borders, 72
doublesex gene drive, 112, 142, 292–294
    Kyrou and Hammond research on,
        104–105, 109, 292–294
    licensing and patent on, 292, 293
    resistance to, 105, 107–108
Doudna, Jennifer, 88–89
Drift, and evolution, 80
Drinking water safety, 65
"Driven to Extinction" (ETC Group
    Report), 204, 205
Driving Y, xx, 83–87, 93–94, 99, 104
Drug therapy
    artemisinin in (see Artemisinin)
    atabrine in, 38, 39, 40, 41
    in children, 59, 250

chloroquine in (see Chloroquine)
cost of, 57, 59, 250, 349n46
counterfeit drugs in, 250, 251
ethical issues in, 242, 250–251
hydroxychloroquine (sontochin) in,
    41, 42, 43–44
intermittent, 59, 67
ivermectin in, 256
as magic bullet, 242
and malaria vaccine combination, 74
mass drug administration in, xxxi,
    255, 256
and multidrug resistance, 67, 224,
    348–349n46
primaquine in, 9, 67, 255
resistance to, 62, 69, 251
dsx gene drive. See doublesex gene drive
Dual use problem, 148, 152, 202, 270,
    271–274
    ethical issues in, xxiii, 265, 271–274,
        314
    governance and regulations in, 126
    NASEM report on, 145, 273
    and opposition to gene drives,
        222–223, 225, 226
Duffy bodies, 6, 7, 8, 13, 253
Durable fidelity of malaria
    interventions, 257

East Africa Commission, 171
Easterlin Paradox, 154
Ebers Papyrus, 231
Ebola, 166
Eco, Umberto, 277
Ecological risk assessment, 151. See also
    Environmental concerns
Econexus, 205
Economic issues. See also Funding
    in Africa, 57–58, 59, 158, 171, 172
    in American South, 37
    in colonialism, 240, 243
    as determinant of health, 61, 65, 246,
        248

Economic issues (cont.)
  in endemic malaria, 37
  and ethical issues in malaria
    prevention, 239–241, 258
  importance in malaria eradication,
    111
  inattention to, 35, 36, 50, 54, 244,
    245
  in incidence of malaria, 239–240,
    241
  in India, 33
  and inequality in malaria control
    programs, 51–52, 61
  in Italy, 26, 27, 33–34, 50
  in opposition to gene drives, 225
  in poverty (see Poverty)
  in precautionary approach, 130
  in primary health care, 247
  and profit motivation in gene drives,
    154, 202, 223, 292–294
  in public health, 27, 61, 65, 242–243
  in recession period (1970s), 58
Egalitarianism, 297
Egypt, ancient, 10
Egyptian Expeditionary Force, 30
Ehrlich, Paul, 242
Eichelberger, Robert L., 39
Elephantiasis, 19, 42
Eli Lily, 117
Elliott, Carl, 284
Ellis, Roy, 78
Emerson, Claudia, 187
Employment
  and health of railway workers,
    26–27
  and migration in India, 32
  and safety in coal mines, 177–180
Empowered communities, 145, 158
Endemic malaria, 12, 13, 15, 326n37
  in Africa, 46–47, 52, 71
  immunity in, 46, 47, 328n86
  in Palestine, 32
  social and economic factors in, 37

Endonuclease
  homing, xx, xxii, 82, 84, 85–87,
    90, 93
  restriction, 114
Endy, Drew, 264
Engagement
  of community (see Community
    engagement)
  NASEM report on, 145–147
  of stakeholders (see Stakeholder
    engagement)
Engelhardt, H. Tristram, Jr., 130
Engineering biology, 225, 263, 349n52.
  See also Synthetic biology
Enhancements, genetic interventions
  for, 225
  compared to therapy, 123, 270–271,
    286, 292
  ethical issues in, 225, 270–271,
    286
Environmental, Social, and Health
  Impact Assessment (ESHIA), 101,
    188
Environmental concerns
  in African Union, 159–160, 183
  biodiversity in (see Biodiversity)
  Burt on, 153
  in climate change (see Climate
    change)
  in DDT use, 49, 50–51, 248–249
  of ETC Group, 204, 205
  food web in, 208, 248, 288, 290
  in horizontal transfer of gene drive,
    109
  invasive species in (see Invasive
    non-native species)
  NASEM report on, 151
  in opposition to gene drives, 201–202,
    203, 208, 232, 287–291
  in Target Malaria, 151, 195–196
  uncertainties in, 146
Environmental Protection Agency, 119,
    125, 249

Epidemic malaria, 5, 13, 15
  in Africa, 57, 58
  death rate in, 15
  malnutrition as factor in, 33
  mathematical model of MacDonald
    on, 50
  in post-WWI period, 35
Epistemic uncertainty, 146, 303, 307,
  312, 315
Epistemology and power, Thompson
  on, 155
Eradication of malaria, xxvi, 5, 206
  ethical issues in gene drives for, 5, 291
  Greenpeace opposition to gene drives
    for, 232
  in Italy, xvi
  limited efforts in Africa for, 46, 62
  MacDonald mathematical model on,
    50, 244–245
  military approach to, 22, 28, 34, 45,
    53, 63
  monoclonal antibody research on,
    111
  multiplex genome editing for, 108
  in Palestine, 36
  in Panama, 29
  and screwworm project compared,
    219
  social and economic issues affecting,
    111, 245, 250
  in United States, xxvi, 25, 48
  in WHO anti-malaria campaign, 48,
    49, 50, 52
Escherichia coli, 114, 224, 266, 269, 281,
  282
Esvelt, Kevin, 138, 139, 154, 278, 336n1
  mice research of, 90, 110
  NASEM presentations of, 143
  STS Association presentation,
    151–152
ETC Group, 200–205, 210, 213
Ethics Advisory Committee of Target
  Malaria, xxxiii, 99, 111, 292

Ethics of Gene Therapy, The (Walters &
  Palmer), 122–123
Eucalyptus trees, 30, 31
Eugenics, 83
Eukaryotes, 89
European Medicines Agency, 72
European Union
  precautionary principle in,
    127–129, 131, 141, 142, 232,
    311, 337–338n27
  regulation of GMOs in, 141–143, 232
European Union Community Treaty,
  129
European Way, 24
Evans, Sam Weiss, 156
Evolution, 78–82, 267
  accommodation in, 7–8, 325n15
  fifth force in, xxii, 80–81, 90
  of mosquitoes, Plasmodium, and
    humans, 1–9, 325n15
  and opposition to gene drives, 201
"Evolution of Fitness, The" (Burt), 79
"Existing scholarly commentary," as
  concern in NASEM report, 145–146
Extinction and extermination, 79, 206,
  207
  and eradication of malaria (see
    Eradication of malaria)
  ETC Group concerns on, 204, 205
  and ethical issues in gene drives, 206,
    291
  as risk in horizontal transfer of gene
    drive, 109
  in screwworm project, 217–219

Fabian, Johannes, 211
Faith, and gene drive opposition,
  226–227, 229
Famine, 33, 34, 35, 171, 243
Farmer, Paul, 166–167, 169, 343n8
Fearnley, Lyle, 164
Federal Trade Commission, 119
Felling Colliery accidents, 177

Female mosquitoes, xxi, 6, 23, 24
  accidental release of, 135, 136
  bites of (*see* Bites of female
    mosquitoes)
  gene targeting fertility of, 84,
    103–105
  landing catches in research, 259–260
  life cycle of, 2, 6, 18, 24
Fertility of female mosquitoes, genetic
    targeting of, 84, 103–105
Fever, 10–13, 72, 75, 253
  as syphilis therapy, 43–44, 260
Fever, The (Shah), 4
Fidelity, 257, 258, 317, 318–321
Field studies, 98, 99, 100, 103
  accidental release of females in, 135,
    136
  community concerns in, 135–136
  consent to, 185–186
  core commitments for, 160
  insecticides in, 135, 136
  NASEM report on, 146
  Scientist Working Group on
    regulation of, 139, 140
  stakeholder engagement in, 180–189
Fifth force, xxii, 80–81, 90
Filariasis, 19, 135, 136, 256
Finland, malaria in, 15
First Aliyah, 29
Fish nets, mosquito netting used as, 60,
    195, 248
Fletcher, John, 269
Fletcher, Joseph, 269
Food and Drug Administration, 118,
    119, 121, 122, 125, 154
Food webs, 208, 248, 288, 290
Ford Foundation, 248
Foucault, Michel, 165
Four Pests campaign in China, 55
France, in colonial Africa, 167, 174
Freedom, 317, 319
Freud, Sigmund, 267
Friends of the Earth, 205

Fruit flies, 89, 101, 103, 202
Funding
  and conflict of interests, 122
  from DARPA, 204, 205–206
  and ethical issues in malaria
    prevention, 239–241
  from Gates Foundation, 202,
    204–205, 206, 210, 223
  of gene therapy research, 122, 125
  of health care system, 247
  in high-burden countries, 68, 241
  of malaria vaccine program, 71
  NASEM report on, 145
  of NGOs, 210
  and profit motive in gene drives, 202,
    223
  of Target Malaria, 97–98, 204, 205
  of WHO global campaign, 47, 51, 52
  WHO World Malaria Report on, 68
  World Bank approach to, 58, 60
"Future of Biology, The" (Haldane), 299

Gain of function research, 144, 270
Galileo Galilei, 230
Gambusia (mosquito fish), 31
Gamete killers, 82, 90
Gametocytes of *Plasmodium,* 3, 11
Gantz, Valentino, 89
Gardner, Martha, 65
Gates, Bill, 4
Gates Foundation, 59, 98, 150, 224
  opposition to, 202, 204–205, 206,
    210, 223
  species mapping project of, 290
Gavi, the Vaccine Alliance, 71
GBIRd group, 110, 161, 232
Ge Hong, 56
Geisel, Ted, 40
Gelsinger, Jesse, 121–122, 124, 125
Gender issues, 158–159, 191
"Gene Drives on the Horizon" report of
    NASEM, 78, 90, 143–151, 158, 160,
    331–332n1

Gene editing, 86
  CRISPR-Cas9 technique in
    (*see* CRISPR-Cas9 technique)
Genentech, 117
Genes in Conflict (Burt), xxii
Gene therapy, 118–124, 125, 134
  compared to non-therapeutic
    enhancements, 270–271, 286,
    292
  use of term, 349n52
Genetically modified organisms, 114
  in agriculture, 119, 125, 131, 134,
    137, 192, 202
  golden rice as, 192, 205, 231–232,
    233–234
  grapes as, 283–284
  House of Lords on, 131, 141–143
  NASEM report on, 144, 149
  opposition to, 200, 209, 220, 233
  WHO on, 149, 185, 187
Genetic engineering, xx, 87, 88,
    269–274
  consent in, 124
  creation of gene drives in, 113,
    282–285
  CRISPR-Cas9 technique in (*see*
    CRISPR-Cas9 technique)
  dual-use problem in (*see* Dual use
    problem)
  safety in, 94, 124
  transgressive nature of, 268
  use of term, 349n52
Genetic pollution, gene drives as,
    208
Genetic technology
  four questions in ethical assessment
    of, xxiii, 124, 234–235, 313–315
  use of term, 349n52
Gene Transfer Safety Advisory Board,
    120
Genome editing, 148
Genotaxis, 82
Geoengineering, 209

Geospatial information system (GIS)
    mapping, 196
Gerasol, 41–42. *See also* DDT
Germany
  in colonial history of Africa, 166,
    167
  incidence of malaria in, 34–35
  and Nuremberg trials, xxii–xxiii,
    xxiv, 44, 116, 147, 237–238,
    240
  scientific hygiene in, 33
Germline modification, 123, 286
Germ theory, 17, 64, 65
Ghana
  malaria vaccine in, 71, 73
  Target Malaria in, 103, 106, 163, 180,
    193–196
Ghebreyesus, Tedros Adhanom, 73
GIS mapping, 196
Global anti-malaria campaign of WHO,
    46–54. *See also* WHO global
    anti-malaria campaign
Global Fund to Fight AIDS, Tuberculosis
    and Malaria, 59, 71
Global Infectious Diseases and
    Epidemiological Network
    (GIDEON), 294
Global North, 49, 238, 257
Global South, 49, 51
Global Technical Strategy for Malaria
    (WHO report), xxvii, 66, 153
Glossary project in Target Malaria,
    183–184, 192
Glucose-6-phosphate dehydrogenase
    (G6PD), 9, 255
Glyphosate resistance, 202
Golden rice, 192, 205, 231–232,
    233–234
Goodall, Jane, 203
Gordon Research Conference, 114–115
Gorgas, William, 28–29
Governing the Commons (Ostrom),
    189

Grapes, genetically modified, 283–284
Grassi, Giovanni, 19, 20
Great Britain
  in Africa, 167, 171, 172, 198
  coal mine accidents in, 177–180
  House of Lords in, 101, 113, 131,
    141–143, 147, 160
  in India, 32, 243, 251
  in North America, 12
  in Palestine, 30–32
Great Expectations (Dickens), 15
Greece, ancient, parrhesia concept in,
  314–315
Greenpeace, 148, 232, 233
Green Revolution, 206, 207, 210
Gregory XII, Pope, xvi
Greider, Carol, 265
gRNA (guide RNA), 93, 108, 125
Gross domestic product, 158, 174,
  239–240, 241
GSK, in malaria vaccine development,
  71, 73, 74
Guadalcanal, military impact of malaria
  in, 38, 39
Guide RNA (gRNA), 93, 108, 125
Guterres, António, 238

Habitat of mosquitoes, 22–23, 24, 26,
  310
  in American South, 36–37
  climate change affecting, 251–252
  in Panama Canal construction, 29
  swamps as (see Swamp/marsh areas)
  warfare affecting, 35–36
H3Africa data set, 176
Hailey, William Malcolm, 170–171
Haldane, J. B. S., 299–300
Hamilton, W. D., 83–84
Hammond, Andrew, 104–105, 106, 109,
  111, 193, 292–294
Handler, Philip, 114
HapMap project, 176
Hardin, Garrett, 189

Harms and benefits compared, 278,
  309–310
  in House of Lords report, 142
  in NASEM report, 144–145
  uncertainties in, 309–310
Harrison, Gordon, 4, 7, 22, 23, 36, 53
Hawai'i, mongoose in, 223
Hawai'i SEED, 205
Health
  definition of, 244, 246
  economic and social factors as
    determinants of, 61, 65, 246, 248
  as human right, 244, 246
Health-care system, 242–251
  in Africa, 52–53, 57, 58
  in China, 55–57
  Declaration of Alma-Ata on, 245–247
  funding of, 247
  infrastructure problems in, 250–251
Heisenberg effect, 312
He Jiamkui, 123–124
Hemolysis, 10
Hepatitis, Willowbrook experiment on,
  116
Herd immunity, xxv, 255
Hickey, W. A., 83
Hippocratic School, 10
Histidine-rich protein (HRP2), 69
History of malaria, xxx, xxxiii–xxxiv
  in Africa, 5–7, 166–175
  in China, 6, 10, 54–57
  evolution of mosquitoes, Plasmodium,
    and humans in, 1–9
  global spread in, 6
  importance of, 63–64
  language of conquest in, 16–37
  in medieval period, 10
  modernity and mortality in, 37–48
  nature of disease in, 1–16
  origin of term in, 17
  in Rome, ancient, xv, xvi, 9–10
  in United States, 12, 13–15, 25–26,
    36–37

vaccine in, 70–75
WHO anti-malaria campaign in, 46–54
in World War I, 34–36
in World War II, 36, 37–45
HIV infection and AIDS, 57, 58, 59, 166, 167
Hofmeyr, Jan, 169
Homing drives, 85–86, 93, 104
Homing endonuclease genes, xx, xxii, 82, 84, 85–87, 90, 93
Homologous repair, 86
Horizontal transfer in gene drives, 109–110, 142, 160, 203, 336n75
Hospitality, theory of, 321–322
House of Lords, 101, 113, 131, 141–143, 147, 160
Housing, 140
    DDT spraying of, 245, 261
    in Italy, 26, 27
    window screens of, 22, 26, 27, 40
HRP2 (histidine-rich protein), 69
Human Gene Therapy Working Group, 118
Human rights issues, 208, 244, 246, 271
Humans
    evolution of mosquitoes, Plasmodium, and, 1–9
    as machines, 280
    as plighted, 304, 311
    preference of mosquitoes for, 4, 5–6, 91
Human waste disposal, 54, 55, 64–65
Humility, commitment to virtue of, 317, 318
Humulin, 117
al-Husseini. Amin, 31
Husserl, Edmund, 262, 263, 268
Huxley, Aldous, 271
Hydroxychloroquine (sontochin), 41, 42, 43–44
Hygiene
    in African colonies, 167
    in China, 54–55

in sanitation campaigns, 25–26, 37, 54–55, 168
scientific, 33

Immune response to Plasmodium, 2, 3–4, 7, 9, 13, 23, 253–254
acquired immunity in (see Acquired immunity)
Duffy bodies in, 6, 7, 8, 13, 253
in endemic malaria, 46, 47, 256–257, 328n86
in syphilis therapy, 43
Imperial College London, 88
    Burt laboratory at, xxx, xxxiv, 84, 88, 113, 141
    Crisanti laboratory at, xxxiv, 84, 94, 113
    doublesex gene drive licensing, 292, 293
    female mosquito fertility research in, 103–105
    regulations on research in, 113
    and Target Malaria, xxx, 99
Imwong, Mallika, 254
Incidence of malaria, 66–70, 261
    in Africa, 60, 62, 67–68, 173
    climate change affecting, xxviii–xxix, 248, 251–252, 294
    in COVID-19 pandemic, xxvii–xxviii, 60, 70
    economic and social factors in, 239–240, 241
    high-burden areas in, 67–68, 173, 241
    in India, 68, 173
    post-WWI, 34–36
    in Thailand, 63
    WHO anti-malaria campaign affecting, 48
    WHO reports on, 66–67, 68, 70, 261
    in World War II, 38–39
India
    agriculture in, 32–33
    colonialism in, 32–33, 169, 243, 251

India (cont.)
   history of malaria in, 10
   incidence of malaria in, 68, 173
   rice problem in, 243
   Ross research on malaria in, 20–21, 32
   WHO anti-malaria campaign in, 48
Inheritance
   gene drives affecting, xx, 77–78
   Mendelian, 80
   selfish genes affecting, xx, xxii, 80–82
Inquiry process, Dewey on, 165
Insecticides, xxvii, xxx
   in American South, 37
   in bug bombs during WWII, 39
   DDT (see DDT)
   ethical issues in use of, 248–250, 261
   nets treated with, xxvii, xxxi, 59, 60,
     69, 248
   regulation of, 239, 248, 249
   resistance to, 49–50, 51, 60, 66, 69,
     108, 182, 314
   in Target Malaria, 135, 136
Institute de Recherche en Sciences de la
     Sante (IRSS), 187
Institutional Biosafety Committees
     (IBCs), 119, 120, 150, 272, 273
Institutional Review Boards (IRBs), xxiv,
     73, 119, 120, 125, 269
Insuco, 188
Insulin, recombinant, 117
Integrated Improvements of Mussolini,
     27–28
Integrated Vector Management, 249
Intermittent treatment, 59, 67
International African Association, Berlin
     Conference of (1884), 169
International Forum on Globalization,
     208
International Monetary Fund, 58
International Rice Research Institute,
     231
International Union of Conservation
     and Nature, 203

Invasive non-native species, 274, 288
   mice as, 110, 146, 161, 232, 292
   mongoose as, 223, 288, 290
   rabbits as, 214, 223, 290
Iron Rule of science, 300–301, 303
Island Conservation, 203
Isoprenoids, 224
Italy, 13, 18, 19–21
   Celli approach to malaria in, 26–27,
     65, 111, 239
   DDT use in, 41–42
   eradication of malaria in, xvi
   history of malaria in, xv, xvi, 9–10
   large-cage research in, xvi, 95, 99, 106
   Marmore Falls in, xv–xvii, 10
   mortality rate from malaria in, 34
   Mussolini approach to malaria in,
     27–28
   swamp drainage in, xv–xvii, 9–10
   Target Malaria research in, 96, 99,
     106
Ivermectin, 256

James, Anthony, 87, 89, 101, 139
Jamestown, Ghana, 194, 197
Jamrozik, Euzebuisz, 241, 248, 255
Jefferson, Thomas, 271
Jerusalem, malaria in, 32
Jesuits in Brazil, and cinchona tree
     powder, 12–13
Jews
   in Nazi Germany, 44
   in Palestine, 29–32
Jonson, Albert, 269
Jotterand, Fabrice, 130
Journal of Responsible Innovation, 151,
     152–154, 158
Justice, 239–241, 294–297
   and burden of disease, 311
   in climate change, 248
   NASEM report on, 145
   and opposition to gene drives,
     224–225

Kaiser, M., 290
Kant, Immanuel, 133
Kass, Leon, 221
Keasling, Jay, 224
Kennedy, Edward, 117
Kenya, malaria vaccine in, 71, 73
Kenya Medical Research Institute, 185
Kibbutz communities, 29–30
Kidwell, Margaret, 87
Killer X chromosomes, 333n22
Killer Y chromosomes, 84–85
Kirk, Norman T., 39
Kligler, Israel Jacob, 30–32
Knipling, Edward, 217
Knock-in genes, 88, 91, 93
Knock-out genes, 88, 91, 93, 104
Knowledge Machine, The (Strevens), 300
Koch, Robert, 17–18, 21, 61, 65
Kopelman, Loretta, 130
Kudzu vine, 288
Kuhn, Thomas, 271
Kuzma, J., 154
Kyrou, Kyros, 104–105, 109, 193, 292–294

Laboratory facilities
  biosafety in, 94–96, 117, 282, 288
  caged mosquitoes in, xvi, 95, 99, 105–106
Landes, Richard, 229
Land reform, 50, 54
Language
  of genetic regulation, 113–124
  and glossary project in Target Malaria, 183–184, 192
  and linguistic uncertainty, 146
  and military terms in malaria control, 22, 34, 35, 36, 53, 63, 242
  nature as term in, 164
  of risk, benefit, and precaution, 124–134
  in stakeholder engagement, 182, 183–184, 192, 193

Laos, 62
Large-cage experiments, xvi, 95, 99, 106
Larvicides, 140, 239
  in American South, 37
  in Italy, 27
  in Panama Canal construction zone, 29
  Paris Green as (see Paris Green)
Last mile problem, xxvi–xxvii, 63
Laveran, Alphonse, 16–19, 20, 21
League of Nations, 35
Legal issues, 129–130, 188
Leishmaniasis, 55
Leitenberg, Milton, 272
Leopold and Loeb case, xxvi, 44
Leukemia, 125
Levinas, Emmanuel, 228
Lewis, C. S., 268
Libchaber, Albert J., 354n55
Liberation theology, 297
Liberia, 52
Libertarianism, 58, 297
Life cycle of Plasmodium, 2–5, 9, 11, 13
  climate change affecting, 251
  immune response to, 253
  liver in, 2, 11, 71
  in low-level infections, 253–254
  red blood cells in, 2, 3, 5–6, 7, 8, 10, 18, 71, 255
  Ross research on, 21
  as vaccine target, 255, 256, 258
Life span of mosquitoes, 23–24
Lindquist, Alfred, 217
Linguistic uncertainty, 146
Liver, Plasmodium in, 2, 11, 71
L9LS antimalarial antibody, 111
Locke, John, 64
Loeb, Leopold, xxvi, 44
Logic of bioethics, 285–298
London School of Hygiene and Tropical Medicine, 71
Longino, Helen, 126–127
Louisiana, 48

Lunshof, Jeantine, 286
Lycorma delicatula (spotted lanternfly), 274
Lyme disease, 110, 152

Macaques, *Plasmodium* infection in, 1
MacArthur, Douglas, 39
Macbeth (Shakespeare), 11
MacDonald, George, 50, 244–245, 251
Madagascar, 58–59, 173
Malaise traps, 196
Malaney, Pia, 239, 241
Malaria Commission (League of Nations), 35, 36
MalariaGEN, 176
Malaria Policy Advisory Group, 73
Malaria Project, 41, 42, 43
Malaria Research Institute, 31
Malaria vaccine, xxxi, 70–75, 294
    clinical trials on, 71–75, 260
    in combination with other control
        strategies, 140, 258–259
    dose schedule in, 71, 74
    ethical issues in, 72–73, 255, 256–259
    funding of, 71
    immunity from, 71, 74, 256–257
    price of, 73
    safety and efficacy of, 72, 73, 75, 258
Malawi, 71, 167
Male mosquitoes
    life cycle of, 2, 3, 6, 18
    in male bias sex ratio, 87, 94, 100,
        103, 188, 192
    mating by, 23, 24
    sterile, release of (*see* Sterile male
        mosquito release)
Male-producing factor in *Aedes*, 83
Mali, 174
    National Ethics Committee in, 197
    Target Malaria in, 96, 103, 105, 163,
        175, 189, 191, 197
Manson, Patrick, 19–21, 168
Mao Tse Tung, 55

Marburg virus, 274
Marchoux, Émile, 35
Marketplace concerns in gene drive
    opposition, 223–224
Mark-release-recapture technique, 187
Marmore Falls (Terni, Italy), xv–xvii, 10
Marsh areas. *See* Swamp/marsh areas
Marsh fever, 11–12, 18
Mass drug administration (MDA), xxxi,
    255, 256
Maternal effect genes, 82
Mating of mosquitoes, 3, 23, 24
Maurer, Stephen, 270, 271
McNamara, Robert, 248
McRoberts, Neil, 154
Mealybug, cassava, biological control of,
    96, 213–216
Measles, xxv, 70
Medieval period, 229
Mefloquine, 62
Meiosis, 82
Mendel, Gregor, 80
Mendelian inheritance, 78, 80
Merozoites of *Plasmodium*, 2–3
Miasmas, 17
Mice
    GBIRd project on, 110, 161
    gene drives in, 143, 146, 161, 203,
        232
    t-haplotype in, 83, 90
    as threat to native birds, 110, 146,
        161, 232, 292
Migration, 29–32, 35, 240
    in climate change, 251, 252
    and evolution, 80
    and WHO anti-malaria campaign,
        53, 245
Military
    in colonial period, 16–18, 63, 167,
        169, 170
    funding of gene drives from, 202
    in India, 20
    in Italy, 27, 28

and language of war in malaria
control, 22, 34, 35, 36, 53, 63, 242
in Palestine, 30, 32
in Panama Canal zone, 28–29
in United States, 22
in WHO anti-malaria campaign, 49
in World War II, 37–45
Millennialism, 229
Misogyny in military anti-malaria liter-
ature, 40
Mitchell, Paul, 154
Mitochondrial DNA transfer, 124
Modernity, 227, 230, 233
Modification drives, 90–91, 92–93, 101,
102, 107
Molecular engineering, 225, 349n52
Moloo, Zahra, 205
Mongoose, 223, 288, 290
Monkeypox, 274
Monoclonal antibody against malaria,
111
Monsanto, 125, 202
Moral issues
in dilemmas, 304, 305
in precautionary principle, 132–133
uneasy/uncanny feeling in, 267–269
Moreno, Jonathan, 305
Morgan, Julia, 115
Mortality rate in malaria, xxi,
xxvii–xxviii, 261
in COVID-19 pandemic, 70
in epidemics, 15
ethical issues in, 284–285
in Italy, 34
in kibbutz communities, 29–30
in malaria vaccine trials, 72, 73
in Palestine, 29–30
from *Plasmodium falciparum*, 7, 12,
13, 14, 60
in post-WWI period, 35, 36
in Russia, 35
in United States, 14, 22, 25
WHO reports on, 70

Mosaicism, 89, 91
Mosquirix malaria vaccine, xxxi, 70–75.
See also Malaria vaccine
Mosquito Coast (Panama), 15
Mosquitoes. *See also specific species*
in climate change, 251–252
DDT for control of (*see* DDT)
early research on, 18, 19, 20–21
ecosystem role of, 201–202
evolution of *Plasmodium*, humans
and, 1–9, 325n15
female (*see* Female mosquitoes)
habitat of (*see* Habitat of mosquitoes)
insecticide resistance, 49–50, 51, 60,
66, 69, 108, 182, 314
life span of, 23–24
male (*see* Male mosquitoes)
Mosquito fish *(Gambusia)*, 31
Mozambique, 158, 173
Mueller, Hermann, 217
Multidrug resistance, 67, 224,
348–349n46
Multinational corporations, stakeholder
engagement of, 181
Multiplex gnome editing, 108
Mummies, ancient, antigens to
Plasmodium in, 10
Mussolini, Benito, 27–28

Namibia, 158
Nanotechnology, 209
Narrative theory in ethical issues,
237
National Academies of Sciences,
Engineering, and Medicine
(NASEM)
on dual use problem, 144, 273
"Gene Drives on the Horizon"
report, 78, 90, 143–151, 158, 160,
331–332n1
on mitochondrial DNA transfer,
124
National Academy of Medicine, 115

National Academy of Sciences, xx, 114, 120, 269
  Burt presentations at, 77–78, 90–94, 213
  Charo at meeting of, 126
  on dual-use problem, 273
National Biosafety Agency, 187
National Commission on the Protection of Human Subjects, 117
National Environmental Policy Act, 126
National Institutes of Health, xxiv, 125, 269, 272
  on dual-use problem, 273
  in gene therapy review, 117, 119, 122
  in Target Malaria funding, 98
National Research Council (NRC), 148
National Science Advisory Board for BioSecurity (NSABB), 273
National Science Foundation, 119
Natural immunity, 47, 257
Natural law, 132–133
Nature
  DNA alteration in, 220–221
  and ethical issues in genetic engineering, 263, 264, 268, 283, 287–291, 353n51
  fascism in writing about, 211–212
  as normative, 221
  and opposition to gene drives, 204–212, 221, 227, 228
  romantic concept of, 210, 211, 212
  use of term, 164, 210
Nature, 78
Navdanya Foundation, 205
Nazi Germany
  gene drives compared to extermination camps in, 206
  Nuremberg trials on, xxii–xxiii, xxiv, 44, 116, 147, 237–238, 240
Neoliberalism, 167
Netting, mosquito. See Bed nets
Newbottle Colliery, 178
New England Journal of Medicine, 74, 111

Newgate Prison, Davy study of ventilation in, 178
New Guinea, military impact of malaria in, 38–39
New Partnership for Africa's Development (NEPAD), 157, 205
Nickase, 103
Nigeria, 57, 173, 230
Nirenberg, Marshall, 269
Nonbeing and being categories, 276
Nongovernmental organizations, 59
  compliance with guidelines from, 98
  ETC Group as, 200–205
  funding of, 210
  in gene drive opposition, 161, 200–209, 210, 218, 219, 227, 231, 234
  in GMO opposition, 141
  Greenpeace as, 148
  and screwworm control, 219
  as visitors in Target Malaria communities, 192
Norgaard, Richard, 215
North America, spread of malaria to, 12, 13
Northumberland collieries, 177–180
Norway maple, 288–289
Novartis, 57
Nuremberg trials, xxii–xxiii, xxiv, 44, 116, 147, 237–238, 240
Nutrition
  cassava in, 214–215
  golden rice in, 231–232, 233–234
  and susceptibility to disease, 25, 33, 34, 171, 172, 241

Obokato, Haruko, 305
Office of Science and Technology Policy (OSTP), 125
Office of Technology Assessment, 120
Onchocerciasis, 256
1,000 Genomes Project, 176
OneWorld Health, 224
O'nyong'nyong virus, 135, 136

Open Philanthropy Project, 98, 205
Oppenheimer, J. Robert, 156
Opposition to gene drives, xxxi,
    xxxiv–xxxv, 186, 191–192,
    199–235
  and DNA alteration, 220–221
  dual use concerns in, 222–223
  in ecological risks, 201–202, 203, 208,
    232, 287–291
  of ETC Group, 200–205, 210
  ethical problem of judgments in, 234
  fear and anxiety as basis of, 212–213
  funding concerns in, 202, 204–205,
    206, 210, 223
  of Greenpeace, 232
  historical errors as basis of, 223, 288
  justice and resource allocation as
    issues in, 224–225
  marketplace as concern in, 223–224
  nature concept in, 204–212, 221, 227,
    228
  precautionary principle in, 208, 232
  religion and faith in, 226–227, 228,
    229
  of Shiva, 205–209, 210
  slippery slope argument in, 222,
    291–294
  species extinction as concern in, 206,
    291
  suffering as belief in, 221–222,
    228–229
  and synthetic biology, 203, 204, 205,
    208, 209, 220, 225
Organization of African Unity, 157
Origin of Species (Darwin), 78–79
Ornithine transcarbamylase *(OTC)* gene,
    121–122, 125
Oryx Expertise, 188
Ostrom, Elinor, 189–190
OTC gene, 121–122, 125
Others, in ethical concerns, 317, 318, 319
Otokuor, Peter Boamah, 195
Ottoman Empire, 35

Overpopulation concerns in malaria
    control, 48, 51, 154, 172, 222
Oxitec, 141, 219

Paarlberg, Robert, 126
Pacific Islands
  malaria impact during WWII, 38
  mice as threat to birds in, 110, 161,
    232, 292
Packard, Randall, 2, 53–54, 61, 62, 65,
    242, 243
Pal, Priya, 69
Palestine, 29–32, 36
Palmer, Julie Gage, 122–123
Palmer, Megan, 156
Palmer amaranth, 146, 202
Pan-African Mosquito Control
    Association, 158, 185
Panama, 14–15, 28–29, 48, 217–218
Panama Canal, xxvi, 28–29
Papua, 38–39, 48
Parent, Brendan, 286
Paris Green, 24, 27, 28, 37, 310
  in China, 55
  mosquito resistance to, 108
  in World War II, 40, 41
Parrhesia, 314
Pasteur, Louis, 17, 21, 33, 242
Patents on gene drives, 293
PATH, in malaria vaccine development,
    71
Paul III, Pope, xvi
PCR technique, 84, 254
Permissible actions, ethical assessment
    of, xxiii, 124, 235, 313, 314–315
Persistent Organic Pollutants (POPs),
    249
Peru, 50
Phagocytes, 2–3
Philadelphia, malaria in, 12
Philippines, 38, 243
Photography, and genetic modification
    compared, 278

Phronesis, 274
Pierce, Charles Taylor, 165
Piperaquine, 62
Pirbright Institute report, 141
Plague, 55, 64
Plants, genetically modified, 119, 125,
    134, 192
  golden rice, 192, 205, 231–232,
    233–234
  grapes, 283–284
  tomatoes, 119, 125, 134, 266
Plants, invasive non-native, 288–289
Plasmids, 114
Plasmochin (SN7618), 50
Plasmodium, 1–14
  in climate change, 251
  drug resistance of, 51, 56, 62, 66, 67
  evolution of mosquitoes, humans
    and, 1–9, 325n15
  historical references to, xvi, 10
  immune response to (see Immune
    response to Plasmodium)
  life cycle of (see Life cycle of
    Plasmodium)
  species of, 1
  World War I affecting distribution
    of, 34, 35
Plasmodium falciparum, 7, 9, 11
  in Africa, 9, 46, 62
  artemisinin in, 56
  in Cambodia, 62
  cerebral malaria from, 56, 60, 69
  chloroquine in, 58
  deaths from, 7, 12, 13, 14, 60
  drug resistance of, 62, 67
  in ecological risk assessment, 196
  evolution of, 7–8, 325n15
  fever from, 10–11, 12
  histidine-rich protein 2 in, 69
  historical references to, 10
  immune response to, 253
  incubation period between bite and
    illness in, 11

  in North America, 12, 14
  rapid diagnostic test for, 254
  in Russia, 34
  in slave trade, 12
  in Target Malaria, 135, 136, 196
Plasmodium malariae, 11
Plasmodium ovale, 10–11, 67
Plasmodium vivax, 5, 7, 9, 11
  chloroquine in, 58–59, 67
  Duffy bodies in resistance to, 6, 13,
    253
  in Europe, 10
  fever from, 10–11, 12, 43
  historical references to, 10
  incubation period between bite and
    illness in, 11
  in North America, 12
  primaquine in, 67
  in syphilis therapy, 43
Plunkett, Carolyn, 286
Poland, 65
Polio vaccine, 72, 74, 230, 258, 274
Political issues in malaria, 51, 53, 61, 111
Polymerase chain reaction technique,
    84, 254
Pontine Marshes (Italy), 27, 41–42
Population growth, as concern in
    malaria control, 48, 51, 154, 172,
    222
Population modification, 90–91, 92–93,
    101, 102, 107
Population suppression, 90–92, 93,
    106–107
  Bier on, 102
  in Kyrou and Hammond research,
    105
  male biased sex ratio in, 87
  male-producing factor in, 83
  mosquito resistance to, 102, 107, 108
  selfish genetic elements in, 81, 82, 86
  sterile males in, 83
  in Target Malaria, 99, 100
  Y drive in, 84–85, 87

Portugal, in colonial Africa, 12, 197–198, 215

Poverty
   in Africa, 158, 174, 175
   and climate change, xxix, 251–252
   and ethical issues in malaria prevention, 239–241
   Greenpeace on, 233
   inattention to, in WHO global campaign, 51, 52
   in India, 33
   in Italy, 27
   last mile problem in, xxvi–xxvii
   malaria as disease of, xxi, 61, 239–241
   and opposition to gene drives, 204
   in post-WWI period, 35
   in United States, xxix, 25
   vitamin A deficiency in, 231

Precautionary principle, 127–134, 151, 311
   burden of proof in, 130, 132
   in Europe and US compared, 131–132
   fidelity principle compared to, 321
   moral issues in, 132–133
   in opposition to gene drives, 208, 232
   and prudent vigilance, 290

Pregnancy
   ACT in, 59
   asymptomatic malaria in, 254
   impact of malaria in, 294
   intermittent therapy in, 67
   primaquine in, 255

Premunition, 47, 253

President's Commission for the Study of Ethical Problems in Medical and Behavioral Research, 117–118

President's Fund, 59

Primaquine, 9, 67, 255

Primary health care, 246, 247

Principles, in ethical assessment of technology, xxiii, 124, 234, 313

"Principles of Effective Occupation" on Africa, 166

Principlism, 237

Prison, research in, xxvi, 43–44
   in Newgate Prison study of Davy, 178
   in Stateville Penitentiary, 43–44, 191, 260

Privacy issues, 253, 271

Problem mapping in stakeholder engagement, 182

Profit motivation in gene drives, 154, 202, 223, 292–294

Prognostication in ethical issues, 306–307

Project Jefferson, 273

Prostitution, 65

Prudent vigilance, 290

Public health, 64–66
   in Africa, 52–53
   in American South, 25.37
   in China, 37, 54–55
   definition of, 243
   ethical issues in, xxiv–xxv, 241–251
   Gorgas approach to, 28, 29
   in Italy, 26–28
   NASEM report on gene drives for, 144
   in Palestine, 30–32
   Rockefeller Foundation approach to, 24–25, 37
   in targeted biomedical model, 61
   in WHO model, 241, 242–243, 244–246

Punjab region of India, xxvi, 32–33

Pyrethroids, 60, 69

Quinacrine (atabrine), 38, 39, 40, 41

Quinghaosu (Chinese wormwood), 56. *See also* Artemisinin

Quinine, 13, 18, 34, 38
   as European Way, 24
   in India, 32
   in Italy, 26, 27, 28
   overdose of, 24
   in Palestine, 31
   resistance to, 24, 51
   WWI affecting availability of, 35

Rabbits
  in Australia, 214, 223, 290
  in laboratory research, 18
RAC. *See* Recombinant DNA Advisory
    Committee
Racism, 40, 51
Rainfall
  crop failure and malnutrition in lack
    of, 33
  and mosquitoes, 32–33, 46–47, 74,
    251, 257
  and prophylactic antimalarials, 74
Rapid diagnostic test for *Plasmodium*, 254
Rats, mongoose introduced for control
    of, 223, 288
Rawl, John, 297
Rebound effect, 47, 160
"Reckless Driving" (ETC Group report),
    203, 204
Recombinant DNA
  Appendix M on, 117, 118
  Asilomar meeting on, xxiii, 115–116,
    269
  ethical issues in, 275–276
  in gene therapy, 118–124 (*see also*
    Gene therapy)
  regulation of, 114–121, 269–270
  safety concerns in, 116–117, 118,
    119, 269–270, 282
Recombinant DNA Advisory Committee
    (RAC), 117–119, 275
  Clinical Gene Transfer Research
    committee of, 119, 120
  disbanding of, 125
  on dual use problem, 269–270, 273
  in research review, xxiv, 117–119,
    120, 122
  safety recommendations of, 288
Red blood cells
  Duffy bodies of, 6, 7, 8, 13, 253
  Plasmodium entering, 2, 3, 5–6, 7, 10,
    18, 71, 255
  in sickle cell disease, 8–9

Redford, Kent, 161
Red Queen theory, 78, 79–80
"Red Queen versus Tangled Bank
    Models" (Burt & Bell), 78
Regulations, 113–162
  African Union report on, 157–160
  agencies involved in, 119–120,
    125–126
  ethical issues in, xxiii, 124, 235, 278,
    280, 286, 313, 315
  in European Union, 141–143, 232
  on gene drives, xxx, xxxiv, 134–162,
    181
  on genetic engineering, 269–271,
    272–274
  House of Lords report on, 141–143
  on insecticide use, 239, 248, 249
  language of, 113–124
  NASEM report on, 143–151
  Paarlberg taxonomy of, 126
  precautionary principle in, 127–134
  on recombinant DNA, 114–121,
    269–270
  Scientist Working Group report on,
    139–140
  and self-regulation, 116, 126–127,
    139, 147
  stakeholder engagement in, 181, 183
  in Target Malaria, 98–99, 106,
    134–137, 138
Regulatory capture, xxxiii
Relapsing fever, 35
Religion
  and gene drive opposition, 226–227,
    228, 229
  and liberation theology, 297
  on sacrifice needed in just and decent
    society, 320
Replacement or reversal drives, 92, 93,
    102, 152, 283
Resistance, xxx, 84
  to artemisinin, 59, 62, 67, 251
  to chloroquine, 51, 56, 67, 252

community concerns about, 135, 182
to DDT, 49–50, 51, 108, 314
in *doublesex* gene drive, 104, 105, 107–109
in homing drives, 104
in mass drug administration, 255
to mefloquine, 62
in modification drives, 92, 107
multidrug, 67, 224, 348–349n46
mutations in, xxvi, xxxi, 5, 8, 24, 104, 107
nutrition affecting, 25, 33
and opposition to gene drives, 201
plasmids in, 114
of *Plasmodium falciparum,* 62, 67
to pyrethroids, 60, 69
to quinine, 24, 51
red blood cell characteristics in, 5–6
in suppression drives, 92, 102, 107
in WHO anti-malaria campaign, 245
WHO reports on, xxviii, 66, 67
Resource allocation, 257
Restriction endonucleases, 114
Reversal or replacement drives, 92, 93, 102, 152, 283
Ribeiro, Jose, 87
Rice, 192, 205, 231–232, 233–234, 243
Rice, William, 79
Rio Declaration (1992), 128
Risks
African Union report on, 159
courage in, 318
environmental (*see* Environmental concerns)
ethical issues in, 277–278, 307–308
House of Lords report on, 141–143
NASEM report on, 146, 149
precautionary principle in, 127–134
in Target Malaria, 134–137, 151
Thompson on, 155
truthfulness about, 317
uncertain, consent issues in, 307–308

RNA
functions of, 266
guide (gRNA), 93, 108, 125
in vaccines, 314, 358n27
Rockefeller Foundation, 24, 25, 37, 38, 39, 248
Rohwer, Sievert, 45
Roll Back Malaria, 59
Roman fever, 13, 19
Rome, ancient, xv–xvii, 9–10
Roosevelt, Franklin D., 37
Roosevelt, Theodore, 29
Ross, Richard, 20–21, 32, 138, 168
challenge trials of, 259
mosquito dissection studies of, 21, 110
on sanitation campaigns, 25, 168
targeted approach of, 36, 61
Rothschild family, 29
RTS,S vaccine, 71, 258
Rubin, Susan, xxxiii
Rural Advancement Foundation International (RAFI), 200
Russell, Paul, 242
Russia
malaria incidence in, 34–35
migration to Palestine from, 29–32

Sachs, Jeffrey, 239, 241
Safety issues, 94–96
Asilomar meeting on, 118, 134, 144, 269, 282, 288
in Bier research, 102
Cartagena Protocol in, 129, 134–135
containment protocols in, 94–95, 288 (*see also* Containment protocols)
in DDT use, 49, 50–51
in dual use problem (*see* Dual use problem)
in ethics of gene drives, 282–283
in genetic engineering, 94, 124
in horizontal transfer of gene drives, 109–110, 336n75

Safety issues (cont.)
  House of Lords report on, 141–143
  precautionary principle in, 127–134
  in recombinant DNA research,
    116–117, 118, 119, 269–270, 282
  reversal of gene drives in, 283
  in Target Malaria, 99–100, 106,
    134–137, 151
  in uncertainties, 311–312
Sanitation campaigns, 25–26, 37, 54–55,
  168
Sanofi, 224
Schieffelin, Eugene, 289
Schistosomiasis, 55
Schultz, Kathryn, 211–212
Science
  deceit in, 305–306
  essential premises of, 306
  Iron Rule of, 300–301
  trends in trust of, 301, 357n8
  uncertainty in, 300–302, 317
Science, 150, 151, 156, 160, 189
Science and technology studies (STS),
  151, 154
Scientific Council for Africa South of
  the Sahara, 172, 173
Scientific hygiene, 33
Scientist Working Group, 139–140
Scoping study of Target Malaria, 188
Scramble for Africa, xxvi, 16, 170
Screwworms, 96, 216–219
Second Aliyah, 29
Secretariat of the Basel, Rotterdam,
  and Stockholm Conventions (BRS
  Secretariat), 249
Selective Primary Health Care, 247
Selfish genetic elements, xx, xxii,
  80–83, 90
  Burt on, 80–82, 90, 332n11
  homing endonuclease genes as,
    85–86
  site-specific, 332n11
Self-regulation in research, 116, 126–127

  NASEM report on, 147
  Scientist Working Group report on,
    139
Self-sustaining gene drives, 94, 100,
  111, 283
Serebrovsky, Alexander Sergevich, 83
Severe combined immunodeficiency
  (SCID), 125
Sex determination, doublesex gene in,
  104–105, 109
Sex ratio of offspring, 91
  male bias in, 87, 94, 100, 103, 188,
    192
Sexual reproduction, 3, 79–80, 81
  of Plasmodium, 1, 3
  and Red Queen theory, 79–80
  sterile male mosquitoes affecting (see
    Sterile male mosquito release)
Sexual selection, 80
Shah, Sonia, 8, 54
  on artemisinin in China, 56–57
  on blood testing in India, 49
  on endemic malaria, 326n37
  on epidemic malaria in Africa, 5
  on funding of malaria control, 52, 58
  on immune response, 4, 7
  on military impact of malaria, 39
  on mortality rate from malaria, 4, 5,
    13, 22
  on scramble for Africa, 16
  on slave trade, 14
  on syphilis, 42
Shakespeare, William, 11, 13–14, 168
Shen, Michael, 286
Shiva, Vandana, 205–209, 210, 220,
  346–347n12
Sickle cell disease, 8–9, 125
Silent Spring (Carson), 50–51
Silicon Valley Community Foundation,
  98
Silverman, Richard, 293
Singer, Maxine, 114, 116, 269
Singer, Peter, 286

Slave trade, 12, 13, 14, 166, 169, 215, 240

Sleep, mosquito bites during, 3, 4, 5, 7, 13

bed nets in prevention of (*see* Bed nets)

Manson research on, 19

Sleeping sickness, 168

Slippery slope arguments, 222, 291–294

Smallpox vaccination, 46, 48, 54, 74, 167

SN7618 (plasmochin), 50

Social contracts, 297

Social factors

in Africa, 57, 158–159, 172

as determinant of health, 61, 65, 246, 248

in endemic malaria, 37

and ethical issues in malaria prevention, 239–240, 258

importance in malaria eradication, 61, 111

inattention to, 35, 36, 50, 54, 244, 245

in incidence of malaria, 239–240, 241

in India, 33

in Italy, 26, 27, 33–34, 50

in public health, 27, 65, 242–243

in United States, 37

Soll, Dieter, 114, 116, 269

Sontochin (hydroxychloroquine), 41, 42, 43–44

South, American, xxvi, 25, 36–37

South Africa, 158

South African Association for Science, 169

South America, malaria in, 12, 13

South Carolina, malaria in, 14

Soviet Union, malaria in, 34

Spanish–American War, 28

Spanish explorations, 12

Sparrows, introduction and spread of, 223, 289

Spermatheca, 24

Splicing Life report, 118

Sporozoites of *Plasmodium*, 2, 3, 9, 71, 258

Spotted lanternfly, 274

Sri Lanka, 45, 51, 326n37

Stakeholder engagement, xxxi, xxxiv, 163–198

in Africa, xxxiv, 160, 163–198, 315

African Union report on, 160

consent in, 98, 190–191

evaluation of, 186, 188

generations in, 184

glossary project in, 183–184, 192

in golden rice research, 192

and governance of commons, 189–190

in insect collection, 98, 196

in justice concerns, 296

language in, 182, 183–184, 192, 193

large projects of Target Malaria in, 110

listening to opposition in, 186, 191–192

at local level, 98, 180–184

in multinational corporations, 181

NASEM report on, 146, 147

problem mapping in, 182

reciprocal deliberation or responsive discourse in, 187

at regional and national level, 184

time required for, 187, 191, 192, 193, 197, 234

trust in, 183, 186, 187, 192, 196–197

Stampar, Andrija, 37

Stanford University, 114

Starlings, introduction and spread of, 289

Stateville Penitentiary research, 43–44, 191, 260

Stavrianakis, Anthony, 164

Stem cell research, 161, 206, 212, 226, 292, 295, 305

Sterile female mosquitoes, 103–105
Sterile male mosquito release, 83, 100,
      103, 135, 136
   in Bana village, 135, 136, 186–187
   mark-release-recapture technique, 187
   by Oxitec, 141, 219
   in staged process, 100, 192
   stakeholder engagement in, 186–187
Sterile male screwworms, 96, 216–219
Stockholm Convention on Persistent
      Organic Pollutants, 249
Strachey, William, 14
Strange Natures (Redford & Adams), 161
Strevens, Michael, 300, 303, 307
STS Association, 151
Sturtevant, Alfred, 83
Suffering, belief in need for, 221–222,
      228–229, 230
Suk, Hwang Woo, 305
Suppression drives. *See* Population
      suppression
Sustainable Development Goals of UN,
      66–67
Suzuki, David, 203
Swamp/marsh areas, 18, 19
   DDT used in, 41–42
   drainage of, xv–xvii, 9–10, 23, 24, 27,
      32, 140, 310
   Gambusia (mosquito fish) in, 31
   Paris Green used in, 27, 28, 40
Swaziland, 158
Swiss Tropical and Public Health
      Institute, 188
Symptoms of malaria, 17
   in chronic low-level infection, 48,
      253–254
   fever in, 10–13, 72, 75, 253
Synbal, Inc., 102
SynBio meetings, 201, 270
Synthetic biology, xx
   in artemisinin research, 223–224,
      263, 281, 349n46
   definition of, 263

ethical issues in, 262–264, 290,
      353n51
genetic engineering in, 349n52
   (*see also* Genetic engineering)
opposition to, 161, 203, 204, 205,
      208, 209, 220, 225
safety and security in, 271–272
as self-defined field, 264, 273, 353n51
use of term, 225, 349n52
Syphilis, 42–44
   fever therapy in, 43–44, 260
   social and economic factors in, 65
   Tuskegee experiment on, 116, 155
Szostak, Jack, 265, 266, 267, 281,
      353n55

Takman (fever demon), 10
TALENS (transcription activator-like
      effector nuclease), 88, 125, 301
"Tangled Bank" model, 78
Target Malaria, xxx, xxxii, 96–103, 110
   accidental release of female
      mosquitoes in, 135, 136
   Burt on, 96, 98–101, 103
   co-development approach in, 173,
      176, 184, 186, 191
   community engagement in, 98, 100,
      135, 180, 292
   consent issues in, 98, 176, 187, 188
   containment policies in, 99–100
   ecological risk assessment in, 151,
      195–196
   Ethics Advisory Committee of, xxxiii,
      99, 111, 292
   funding of, 97–98, 204, 205
   GIS mapping in, 196
   glossary project in, 183–184, 192
   horizontal transfer of gene drive as
      concern in, 109
   independent evaluation of, 188
   insect collection sites and methods
      in, 196
   institutions involved with, 173

large cage experiments in, 99
listening to opposition in, 186,
191–192, 199–235
male bias mosquitoes in, 100, 103,
188, 192
oversight of, 101
regulations in, 98–99, 106, 134–137,
138
safety issues in, 99–100, 106,
134–137, 151
scoping study of, 188
as staged process, 99, 100, 103,
188–189, 192
stakeholder engagement in, 163
(see also Stakeholder engagement)
sterile male release in, 100, 103, 135,
136, 186–187, 192
team members in, 96–97
transparency in, 97, 185, 186, 187,
292
Tata Trust, 101
Tay-Sachs disease, 123
Technical uncertainty, 303, 307, 315
Techno-utopianism, 208
Tempest, The (Shakespeare), 13–14
Tennessee Valley Authority, 37
Terni, Italy, xv–xvii, 95, 96, 99, 106
Tertian fever, 11
Thailand, 62, 63
Thaler, Richard, 308
t-haplotype in mice, 83, 90
Thizy, Delphine, 184, 187
Thomas, Jim, 201–205
Thompson, Paul, 155
Tilley, Helen, 169–170, 171, 173, 194,
196
Time and the Other (Fabian), 211
Tomatoes, genetically modified, 119,
125, 134, 266
Trade
of slaves, 12, 13, 14, 166, 169, 215,
240
spread of malaria in, 11, 12, 15

Tragedy of the commons, 189
Transcription activator-like effector
nuclease (TALENS), 88, 125, 301
Transgenes, 89
Transparency
commitment to, 160, 185, 292
Esveldt on, 152
NASEM report on, 150
of NGOs, 210
Scientist Working Group on, 139, 140
in stakeholder engagement, 185, 186
in synthetic biology research, 264
in Target Malaria, 97, 185, 186, 187,
292
Transposable genetic elements, 82, 86
Traore, Ibrahim, 175
Treaty on the Functioning of the
European Union (TFEU), 127
Trivers, Robert, xxii, 81–82, 84, 85,
86–87
Truman, Harry, 244
Trump, Donald, xxix
Trust, and stakeholder engagement,
183, 186, 187, 192, 196–197
Truth
commitment to virtue of, 317–318
opinion and politics affecting, 316
in parrhesia concept, 314
in science, 305–306
Tsetse fly, 171
Tuberculosis, 59
Tuskegee syphilis experiment, 116, 155
Typhus, 35, 65

Uganda
asymptomatic malaria in, 254
incidence of malaria in, 173
Target Malaria in, 96, 97, 103, 163,
189, 191, 196
Uncertainties, 110, 299–322
Burt on, 91–93
consent issues in, 307–308
courage in, 318

Uncertainties (cont.)
  in ecological risk assessments, 146
  epistemic, 146, 303, 307, 312, 315
  ethical issues in, 278, 280, 282, 286,
    303–322
  fidelity in, 318–321
  in gene drives for malaria, 309–322
  House of Lords report on, 141
  humility in, 318
  and Iron Rule of science, 300–301
  linguistic, 146
  methodological, 303
  in modification drives, 92
  NASEM report on, 145, 146, 148
  precautionary principle in, 129, 130,
    132, 133, 311
  in research, 310–312
  technical, 303, 307, 315
  teleological, 303
  truthfulness in, 317–318
  types of, 146, 303–304
Uneasy/uncanny feeling, 267–269, 276
UNICEF, 71
Unitaid, 71
United Nations
  Commission on Poverty, xxix
  Convention on Biological Diversity,
    149, 203, 204, 205
  definition of health, 246
  Environment Programme, 149
  Intergovernmental Panel on Climate
    Change, xxviii
  on precautionary approach, 128
  Relief and Rehabilitation
    Administration, 45, 242
  Rio Declaration (1992), 128
  Sustainable Development Goals,
    66–67
United States
  and American way in malaria control,
    24–26
  in Cuba, 28
  eradication of malaria in, xxvi, 25, 48

history of malaria in, 12, 13–15,
    25–26, 36–37
  mortality rate from malaria in, 14,
    22, 25
  NASEM report in, 143–157
  Panama Canal construction, xxvi,
    28–29
  poverty in, xxix, 25
  precautionary approach in, 131–132
  sanitation campaigns in, 25–26
  screwworms as pest in, 216–219
  southern states in, xxvi, 25, 36–37
  vaccination resistance in, 230
  WHO anti-malaria campaign in, 48
United States Department of Agriculture
    (USDA), 45, 119, 125, 154, 217,
    218
University of California, Berkeley, 224,
    270
University of California, Irvine, xxxiv,
    101, 110
University of California, San Diego,
    xxxiv, 101, 110
University of California, San Francisco,
    114
University of Chicago, 43–44
University of Pennsylvania, 121, 122,
    125
Utilitarianism, 247, 296, 297

Vaccinations
  in China, 54
  COVID-19, 75, 238
  herd immunity in, xxv
  malaria (see Malaria vaccine)
  measles, xxv
  polio, 72, 74, 230, 258, 274
  resistance in US to, 230
  RNA, 314, 358n27
  in Selective Primary Health Care, 247
  smallpox, 46, 48, 54, 74, 167
Vanderbilt, R. C., 83
Vaughan, Megan, 167–168, 169

Vedic texts, 10
Vesalius, Andreas, 230
Vietnam, 62
Viral vectors, 88, 89, 115, 123, 162
    in *OTC* gene therapy, 121, 122
Virchow, Rudolf, 65
Virginia Company, 14
Vitamin A, 231, 233
Vulnerable populations
    climate change affecting, 251–252
    in precautionary approach, 133
    as research subjects, 116, 118, 191,
        260

Wagner-Jauregg, Julius, 42, 43
Walters, Leroy, 117, 119, 122–124, 305
War
    gene technology potential as weapon
        in, 148, 152, 272, 273
    and incidence of malaria, 35–36,
        158
    malaria control as, military language
        in, 22, 34, 35, 36, 53, 63, 242
Wasps for biological control of cassava
    mealybug, 96, 213–216
Water, and mosquitoes
    in Africa, 46–47, 257
    in American South, 37
    in Celli public health interventions,
        26
    in India, 32–33
    Kligler research on, 31, 32
    in life cycle, 19–20, 23, 24
    Manson research on, 19, 21
    in Palestine, 29–30, 31
    Paris Green spray in control of, 24,
        27, 28, 40, 55
    pesticide contamination of, 248–249
    petroleum spray in control of, 23, 24
    in rain, 32–33, 46–47, 74, 251, 257
    in swamp areas (*see* Swamp/marsh
        areas)
    in WWII, 41–42

Weapons, gene technology potential as,
    148, 152, 272, 273. *See also* Dual
    use problem
Webb, James L. A., Jr., 54
Weiner, Jonathan, 131–132
Wellcome Trust, 98, 113
West Africa, 163, 166–167, 173
    Burkina Faso in (*see* Burkina Faso)
West African Integrated Vector
    Management Group, 158
West Nile virus, 189
WHO global anti-malaria campaign,
    46–54
    in Africa, 46–47, 48, 52, 53–54, 62
    blood sampling in, 49
    consent issues in, 49, 53
    DDT in, 46, 49–51
    failure of, 53–54
    funding of, 47, 51, 52
    inattention to social and economic
        factors in, 50, 54, 245
    local resistance to, 245
    migration affecting, 53, 245
    official end of, 52
    overpopulation concerns in, 48, 51
    political issues affecting, 51, 53
Wilcocks, Charles, 172
Willowbrook hepatitis studies, 116
Wilson, D. Bagster, 46, 47, 122, 250,
    257
Wilson, Margaret, 46, 47, 250, 257
Window screens, 22, 26, 27, 40, 326n37
Wong, Alan, 65–66
Wood, Gaby, 278
World Bank, 58, 60, 248
World Health Organization, 113
    artemisinin approved by, 56, 59
    on consent in malaria vaccine trials,
        72–73
    on DDT use, 249
    and Declaration of Alma-Ata,
        245–247
    definition of health, 244, 246

World Health Organization (cont.)
  economic and social concerns of, 50,
      54, 242–243, 244
  on eradication of malaria in Italy,
      xvi
  and ethical issues in malaria control,
      241, 242–243, 244–246
  on funding of malaria control, 241
  gene drive report, 160
  global anti-malaria campaign, 46–54
      (see also WHO global anti-malaria
      campaign)
  Global Technical Strategy for Malaria,
      xxvii, 66, 153
  on GMOs, 149, 185, 187
  on incidence of malaria, 66–67, 68,
      70, 261
  Malaria Report (2018), xxvii, 68
  Malaria Report (2021), 70
  malaria vaccine administered by, 71
  on mortality rate in malaria, xviii,
      xxvii
  pilot anti-malaria programs in Africa,
      48, 52, 54
  on precautionary approach, 129
  public health model, 241, 242–243,
      244–246
  smallpox vaccination campaign,
      46, 48
World Malaria Day, xxvii
World Malaria Report (2018), xxvii, 68
World Malaria Report (2021), 70
World War I, 30, 33, 34, 171
  incidence of malaria after, 34–36
World War II, 36, 37–45, 173
Worldwide Threat Assessment report,
      148
Wormwood, Chinese, 56, 223–224.
      See also Artemisinin

X chromosome, xxi, 84–85, 87, 188,
      333n22

Yaws, 42
Y chromosome, xx–xxi, 83–87, 93–94,
      104, 188
Yellow fever, 28, 29, 70, 101, 146, 245

Zambia, 158
Zhang, Feng, 89
Zika virus, xxix, 101, 146, 201
Zimbabwe, 158, 230
Zinc finger nucleases, 88
Zionist movement, 30, 31
Zoo of genetic elements, 82, 84, 90

Basic Bioethics

Arthur Caplan, editor

Books Acquired under the Editorship of Glenn McGee and Arthur Caplan

Peter A. Ubel, *Pricing Life: Why It's Time for Health Care Rationing*

Mark G. Kuczewski and Ronald Polansky, eds., *Bioethics: Ancient Themes in Contemporary Issues*

Suzanne Holland, Karen Lebacqz, and Laurie Zoloth, eds., *The Human Embryonic Stem Cell Debate: Science, Ethics, and Public Policy*

Gita Sen, Asha George, and Piroska Östlin, eds., *Engendering International Health: The Challenge of Equity*

Carolyn McLeod, *Self-Trust and Reproductive Autonomy*

Lenny Moss, *What Genes Can't Do*

Jonathan D. Moreno, ed., *In the Wake of Terror: Medicine and Morality in a Time of Crisis*

Glenn McGee, ed., *Pragmatic Bioethics, 2d edition*

Timothy F. Murphy, *Case Studies in Biomedical Research Ethics*

Mark A. Rothstein, ed., *Genetics and Life Insurance: Medical Underwriting and Social Policy*

Kenneth A. Richman, *Ethics and the Metaphysics of Medicine: Reflections on Health and Beneficence*

David Lazer, ed., *DNA and the Criminal Justice System: The Technology of Justice*

Harold W. Baillie and Timothy K. Casey, eds., *Is Human Nature Obsolete? Genetics, Bioengineering, and the Future of the Human Condition*

Robert H. Blank and Janna C. Merrick, eds., *End-of-Life Decision Making: A Cross-National Study*

Norman L. Cantor, *Making Medical Decisions for the Profoundly Mentally Disabled*

Margrit Shildrick and Roxanne Mykitiuk, eds., *Ethics of the Body: Post-Conventional Challenges*

Alfred I. Tauber, *Patient Autonomy and the Ethics of Responsibility*

David H. Brendel, *Healing Psychiatry: Bridging the Science/Humanism Divide*

Jonathan Baron, *Against Bioethics*

Michael L. Gross, *Bioethics and Armed Conflict: Moral Dilemmas of Medicine and War*

Karen F. Greif and Jon F. Merz, *Current Controversies in the Biological Sciences: Case Studies of Policy Challenges from New Technologies*

Deborah Blizzard, *Looking Within: A Sociocultural Examination of Fetoscopy*

Ronald Cole-Turner, ed., *Design and Destiny: Jewish and Christian Perspectives on Human Germline Modification*

Holly Fernandez Lynch, *Conflicts of Conscience in Health Care: An Institutional Compromise*

Mark A. Bedau and Emily C. Parke, eds., *The Ethics of Protocells: Moral and Social Implications of Creating Life in the Laboratory*

Jonathan D. Moreno and Sam Berger, eds., *Progress in Bioethics: Science, Policy, and Politics*

Eric Racine, *Pragmatic Neuroethics: Improving Understanding and Treatment of the Mind-Brain*

Martha J. Farah, ed., *Neuroethics: An Introduction with Readings*

Jeremy R. Garrett, ed., *The Ethics of Animal Research: Exploring the Controversy*

Books Acquired under the Editorship of Arthur Caplan

Sheila Jasanoff, ed., *Reframing Rights: Bioconstitutionalism in the Genetic Age*

Christine Overall, *Why Have Children? The Ethical Debate*

Yechiel Michael Barilan, *Human Dignity, Human Rights, and Responsibility: The New Language of Global Bioethics and Bio-Law*

Tom Koch, *Thieves of Virtue: When Bioethics Stole Medicine*

Timothy F. Murphy, *Ethics, Sexual Orientation, and Choices about Children*

Daniel Callahan, *In Search of the Good: A Life in Bioethics*

Robert Blank, *Intervention in the Brain: Politics, Policy, and Ethics*

Gregory E. Kaebnick and Thomas H. Murray, eds., *Synthetic Biology and Morality: Artificial Life and the Bounds of Nature*

Dominic A. Sisti, Arthur L. Caplan, and Hila Rimon-Greenspan, eds., *Applied Ethics in Mental Healthcare: An Interdisciplinary Reader*

Barbara K. Redman, *Research Misconduct Policy in Biomedicine: Beyond the Bad-Apple Approach*

Russell Blackford, *Humanity Enhanced: Genetic Choice and the Challenge for Liberal Democracies*

Nicholas Agar, *Truly Human Enhancement: A Philosophical Defense of Limits*

Bruno Perreau, *The Politics of Adoption: Gender and the Making of French Citizenship*

Carl Schneider, *The Censor's Hand: The Misregulation of Human-Subject Research*

Lydia S. Dugdale, ed., *Dying in the Twenty-First Century: Towards a New Ethical Framework for the Art of Dying Well*

John D. Lantos and Diane S. Lauderdale, *Preterm Babies, Fetal Patients, and Childbearing Choices*

Harris Wiseman, *The Myth of the Moral Brain*

Arthur L. Caplan and Jason Schwartz, eds., *Vaccine Ethics and Policy: An Introduction with Readings*

Tom Koch, *Ethics in Everyday Places: Mapping Moral Stress, Distress, and Injury*

Nicole Piemonte, *Afflicted: How Vulnerability Can Heal Medical Education and Practice*

Abigail Gosselin, *Mental Patient: Ethics from a Patient's Perspective*

Laurie Zoloth, *May We Make the World?*